READINGS IN HEALTH SCIENCE

Benjamin A. Kogan received his M.D. from Wayne State University College of Medicine and his M.S.P.H. and Dr. P.H. from the University of Michigan. He is Director of the Bureau of Medical Services of the County of Los Angeles Health Department. An experienced classroom teacher, Dr. Kogan holds the following appointments: Associate Clinical Professor of Community Medicine and Public Health, University of Southern California School of Medicine; Professor of Health Science, San Fernando Valley State College; Lecturer in Public Health, University of California at Los Angeles; Lecturer in Preventive Medicine, University of California at Irvine, College of Medicine. Dr. Kogan has made frequent television appearances and has written a number of articles on public health. He is the author of *Health: Man in a Changing Environment.*

Readings
in Health Science

edited by
Benjamin A. Kogan, M.D., Dr. P.H.

HARCOURT BRACE JOVANOVICH, INC.
New York   Chicago   San Francisco   Atlanta

COVER DRAWING: Louis Efstathiou, *Untitled*, 1969. Pen and ink, 24″ x 18″.

ISBN: 0-15-575841-1

Library of Congress Catalog Card Number: 70-157877

PRINTED IN THE UNITED STATES OF AMERICA

Preface

Modern health problems are complex. Many are poorly defined. Like an iceberg, only a small part of a hazard may be visible on the surface. This book of readings has been compiled to provide a more revealing view of some of the threats to man's well-being. Its selections have been chosen because they offer fresh ways of viewing these threats and, even more important, will stimulate discussion about them. Only through such discussion can the depth of the problems be appreciated and the first steps toward solutions be taken.

The selections have been grouped in four sections: "Man and His Environment," "Man and Society," "Man's Mind and Body," and "Man's Future." These divisions are not intended to fragment man. Mind and body cannot be considered apart from each other, nor are they separable from the society and the environment in which they exist and with which they interact. This book is about man as a whole being. Its divisions are merely for the reader's convenience. He may rearrange their contents to suit his own needs.

The basic thesis of this volume is that man has created an imbalance between himself and his environment. This imbalance makes him sick. When he deserted the fields for the towns, man exchanged the bondage of the seasons for the bondage of technology. Now he is separated from nature, his source of origin. But this separation is only part of the reason for the imbalance. Compared with social evolution, genetic evolution is slow. Man's internal environment, governed by the subtly operating genetic mechanisms within his cells, has changed little in the past twenty thousand years. But the changes in his external environment have been both rapid and drastic. This vast difference in evolutionary speed between man's internal and external ecosystems poses critical problems of adaptation. Man's hope for a return to physical and emotional well-being depends on whether he can control his present assault on nature, heal both his wounds and those of his natural world, and, finally, maintain a harmonious balance between his internal and external environments.

Drugs, violence, poverty, pollution, alienation—these are but a few of the dilemmas confronting the health scientist. The articles in this book explore many facets of the problems. But underlying them all is the most relevant question of this era: Can man learn to control the scientific forces he has unleashed, or will he, ultimately, bring about his own extinction?

If this book helps to create an atmosphere of calm contention and constant questioning in which learning about health can take place, it will have achieved its primary purpose.

B. A. K.

Contents

Preface   v

MAN & HIS ENVIRONMENT   1

The fog
BERTON ROUECHÉ   5

Mortgaging the old homestead
LORD RITCHIE-CALDER   17

Human ecology
RENÉ DUBOS   28

Where will we put all that garbage?
TOM ALEXANDER   36

It's time to turn down all that noise
JOHN M. MECKLIN   46

Secrecy and safety at rocky flats
ROGER RAPOPORT   58

Medicine in the ghetto
JOHN C. NORMAN, M.D.   68

Contents

The health of haight-ashbury
DAVID E. SMITH, JOHN LUCE, and
ERNEST A. DERNBURG   77

The world of the haight-ashbury speed freak
ROGER C. SMITH   93

The first probe
CHARLES C. BRAUNER   105

MAN & SOCIETY   121

The world of migratory workers
JOHN STEINBECK   127

THE HUMAN CONDITION   131

**If hitler asked you to electrocute a stranger,
would you?**
PHILIP MEYER   133

Paranoia and high office
ROBERT E. KANTOR and WILLIAM G. HERRON   146

A psychohistorical perspective of the negro
ROBERT H. SHARPLEY, M.D.   152

The culture of poverty
OSCAR LEWIS   160

An informal history of love u.s.a.
ARTHUR SCHLESINGER, JR.   169

THE DRUG CULTURE   181

Runaways, hippies, and marihuana
JOSHUA KAUFMAN, JAMES R. ALLEN, M.D., and
LOUIS JOLYON WEST, M.D.   183

viii

No marijuana for adolescents
KLAUS ANGEL
189

THE GENERATION GAP 195

What generation gap?
JOSEPH ADELSON
197

What troubles our troubled youth?
ROY MENNINGER, M.D.
207

Alienated youth
WILLIAM NEAL BROWN
216

Breaking isn't everything
SUBHAS MUKHOPADHYAY, translated by Kshitis Roy
224

MAN'S MIND & BODY 227

The bound man
ILSE AICHINGER
231

Infant malnutrition and adult learning
NEVIN S. SCRIMSHAW
241

Atherosclerosis
DAVID M. SPAIN
249

Of viruses and cancers
LIN ROOT
259

The many clocks of man
JOHN D. PALMER
267

Chromosomes and crime: some tentative thoughts
MARY A. TELFER
276

Recently exploded sexual myths
LEON SALZMAN, M.D.
280

Contents

Sex and the work of masters and johnson
HARVEY D. STRASSMAN, M.D.   289

Drug addiction—facts and folklore
OLIVER GILLIE   296

Igor stravinsky: on illness and death
ROBERT CRAFT   305

MAN'S FUTURE   321

The scientific urgencies of the next ten years
DR. JOHN PLATT   325

On living in a biological revolution
DONALD FLEMING   331

The desexualized society
CHARLES WINICK   341

The beckwith letter   346

This book is for Esther, Becky, and Kay

Man &
his environment

*M*ore than twenty years ago Berton Roueché wrote his vivid warning "The Fog," the first essay in this section. His description of the smog that enveloped the residents of Donora, Pennsylvania, did much to make the nation aware of a growing menace. But pollution problems are not always so striking. Too often forgotten are the people who survive disasters like the Donora smog but suffer chronically or die prematurely from less dramatic exposures to pollution. In the cities many people now count their clear days as if they were to be hoarded and remembered. And on days when the smog is not thick enough to cause discomfort most people understandably ignore or dismiss the possible dangers. But it is this low-level exposure to smog that is now worrying so many medical men.

In his article "Mortgaging the Old Homestead," Lord Ritchie-Calder discusses the many kinds of pollution of the ecosystem. His first and last sentences, which suggest the dangers inherent in man's continuing abuse of the world in which he lives, are the keys to a provocative discussion. René Dubos draws on many disciplines for his essay "Human Ecology." But whether he uses elements of history or biology or anthropology or sociology is irrelevant; the result is an urbane and thoughtful approach to the future. Each of the next three essays examines a specific pollution problem. In "Where Will We Put All That Garbage?" Tom Alexander not only points to the dangerously inadequate methods of solid-waste disposal in this country, but suggests improvements. Noise, as John M. Mecklin hears it in "It's Time to Turn Down All That Noise," is more than a nuisance—it is a serious health hazard that is all the more dangerous because it is insidious. But Roger Rapoport raises the most disturbing questions in his "Secrecy and Safety at Rocky Flats." Although he concedes that security is essential at the plutonium factory near Denver, Rapoport wonders, first, if there is not excessive risk-taking there and, second, if the secret nature of the work is not being used to obscure public knowledge about a possible peril. A recent serious fire in the plant, preceded by numerous small fires, the too-frequent radioactive contamination of workers at the plant, and the possibility of an increased incidence of cancer among these workers are some of the matters Rapoport discusses. As Lord Ritchie-Calder reminds his readers, those who first decided to use the atom bomb knew little or nothing about its genetic effects. Today's scientist may not enjoy the quiet retreat of his laboratory. He must speak out; he must tell it as it is. He must inform—and warn. Not only human health, but the very survival of humanity may depend on his willingness to carry out this responsibility (see "The Beckwith Letter," page 346).

For centuries poverty has been known as "the mother of disease." How bigotry condemns people to environmental poverty and, therefore, to sickness is described by John C. Norman in "Medicine in the Ghetto." Although money is needed to care for the sick poor, money alone cannot solve the problem. As Norman makes clear, the roots of the problem lie in the racism among the people of this country.

Poverty among a group of young people is considered in two articles about San Francisco's Haight-Ashbury district. Hippies are not a new phenomenon. Sixteen centuries ago the Roman emperor Julian complained that

"Nowadays, any young man who does not choose to study or to work grows a beard, insults the gods, and calls himself Cynic." In San Francisco there once was a brisk business in Haight-Ashbury street signs and other such souvenirs. The tourists who bought these on the way back to their hotels felt a sense of romance about the Haight—all that love and pot and nothing to do but stroll free in the San Francisco wind. But David Smith and the coauthors of "The Health of Haight-Ashbury," see conditions more realistically. If, as they write, San Francisco officials have been slow to alleviate the agony of those in the Haight, there has been a dividend. Other communities have learned from the San Francisco experience. To the south, the County of Los Angeles now spends hundreds of thousands of dollars annually for youth and drug-abuse clinics. Despair and death are only too common in the Haight. "When we are at the end of life, to die means to go away; when we are at the beginning, to go away means to die." Those who work in the Haight-Ashbury district may be haunted by these words of Victor Hugo's. For the Haight-Ashbury wanderer is not old; he is young. And if he has gone away, must he die? Can he not come back? Roger Smith adds to the grim picture of the area with his "The World of Haight-Ashbury Speed Freak." Smith's article provides a revealing look at a declining phase of drug abuse in the district. Not many in the Haight shoot speed anymore. It was too much, a hassle. Now it's heroin. The young people of the Haight-Ashbury district are often voluntarily poor. Rejecting materialism, they have no interest in possessions. Many have wandered off from the district to hallucinate along the Pacific coast.

Charles C. Brauner's "The First Probe" describes a fascinating experimental course given to first-year architecture students at the University of British Columbia. The students were exposed to unexpected and unusual social experiences and widely varying and rapidly changing ecological stimuli. Their reactions—on a desolate island, on a glacier, in an industrial town, on a skid row, and in an abandoned brick kiln—are not only of psychological interest; they are a moving testament to man's ingenuity and to his probing search for a more meaningful architecture and human ecology.

The fog

BERTON ROUECHÉ

The Monongahela River rises in the middle Alleghenies and seeps for a hundred and twenty-eight miles through the iron and bituminous-coal fields of northeastern West Virginia and southwestern Pennsylvania to Pittsburgh. There, joining the Allegheny River, it becomes the wild Ohio. It is the only river of any consequence in the United States that flows due north, and it is also the shortest. Its course is cramped and crooked, and flanked by bluffs and precipitous hills. Within living memory, its waters were quick and green, but they are murky now with pollution, and a series of locks and dams steady its once tumultuous descent, rendering it navigable from source to mouth. Traffic on the Monongahela is heavy. Its shipping, which consists almost wholly of coal barges pushed by wheezy, coal-burning stern-wheelers, exceeds in tonnage that of the Panama Canal. The river is densely industrialized. There are trucking highways along its narrow banks and interurban lines and branches of the Pennsylvania Railroad and the New York Central and smelters and steel plants and chemical works and glass factories and foundries and coke plants and machine shops and zinc mills, and its hills and bluffs are scaled by numerous blackened mill towns. The blackest of them is the borough of Donora, in Washington County, Pennsylvania.

Donora is twenty-eight miles south of Pittsburgh and covers the tip of a lumpy point formed by the most convulsive of the Monongahela's many horseshoe bends. Though accessible by road, rail, and river, it is an extraordinarily secluded place. The river and the bluffs that lift abruptly from the water's edge to a height of four hundred and fifty feet enclose it on the north and east and south, and just above it to the west is a range of rolling but even higher hills. On its outskirts are acres of sidings and rusting gondolas, abandoned mines, smoldering slag piles, and gulches filled with rubbish. Its limits are marked by sooty signs that read, "Donora. Next to Yours the Best Town in the U.S.A." It is a harsh, gritty town, founded in 1901 and old for its

THE FOG Reprinted by permission; Copr. © 1950 The New Yorker Magazine, Inc. *The New Yorker*, September 30, 1950.

age, with a gaudy main street and a thousand identical gaunt gray houses. Some of its streets are paved with concrete and some are cobbled, but many are of dirt and crushed coal. At least half of them are as steep as roofs, and several have steps instead of sidewalks. It is treeless and all but grassless, and much of it is slowly sliding downhill. After a rain, it is a smear of mud. Its vacant lots and many of its yards are mortally gullied, and one of its three cemeteries is an eroded ruin of gravelly clay and toppled tombstones. Its population is 12,300. Two-thirds of its men, and a substantial number of its women, work in its mills. There are three of them—a steel plant, a wire plant, and a zinc-and-sulphuric-acid plant—all of which are operated by the American Steel & Wire Co., a subsidiary of the United States Steel Corporation, and they line its river front for three miles. They are huge mills. Some of the buildings are two blocks long, many are five or six stories high, and all of them bristle with hundred-foot stacks perpetually plumed with black or red or sulphurous yellow smoke.

Donora is abnormally smoky. Its mills are no bigger or smokier than many, but their smoke, and the smoke from the passing boats and trains, tends to linger there. Because of the crowding bluffs and sheltering hills, there is seldom a wind, and only occasionally a breeze, to dispel it. On still days, unless the skies are high and buoyantly clear, the lower streets are always dim and there is frequently a haze on the heights. Autumn is the smokiest season. The weather is close and dull then, and there are persistent fogs as well. The densest ones generally come in October. They are greasy, gagging fogs, often intact even at high noon, and they sometimes last for two or three days. A few have lasted as long as four. One, toward the end of October, 1948, hung on for six. Unlike its predecessors, it turned out to be of considerably more than local interest. It was the second smoke-contaminated fog in history ever to reach a toxic density. The first such fog occurred in Belgium, in an industrialized stretch of the Meuse Valley, in 1930. During it several hundred people were prostrated, sixty of them fatally. The Donora fog struck down nearly six thousand. Twenty of them—five women and fifteen men—died. Nobody knows exactly what killed them, or why the others survived. At the time, not many of the stricken expected to.

The fog closed over Donora on the morning of Tuesday, October 26th. The weather was raw, cloudy, and dead calm, and it stayed that way as the fog piled up all that day and the next. By Thursday it had stiffened adhesively into a motionless clot of smoke. That afternoon, it was just possible to see across the street, and, except for the stacks, the mills had vanished. The air began to have a sickening smell, almost a taste. It was the bittersweet reek of sulphur dioxide. Everyone who was out that day remarked on it, but no one was much concerned. The smell of sulphur dioxide, a scratchy gas given off by burning coal and melting ore, is a normal concomitant of any durable fog in Donora. This time, it merely seemed more penetrating than usual.

At about eight-thirty on Friday morning, one of Donora's eight physicians, Dr. Ralph W. Koehler, a tense, stocky man of forty-eight, stepped to his bathroom window for a look at the weather. It was, at best, unchanged. He could see nothing but a watery waste of rooftops islanded in fog. As he was turning away, a shimmer of movement in the distance caught his eye. It was a freight train creeping along the riverbank just south of town, and the sight of it shook him. He had never seen anything quite like it before. "It was the smoke," he says. "They were firing up for the grade and the smoke was belching out, but it didn't rise. I mean it didn't go up at all. It just spilled out over the lip of the stack like a black liquid, like ink or oil, and rolled down to the ground and lay there. My God, it just lay there! I thought, Well, God damn—and they talk about needing smoke control up in Pittsburgh! I've got a heart condition, and I was so disgusted my heart began to act up a little. I had to sit down on the edge of the tub and rest a minute."

Dr. Koehler and an associate, Dr. Edward Roth, who is big, heavyset, and in his middle forties, share an office on the second floor of a brownstone building one block up from the mills, on McKean Avenue, the town's main street. They have one employee, a young woman named Helen Stack, in whom are combined an attractive receptionist, an efficient secretary, and a capable nurse. Miss Stack was the first to reach the office that morning. Like Dr. Koehler and many other Donorans, she was in uncertain spirits. The fog was beginning to get on her nerves, and she had awakened with a sore throat and a cough and supposed that she was coming down with a cold. The appearance of the office deepened her depression. Everything in it was smeared with a kind of dust. "It wasn't just ordinary soot and grit," she says. "There was something white and scummy mixed up in it. It was just wet ash from the mills, but I didn't know that then. I almost hated to touch it, it was so nasty-looking. But it had to be cleaned up, so I got out a cloth and went to work." When Miss Stack had finished, she lighted a cigarette and sat down at her desk to go through the mail. It struck her that the cigarette had a very peculiar taste. She held it up and sniffed at the smoke. Then she raised it to her lips, took another puff, and doubled up in a paroxysm of coughing. For an instant, she thought she was going to be sick. "I'll never forget that taste," she says, "Oh, it was awful! It was sweet and horrible, like something rotten. It tasted the way the fog smelled, only ten times worse. I got rid of the cigarette as fast as I could and drank a glass of water, and then I felt better. What puzzled me was I'd smoked a cigarette at home after breakfast and it had tasted all right. I didn't know what to think, except that maybe it was because the fog wasn't quite as bad up the hill as here downstreet. I guess I thought my cold was probably partly to blame. I wasn't really uneasy. The big Halloween parade the Chamber of Commerce puts on every year was to be held that night, and I could hear the workmen down in the street putting up the decorations. I knew the committee wouldn't be going ahead with the parade if they thought anything was wrong. So I went on with my work, and pretty soon the Doctors came in from their early calls and it was just like any other morning."

The office hours of Dr. Koehler and Dr. Roth are the same, from one to three in the afternoon and from seven to nine at night. Whenever possible in the afternoon, Dr. Koehler leaves promptly at three. Because of his unsteady heart, he finds it desirable to rest for a time before dinner. That Friday afternoon, he was just getting into his coat when Miss Stack announced a patient. "He was wheezing and gasping for air," Dr. Koehler says, "but there wasn't anything very surprising about that. He was one of our regular asthmatics, and the fog gets them every time. The only surprising thing was that he hadn't come in sooner. The fact is, none of our asthmatics had been in all week. Well, I did what I could for him. I gave him a shot of adrenalin or aminophyllin—some anti-spasmodic—to dilate the bronchia, so he could breathe more easily, and sent him home. I followed him out. I didn't feel so good myself."

Half an hour after Dr. Koehler left, another gasping asthmatic, an elderly steelworker, tottered into the office. "He was pretty wobbly," Miss Stack says. "Dr. Roth was still in his office, and saw him right away. I guess he wasn't much better when he came out, because I remember thinking, Poor fellow. There's nothing sadder than an asthmatic when the fog is bad. Well, he had hardly gone out the door when I heard a terrible commotion. I thought, Oh, my gosh, he's fallen down the stairs! Then there was an awful yell. I jumped up and dashed out into the hall. There was a man I'd never seen before sort of draped over the banister. He was kicking at the wall and pulling at the banister and moaning and choking and yelling at the top of his voice, 'Help! Help me! I'm dying!' I just stood there. I was petrified. Then Dr. Brown, across the hall, came running out, and he and somebody else helped the man on up the stairs and into his office. Just then, my phone began to ring. I almost bumped into Dr. Roth. He was coming out to see what was going on. When I picked up the phone, it was just like hearing that man in the hall again. It was somebody saying somebody was dying. I said Dr. Roth would be right over, but before I could even tell him, the phone started ringing again. And the minute I hung up the receiver, it rang again. That was the beginning of a terrible night. From that minute on, the phone never stopped ringing. That's the honest truth. And they were all alike. Everybody who called up said the same thing. Pain in the abdomen. Splitting headache. Nausea and vomiting. Choking and couldn't get their breath. Coughing up blood. But as soon as I got over my surprise, I calmed down. Hysterical people always end up by making me feel calm. Anyway, I managed to make a list of the first few calls and gave it to Dr. Roth. He was standing there with his hat and coat on and his bag in his hand and chewing on his cigar, and he took the list and shook his head and went out. Then I called Dr. Koehler, but his line was busy. I don't remember much about the next hour. All I know is I kept trying to reach Dr. Koehler and my phone kept ringing and my list of calls kept getting longer and longer."

One of the calls that lengthened Miss Stack's list was a summons to the home of August Z. Chambon, the burgess, or mayor, of Donora. The patient was the Burgess's mother, a widow of seventy-four, who lives with her son and his wife. "Mother Chambon was home alone that afternoon," her daughter-in-law says. "August was in Pittsburgh on business and I'd gone downstreet to do some shopping. It took me forever, the fog was so bad. Even the inside of the stores was smoky. So I didn't get home until around five-thirty. Well, I opened the door and stepped into the hall, and there was Mother Chambon. She was lying on the floor, with her coat on and a bag of cookies spilled all over beside her. Her face was blue, and she was just gasping for breath and in terrible pain. She told me she'd gone around the corner to the bakery a few minutes before, and on the way back the fog had got her. She said she barely made it to the house. Mother Chambon has bronchial trouble, but I'd never seen her so bad before. Oh, I was frightened! I helped her up—I don't know how I ever did it—and got her into bed. Then I called the doctor. It took me a long time to reach his office, and then he wasn't in. He was out making calls. I was afraid to wait until he could get here—Mother Chambon was so bad, and at her age and all—so I called another doctor. He was out, too. Finally, I got hold of Dr. Levin and he said he'd come right over, and he finally did. He gave her an injection that made her breathe easier and something to put her to sleep. She slept for sixteen solid hours. But before Dr. Levin left, I told him that there seemed to be an awful lot of sickness going on all of a sudden. I was coughing a little myself. I asked him what was happening. 'I don't know,' he said. 'Something's coming off, but I don't know what.' "

Dr. Roth returned to his office at a little past six to replenish his supply of drugs. By then, he, like Dr. Levin, was aware that something was coming off. "I knew that whatever it was we were up against was serious," he says. "I'd seen some very pitiful cases, and they weren't all asthmatics or chronics of any kind. Some were people who had never been bothered by fog before. I was worried, but I wasn't bewildered. It was no mystery. It was obvious—all the symptoms pointed to it—that the fog and smoke were to blame. I didn't think any further than that. As a matter of fact, I didn't have time to think or wonder. I was too damn busy. My biggest problem was just getting around. It was almost impossible to drive. I even had trouble finding the office. McKean Avenue was solid coal smoke. I could taste the soot when I got out of the car, and my chest felt tight. On the way up the stairs, I started coughing and I couldn't stop. I kept coughing and choking until my stomach turned over. Fortunately, Helen was out getting something to eat—I just made it to the office and ino the lavatory in time. My God, I was sick! After a while, I dragged myself into my office and gave myself an injection of adrenalin and lay back in a chair. I began to feel better. I felt so much better I got out a cigar and lighted up. That practically finished me. I took one pull, and went into another paroxysm of coughing. I probably should have known better—cigars had tasted terrible all day—but I hadn't had that reaction before. Then I heard the phone ringing. I guess it must have been ringing off and on all along. I thought about answering it, but I didn't have the strength to move. I just lay there in my chair and let it ring."

When Miss Stack came into the office a few minutes later, the telephone was still ringing. She had answered it and added the call to her list before she realized that she was not alone. "I heard someone groaning," she says. "Dr. Roth's door was open and I looked in. I almost jumped, I was so startled. He was slumped down in his chair, and his face was brick red and dripping with perspiration. I wanted to help him, but he said there wasn't anything to do. He told me what had happened. 'I'm all right now,' he said. 'I'll get going again in a minute. You go ahead and answer the phone.' It was ringing again. The next thing I knew, the office was full of patients, all of them coughing and groaning. I was about ready to break down and cry. I had talked to Dr. Koehler by that time and he knew what was happening. He had been out on calls from home. 'I'm coughing and sick myself,' he said,

9

'but I'll go out again as soon as I can.' I tried to keep calm, but with both Doctors sick and the office full of patients and the phone ringing, I just didn't know which way to turn. Dr. Roth saw two or three of the worst patients. Oh, he looked ghastly! He really looked worse than some of the patients. Finally, he said he couldn't see any more, that the emergency house calls had to come first, and grabbed up his stuff and went out. The office was still full of patients, and I went around explaining things to them. It was awful. There wasn't anything to do but close up, but I've never felt so heartless. Some of them were so sick and miserable. And right in the middle of everything the parade came marching down the street. People were cheering and yelling, and the bands were playing. I could hardly believe my ears. It just didn't seem possible."

The sounds of revelry that reached Miss Stack were deceptive. The parade, though well attended, was not an unqualified success. "I went out for a few minutes and watched it," the younger Mrs. Chambon says. "It went right by our house. August wasn't home yet, and after what had happened to Mother Chambon, I thought it might cheer me up a little. It did and it didn't. Everybody was talking about the fog and wondering when it would end, and some of them had heard there was sickness, but nobody seemed at all worried. As far as I could tell, all the sick people were old. That made things look not too bad. The fog always affects the old people. But as far as the parade was concerned, it was a waste of time. You really couldn't see a thing. They were just like shadows marching by. It was kind of uncanny. Especially since most of the people in the crowd had handkerchiefs tied over their nose and mouth to keep out the smoke. All the children did. But, even so, everybody was coughing. I was glad to get back in the house. I guess everybody was. The minute it was over, everybody scattered. They just vanished. In two minutes there wasn't a soul left on the street. It was as quiet as midnight."

Among the several organizations that participated in the parade was the Donora Fire Department. The force consists of about thirty volunteers and two full-time men. The latter, who live at the firehouse, are the chief, John Volk, a wiry man in his fifties, and his assistant and driver, a hard, round-faced young man named Russell Davis. Immediately after the parade, they returned to the firehouse. "As a rule," Chief Volk says, "I like a parade. We've got some nice equipment here, and I don't mind showing it off. But I didn't get much pleasure out of that one. Nobody could see us, hardly, and we couldn't see them. That fog was black as a derby hat. It had us all coughing. It was a relief to head for home. We hadn't much more than got back to the station, though, and got the trucks put away and said good night to the fellows than the phone rang. Russ and I were just sitting down to drink some coffee. I dreaded to answer it. On a night like that, a fire could have been real mean. But it wasn't any fire. It was a fellow up the street, and the fog had got him. He said he was choking to death and couldn't get a doctor, and what he wanted was our inhalator. He needed air. Russ says I just stood there with my mouth hanging open. I don't remember what I thought. I guess I was trying to think what to do as much as anything else. I didn't disbelieve him—he sounded half dead already—but, naturally, we're not supposed to go running around treating the sick. But what the hell, you can't let a man die! So I told him O.K. I told Russ to take the car and go. The way it turned out, I figure we did the right thing. I've never heard anybody say different."

"That guy was only the first," Davis says. "From then on, it was one emergency call after another. I didn't get to bed until Sunday. Neither did John. I don't know how many calls we had, but I do know this: We had around eight hundred cubic feet of oxygen on hand when I started out Friday night, and we ended up by borrowing from McKeesport and Monessen and Monongahela and Charleroi and everywhere around here. I never want to go through a thing like that again. I was laid up for a week after. There never was such a fog. You couldn't see your hand in front of your face, day or night. Hell, even inside the station the air was blue. I drove on the left side of the street with my head out the window, steering by scraping the curb. We've had bad fogs here before. A guy lost his car in one. He'd come to a fork in the road and didn't know where he was, and got out to try and tell which way to go. When he turned back to his car, he couldn't find it. He had no idea where it was until, finally, he stopped and listened and heard the engine. That guided him back. Well, by God, this fog was so bad you couldn't even get a car to idle. I'd take my foot off the accelerator and—bango—the engine would stall. There just wasn't any oxygen in the air. I don't know how I kept breathing. I don't know how anybody did. I found people laying in bed and laying on the floor. Some of them were laying there and they didn't give a damn whether they died or not. I found some down in the basement with the furnace draft open and their head stuck inside, trying to get air that way. What I did when I got to a place was throw a sheet or a blanket over the patient and stick a cylinder of oxygen underneath and crack the valves for fifteen minutes or so. By God, that rallied them! I didn't take any myself. What I did every time I came back to the station was have a little shot of whiskey. That seemed to help. It eased my throat. There was one funny thing about the whole thing. Nobody seemed to realize what was going on. Everybody seemed to think he was the only sick man in town. I don't know what they figured was keeping the doctors so busy. I guess everybody was so miserable they just didn't think."

Toward midnight, Dr. Roth abandoned his car and continued his rounds on foot. He found not only that walking was less of a strain but that he made better time. He walked the streets all night, but he was seldom lonely. Often, as he entered or left a house, he encountered a colleague. "We all had practically the same calls," Dr. M. J. Hannigan, the president of the Donora Medical Association, says. "Some people called every doctor in town. It was pretty discouraging to finally get someplace and drag yourself up the steps and then be told that Dr. So-and-So had just been there. Not that I blame them, though. Far from it. There were a couple of times when I was about ready to call for help myself. Frankly, I don't know how any of us doctors managed to hold out and keep going that night."

Not all of them did. Dr. Koehler made his last call that night at one o'clock. "I had to go home," he says. "God knows I didn't want to. I'd hardly made a dent in my list. Every time I called home or the Physicians' Exchange, it doubled. But my heart gave out. I couldn't go on any longer without some rest. The last thing I heard as I got into bed was my wife answering the phone. And the phone was the first thing I heard in the morning. It was as though I hadn't been to sleep at all." While Dr. Koehler was bolting a cup of coffee, the telephone rang again. This time, it was Miss Stack. They conferred briefly about the patients he had seen during the night and those he planned to see that morning. Among the latter was a sixty-four-year-old steelworker named Ignatz Hollowitti. "One of the Hollowitti girls, Dorothy, is a good friend of mine," Miss Stack says. "So as soon as I finished talking to Dr. Koehler, I called her to tell her that Doctor would be right over. I wanted to relieve her mind. Dorothy was crying when she answered the phone. I'll never forget what she said. She said, 'Oh, Helen—my dad just died! He's dead!' I don't remember what I said. I was simply stunned. I suppose I said what people say. I must have. But all I could think was, My gosh, if people are dying—why, this is tragic! Nothing like this has ever happened before!"

Mr. Hollowitti was not the first victim of the fog. He was the sixth. The first was a retired steelworker of seventy named Ivan Ceh. According to the records of the undertaker who was called in—Rudolph Schwerha, whose establishment is the largest in Donora—Mr. Ceh died at one-thirty Saturday morning. "I was notified at two," Mr. Schwerha says. "There is a note to such effect in my book. I thought nothing, of course. The call awakened me from sleep, but in my profession anything is to be expected. I reassured the bereaved and called my driver and sent him for the body. He was gone forever. The fog that night was impossible. It was a neighborhood case—only two blocks to go, and my driver works quick—but it was thirty minutes by the clock before I heard the service car in the drive. At that moment, again the phone rang. Another case. Now I was surprised. Two different cases so soon together in this size town doesn't happen every day. But there was no time then for thinking. There was work to do. I must go with my driver for the second body. It was in the Sunnyside section, north of town, too far in such weather for one man alone. The fog, when we got down by the mills, was unbelievable. Nothing could be seen. It was like a blanket. Our fog lights were useless, and even with the fog spotlight on, the white line in the street was invisible. I began to worry. What if we should bump a parked car? What if we should fall off the road? Finally, I told my driver, 'Stop! I'll take the wheel. You walk in front and show the way.' So we did that for two miles. Then we were in the country. I know that section like my hand, but we had missed the house. So we had to turn around and go back. That was an awful time. We were on the side of a hill, with a terrible drop on one side and no fence. I was afraid every minute. But we made it, moving by inches, and pretty soon I found the house. The case was an old man and he had died all of a sudden. Acute cardiac dilation. When we were ready, we started back. Then I began to feel sick. The fog was getting me. There was an awful tickle in my throat. I was coughing and ready to vomit. I called to my driver that I had to stop and get out. He was ready to stop, I guess. Already he had walked four or five miles. But I envied him. He was well and I was awful sick. I leaned against the car, coughing and gagging, and at last I riffled a few times. Then I was much better. I could drive. So we went on, and finally we were home. My wife was standing at the door. Before she spoke, I knew what she would say. I thought, Oh, my God—another! I knew it by her face. And after that came another. Then another. There seemed to be no end. By ten o'clock in the morning, I had nine bodies waiting here. Then I heard that DeRienzo and Lawson, the other morticians, each had one. Eleven people dead! My driver and I kept looking at each other. What was happening? We didn't know. I thought probably the fog was the reason. It had the smell of poison. But we didn't know."

Mr. Schwerha's bewilderment was not widely shared. Most Donorans were still unaware Saturday morning that anything was happening. They had no way of knowing. Donora has no radio station, and its one newspaper, the *Herald-American*, is published only five days a week, Monday through Friday. It was past noon before a rumor of widespread illness began to drift through town. The news reached August Chambon at about two o'clock. In addition to being burgess, an office that is more an honor than a livelihood, Mr. Chambon operates a moving-and-storage business, and he had been out of town on a job all morning. "There was a message waiting for me when I got home," he says. "John Elco, of the Legion, had called and wanted me at the Borough Building right away. I wondered what the hell, but I went right over. It isn't like John to get excited over nothing. The fog didn't even enter my mind. Of course, I'd heard there were some people sick from it. My wife had told me that. But I hadn't paid it any special significance. I just thought they were like Mother—old people that were always bothered by fog. Jesus, in a town like this you've got to expect fog. It's natural. At least, that's what I thought then. So I was astonished when John told me that the fog was causing sickness all over town. I was just about floored. That's a fact. Because I felt fine myself. I was hardly even coughing much. Well, as soon as I'd talked to John and the other fellows he had rounded up, I started in to do what I could. Something had already been done. John and Cora Vernon, the Red Cross director, were setting up an emergency-aid station in the Community Center. We don't have a hospital here. The nearest one is at Charleroi. Mrs. Vernon was getting a doctor she knew there to come over and take charge of the station, and the Legion was arranging for cars and volunteer nurses. The idea was to get a little organization in things—everything was confused as hell—and also to give our doctors a rest. They'd been working steady for thirty-six hours or more. Mrs. Vernon was fixing it so when somebody called a doctor's number, they would be switched to the Center and everything would be handled from there. I've worked in the mills and I've dug coal, but I never worked any harder than I worked that day. Or was so worried. Mostly I was on the phone. I called every town around here to send supplies for the station and oxygen for the firemen. I even called Pittsburgh. Maybe I overdid it. There was stuff pouring in here for a week. But what I wanted to be was prepared for anything. The way that fog looked that day, it wasn't ever going to lift. And then the rumors started going around that now people were dying. Oh, Jesus! Then I was scared. I heard all kinds of reports. Four dead. Ten dead. Thirteen dead. I did the only thing I could think of. I notified the State Health Department, and I called a special meeting of the Council and our Board of Health and the mill officials for the first thing Sunday morning. I wanted to have it right then, but I couldn't get hold of everybody —it was Saturday night. Every time I looked up from the phone, I'd heard a new rumor. Usually a bigger one. I guess I heard everything but the truth. What I was really afraid of was that they might set off a panic. That's what I kept dreading. I needn't have worried, though. The way it turned out, half the town had hardly heard that there was anybody even sick until Sunday night, when Walter Winchell opened his big mouth on the radio. By then, thank God, it was all over."

The emergency-aid station, generously staffed and abundantly supplied with drugs and oxygen inhalators, opened at eight o'clock Saturday night. "We were ready for anything and prepared for the worst," Mrs. Vernon says. "We even had an ambulance at our disposal. Phillip DeRienzo, the under-taker, loaned it to us. But almost nothing happened. Altogether, we brought in just eight patients. Seven, to be exact. One was dead when the car arrived. Three were very bad and we sent them to the hospital in Charleroi. The others we just treated and sent home. It was really very queer. The fog was as black and nasty as ever that night, or worse, but all of a sudden the calls for a doctor just seemed to trickle out and stop. It was as though everybody was sick who was going to be sick. I don't believe we had a call after mid-night. I knew then that we'd seen the worst of it."

Dr. Roth had reached that conclusion, though on more slender evidence, several hours before. "I'd had a call about noon from a woman who said two men roomers in her house were in bad shape," he says. "It was nine or nine-thirty by the time I finally got around to seeing them. Only, I never saw them. The landlady yelled up to them that I was there, and they yelled right back, 'Tell him never mind. We're O.K. now.' Well, that was good enough for me. I decided things must be letting up. I picked up my grip and walked home and fell into bed. I was dead-beat."

There was no visible indication that the fog was beginning to relax its smothering grip when the group summoned by Burgess Chambon assembled at the Borough Building the next morning to discuss the calamity. It was another soggy, silent midnight day. "That morning was the worst," the Bur-gess says. "It wasn't just that the fog was still hanging on. We'd begun to get some true facts. We didn't have any real idea how many people were sick. That didn't come out for months. We thought a few hundred. But we did have the number of deaths. It took the heart out of you. The rumors hadn't come close to it. It was eighteen. I guess we talked about that first. Then the question of the mills came up. The smoke. L. J. Westhaver, who was general superintendent of the steel and wire works then, was there, and so was the head of the zinc plant, M. M. Neale. I asked them to shut down for the dura-tion. They said they already had. They had started banking the fires at six that morning. They went on to say, though, that they were sure the mills had nothing to do with the trouble. We didn't know what to think. Everybody was at a loss to point the finger at anything in particular. There just didn't seem to be any explanation. We had another meeting that afternoon. It was the same thing all over again. We talked and we wondered and we worried. We couldn't think of anything to do that hadn't already been done. I think we heard about the nineteenth death before we broke up. We thought for a week that was the last. Then one more finally died. I don't remember exactly what all we did or said that afternoon. What I remember is after we broke up. When we came out of the building, it was raining. Maybe it was only drizzling then—I guess the real rain didn't set in until evening—but, even so, there was a hell of a difference. The air was different. It didn't get you any more. You could breathe."

The investigation of the disaster lasted almost a year. It was not only the world's first full-blooded examination of the general problem of air pollution but one of the most exhaustive inquiries of any kind ever made in the field of public health. Its course was directed jointly by Dr. Joseph Shilen, director of the Bureau of Industrial Hygiene of the Pennsylvania Department of Health, and Dr. J. G. Townsend, chief of the Division of Industrial Hygiene of the United States Public Health Service, and at times it involved the entire technical personnel of both agencies. The Public Health Service assigned to the case nine engineers, seven physicians, six nurses, five chemists, three statisticians, two meteorologists, two dentists, and a veterinarian. The force under the immediate direction of Dr. Shilen, though necessarily somewhat smaller, was similarly composed.

The investigation followed three main lines, embracing the clinical, the environmental, and the meteorological aspects of the occurrence. Of these, the meteorological inquiry was the most nearly conclusive. It was also the most reassuring. It indicated that while the situation of Donora is unwholesomely conducive to the accumulation of smoke and fog, the immediate cause of the October, 1948, visitation was a freak of nature known to meteorologists as a temperature inversion. This phenomenon is, as its name suggests, characterized by a temporary, and usually brief, reversal of the normal atmospheric conditions, in which the air near the earth is warmer than the air higher up. Its result is a more or less complete immobilization of the convection currents in the lower air by which gases and fumes are ordinarily carried upward, away from the earth.

The clinical findings, with one or two exceptions, were more confirmatory than illuminating. One of the revelations, which was gleaned from several months of tireless interviewing, was that thousands, rather than just hundreds, had been ill during the fog. For the most part, the findings demonstrated, to the surprise of neither the investigators nor the Donora physicians, that the affection was essentially an irritation of the respiratory tract, that its severity increased in proportion to the age of the victim and his predisposition to cardio-respiratory ailments, and that the ultimate cause of death was suffocation.

The environmental study, the major phase of which was an analysis of the multiplicity of gases emitted by the mills, boats, and trains, was, in a positive sense, almost wholly unrewarding. It failed to determine the direct causative agent. Still, its results, though negative, were not without value. They showed, contrary to expectation, that no one of the several stack gases known to be irritant—among them fluoride, chloride, hydrogen sulphide, cadmium oxide, and sulphur dioxide—could have been present in the air in sufficient concentration to produce serious illness. "It seems reasonable to state," Dr. Helmuth H. Schrenk, chief of the Environmental Investigations

15

Branch of the Public Health Service's Division of Industrial Hygiene, has written of this phase of the inquiry, "that while no single substance was responsible for the ... episode, the syndrome could have been produced by a combination, or summation of the action, of two or more of the contaminants. Sulphur dioxide and its oxidation products, together with particulate matter [soot and fly ash], are considered significant contaminants. However, the significance of the other irritants as important adjuvants to the biological effects cannot be finally estimated on the basis of present knowledge. It is important to emphasize that information available on the toxicological effects of mixed irritant gases is meagre and data on possible enhanced action due to absorption of gases on particulate matter is limited." To this, Dr. Leonard A. Scheele, Surgeon General of the Service, has added, "One of the most important results of the study is to show us what we do not know."

Funeral services for most of the victims of the fog were held on Tuesday, November 2nd. Monday had been a day of battering rain, but the weather cleared in the night, and Tuesday was fine. "It was like a day in spring," Mr. Schwerha says. "I think I have never seen such a beautiful blue sky or such a shining sun or such pretty white clouds. Even the trees in the cemetery seemed to have color. I kept looking up all day."

Mortgaging the old homestead

LORD RITCHIE-CALDER

Past civilizations are buried in the graveyards of their own mistakes, but as each died of its greed, its carelessness or its effeteness another took its place. That was because such civilizations took their character from a locality or region. Today ours is a global civilization; it is not bounded by the Tigris and the Euphrates nor even the Hellespont and the Indus; it is the whole world. Its planet has shrunk to a neighborhood round which a man-made satellite can patrol sixteen times a day, riding the gravitational fences of Man's family estate. It is a community so interdependent that our mistakes are exaggerated on a world scale.

For the first time in history, Man has the power of veto over the evolution of his own species through a nuclear holocaust. The overkill is enough to wipe out every man, woman and child on earth, together with our fellow lodgers, the animals, the birds and the insects, and to reduce our planet to a radioactive wilderness. Or the Doomsday Machine could be replaced by the Doomsday Bug. By gene-manipulation and man-made mutations, it is possible to produce, or generate, a disease against which there would be no natural immunity; by "generate" is meant that even if perpetrators inoculated themselves protectively, the disease in spreading round the world could assume a virulence of its own and involve them too. When a British bacteriologist died of the bug he had invented, a distinguished scientist said, "Thank God he didn't sneeze; he could have started a pandemic against which there would have been no immunity."

Modern Man can outboast the Ancients, who in the arrogance of their material achievements built pyramids as the gravestones of the civilizations. We can blast our pyramids into space to orbit through all eternity round a planet which perished by our neglect.

A hundred years ago Claude Bernard, the famous French physiologist, enjoined his colleagues, "True science teaches us to doubt and in ignorance to refrain." What he meant was that the scientist must proceed from one

MORTGAGING THE OLD HOMESTEAD Excerpted by permission from *Foreign Affairs*, January 1970. Copyright © 1970 by the Council on Foreign Relations, Inc., New York.

17

tested foothold to the next (like going into a mine-field with a mine-detector). Today we are using the biosphere, the living space, as an experimental laboratory. When the mad scientist of fiction blows himself and his laboratory skyhigh, that is all right, but when scientists and decision-makers act out of ignorance and pretend that it is knowledge, they are putting the whole world in hazard. Anyway, science at best is not wisdom; it is knowledge, while wisdom is knowledge tempered with judgment. Because of overspecialization, most scientists are disabled from exercising judgments beyond their own sphere.

A classic example was the atomic bomb. It was the Physicists' Bomb. When the device exploded at Alamogordo on July 16, 1945, and made a notch-mark in history from which Man's future would be dated, the safe-breakers had cracked the lock of the nucleus before the locksmiths knew how it worked. (The evidence of this is the billions of dollars which have been spent since 1945 on gargantuan machines to study the fundamental particles, the components of the nucleus; and they still do not know how they interrelate.)

Prime Minister Clement Attlee, who concurred with President Truman's decision to drop the bomb on Hiroshima, later said:

> We knew nothing whatever at that time about the genetic effects of an atomic explosion. I knew nothing about fall-out and all the rest of what emerged after Hiroshima. As far as I know, President Truman and Winston Churchill knew nothing of those things either, nor did Sir John Anderson who coordinated research on our side. Whether the scientists directly concerned knew or guessed, I do not know. But if they did, then so far as I am aware, they said nothing of it to those who had to make the decision.[1]

That sounds absurd, since as long before as 1927, Herman J. Muller had been studying the genetic effects of radiation, work for which he was awarded the Nobel Prize in 1946. But it is true that in the whole documentation of the British effort, before it merged in the Manhattan Project, there is only one reference to genetic effects—a Medical Research Council minute which was not connected with the bomb they were intending to make; it concerned the possibility that the Germans might, short of the bomb, produce radioactive isotopes as a form of biological warfare. In the Franck Report, the most statesmanlike document ever produced by scientists, with its percipience of the military and political consequences of unilateral use of the bomb (presented to Secretary of War Henry L. Stimson even before the test bomb exploded), no reference is made to the biological effects, although one would have supposed that to have been a very powerful argument. The explanation, of course, was that it was the Physicists' Bomb and military security restricted information and discussion to the bomb-makers, which excluded the biologists.

The same kind of breakdown in interdisciplinary consultation was manifest in the subsequent testing of fission and fusion bombs. Categorical assur-

---

[1] "Twilight of Empire," by Clement Attlee with Francis Williams. New York: Barnes, 1961, p. 74.

ances were given that the fallout would be confined to the testing area, but the Japanese fishing-boat *Lucky Dragon* was "dusted" well outside the predicted range. Then we got the story of radiostrontium. Radiostrontium is an analogue of calcium. Therefore in bone-formation an atom of natural strontium can take the place of calcium and the radioactive version can do likewise. Radiostrontium did not exist in the world before 1945; it is a man-made element. Today every young person, anywhere in the world, whose bones were forming during the massive bomb-testing in the atmosphere, carries this brandmark of the Atomic Age. The radiostrontium in their bones is medically insignificant, but if the test ban (belated recognition) had not prevented the escalation of atmospheric testing, it might not have been.

Every young person everywhere was affected, and why? Because those responsible for H-bomb testing miscalculated. They assumed that the upthrust of the H-bomb would punch a hole in the stratosphere and that the gaseous radioactivity would dissipate itself. One of those gases was radioactive krypton, which quickly decays in radiostrontium, which is a particulate. The technicians had been wrongly briefed about the nature of the troposphere, the climatic ceiling which would, they maintained, prevent the fall-back. But between the equatorial troposphere and the polar troposphere, there is a gap, and the radiostrontium came back through this fanlight into the climatic jet-streams. It was swept all around the world to come to earth as radioactive rain, to be deposited on foodcrops and pastures, to be ingested by animals and to get into milk and into babies and children and adolescents whose growing bones were hungry for calcium or its equivalent strontium, in this case radioactive. Incidentally, radiostrontium was known to the biologists before it "hit the headlines." They had found it in the skin burns of animals exposed on the Nevada testing ranges and they knew its sinister nature as a "bone-seeker." But the authorities clapped security on their work, classified it as "Operation Sunshine" and cynically called the units of radiostrontium "Sunshine Units"—an instance not of ignorance but of deliberate non-communication.

One beneficial effect of the alarm caused by all this has been that the atoms industry is, bar none, the safest in the world for those working in it. Precautions, now universal, were built into the code of practice from the beginning. Indeed it can be admitted that the safety margins in health and in working conditions are perhaps excessive in the light of experience, but no one would dare to modify them. There can, however, be accidents in which the public assumes the risk. At Windscale, the British atomic center in Cumberland, a reactor burned out. Radioactive fumes escaped from the stacks in spite of the filters. They drifted over the country. Milk was dumped into the sea because radioactive iodine had covered the dairy pastures.

There is the problem of atomic waste disposal, which persists in the peaceful uses as well as in the making of nuclear explosives. Low energy wastes, carefully monitored, can be safely disposed of. Trash, irradiated metals and laboratory waste can be embedded in concrete and dumped in the ocean deeps—although this practice raises some misgivings. But high-level wastes, some with elements the radioactivity of which can persist for *hundreds of thousands* of years, present prodigious difficulties. There must be "burial grounds" (or euphemistically "farms"), the biggest of which is at Hanford, Washington. It encloses a stretch of the Columbia River in a tract covering 575 square miles, where no one is allowed to live or to trespass.

There, in the twentieth century Giza, it has cost more, much more, to bury live atoms than it cost to entomb the sun-god Kings of Egypt. The capital outlay runs into hundreds of millions of dollars and the maintenance of the U.S. sepulchres is over $6 million a year. (Add to that the buried waste of the U.S.S.R., Britain, Canada, France and China, and one can see what it costs to bury live atoms.) And they are very much alive. At Hanford they are kept in million-gallon carbon-steel tanks. Their radioactive vitality keeps the accompanying acids boiling like a witches' cauldron. A cooling system has to be maintained continuously. The vapors from the self-boiling tanks have to be condensed and "scrubbed" (radioactive atoms removed); otherwise a radioactive miasma would escape from the vents. The tanks will not endure as long as the pyramids and certainly not for the hundreds of thousands of years of the long-lived atoms. The acids and the atomic ferments erode the toughest metal, so the tanks have to be periodically decanted. Another method is to entomb them in disused salt mines. Another is to embed them in ceramics, lock them up in glass beads. Another is what is known as "hydraulic fraction": a hole is drilled into a shale formation (below the subsoil water); liquid is piped down under pressure and causes the shale to split laterally. Hence the atoms in liquid cement can be injected under enormous pressure and spread into the fissures to set like a radioactive sandwich.

This accumulating waste from fission plants will persist until the promise, still far from fulfilled, of peaceful thermonuclear power comes about. With the multiplication of power reactors, the wastes will increase. It is calculated that by the year 2000, the number of six-ton nuclear "hearses" in transit to "burial grounds" at any given time on the highways of the United States will be well over 3,000 and the amount of radioactive products will be about a billion curies, which is a mighty lot of curies to be roaming around a populated country.

The alarming possibilities were well illustrated by the incident at Palomares, on the coast of Spain, when there occurred a collision of a refueling aircraft with a U.S. nuclear bomber on "live" mission. The bombs were scattered. There was no explosion, but radioactive materials broke loose and the contaminated beaches and farm soil had to be scooped up and taken to the United States for burial.

Imagine what would have happened if the *Torrey Canyon*, the giant tanker which was wrecked off the Scilly Isles, had been nuclear-powered. Some experts make comforting noises and say that the reactors would have "closed down," but the *Torrey Canyon* was a wreck and the Palomares incident showed what happens when radioactive materials break loose. All those oil-polluted beaches of southwest England and the coasts of Brittany would have had to be scooped up for nuclear burial.

II

The *Torrey Canyon* is a nightmarish example of progress for its own sake. The bigger the tanker the cheaper the freightage, which is supposed to be progress. This ship was built at Newport News, Virginia, in 1959 for the Union Oil Company; it was a giant for the time—810 feet long and 104 feet beam—but, five years later, that was not big enough. She was taken to Japan to be "stretched." The ship was cut in half amidship and a mid-body section inserted. With a new bow, this made her 974 feet long, and her beam was extended 21 feet. She could carry 850,000 barrels of oil, twice her original capacity.

Built for Union Oil, she was "owned" by the Barracuda Tanker Corporation, the head office of which is a filing cabinet in Hamilton, Bermuda. She was registered under the Liberian flag of convenience and her captain and crew were Italians, recruited in Genoa. Just to complicate the international triangle, she was under charter to the British Petroleum Tanker Company to bring 118,000 tons of crude oil from Kuwait to Milford Haven in Wales, via the Cape of Good Hope. Approaching Lands End, the Italian captain was informed that if he did not reach Milford Haven by 11 P.M. Saturday night, he would miss highwater and would not be able to enter the harbor for another five days, which would have annoyed his employers. He took a shortcut, setting course between Seven Stones rocks and the Scilly Isles, and he finished up on Pollard Rock, in an area where no ship of that size should ever have been.

Her ruptured tanks began to vomit oil and great slicks spread over the sea in the direction of the Cornish holiday beaches. A Dutch tug made a dash for the stranded ship, gambling on the salvage money. (Where the salvaged ship could have been taken one cannot imagine, since no place would offer harborage to a leaking tanker). After delays and a death in the futile salvage effort, the British Government moved in with the navy, the air force and, on the beaches, the army. They tried to set fire to the floating oil which, of course, would not volatilize. They covered the slicks with detergents (supplied at a price by the oil companies), and then the bombers moved in to try to cut open the deck and, with incendiaries, to set fire to the remaining oil in the tanks. Finally the ship foundered and divers confirmed that the oil had been effectively consumed.

Nevertheless the result was havoc. All measures had had to be improvised. Twelve thousand tons of detergent went into the sea. Later marine biologists found that the cure had been worse than the complaint. The oil was disastrous for seabirds, but marine organic life was destroyed by the detergents. By arduous physical efforts, with bulldozers and flame-throwers and, again, more detergents, the beaches were cleaned up for the holiday-makers. Northerly winds swept the oil slicks down Channel to the French coast with even more serious consequences, particularly to the valuable shellfish industry. With even bigger tankers being launched, this affair is a portentous warning.

Two years after *Torrey Canyon* an offshore oil rig erupted in the Santa Barbara Channel. The disaster to wildlife in this area, which has island nature reserves and is on the migratory route of whales, seals and seabirds, was a repetition of the *Torrey Canyon* oil-spill. And the operator of the lethal oil rig was Union Oil.

III

Another piece of stupidity shows how much we are at the mercy of ignorant men pretending to be knowledgeable. During the International Geophysical Year, 1957–58, the Van Allen Belt was discovered. This is an area of magnetic phenomena. Immediately it was decided to explode a nuclear bomb in the Belt to see whether an artificial aurora could be produced. The colorful draperies and luminous skirts of the aurora borealis are caused by the drawing in of cosmic particles through the rare bases of the upper atmosphere—ionization it is called; it is like passing electrons through the vacuum tubes of our familiar fluorescent lighting. The name Rainbow Bomb was given it in anticipation of the display it was expected to produce. Every eminent scientist in the field of cosmology, radio-astronomy or physics of the atmosphere protested at this irresponsible tampering with a system which we did not understand. And typical of the casual attitude toward this kind of thing, the Prime Minister of the day, answering protests in the House of Commons that called on him to intervene with the Americans, asked what all the fuss was about. After all, they hadn't known that the Van Allen Belt even existed a year before. This was the cosmic equivalent of Chamberlain's remark about Czechoslovakia, at the time of Munich, about that distant country of which we knew so little. They exploded the bomb. They got their pyrotechnics and we still do not know the cost we may have to pay for this artificial magnetic disturbance.

In the same way we can look with misgivings on those tracks—the white tails of the jets, which are introducing into our climatic system new factors, the effects of which are immeasurable. Formation of rain clouds depends upon water vapor having a nucleus on which to form. That is how artificial precipitation is introduced—the so-called rain-making. So the jets, crisscrossing the weather system, playing noughts and crosses with it, can produce a man-made change.

In the longer term we can foresee even more drastic effects from Man's unthinking operations. At the United Nations' Science and Technology Conference in Geneva in 1963 we took stock of the effects of industrialization on our total environment thus far. The atmosphere is not only the air which humans, animals and plants breathe; it is also the envelope which protects living things from harmful radiation from the sun and outer space. It is also the medium of climate, the winds and the rain. Those are inseparable from the hydrosphere—the oceans, covering seven-tenths of the globe, with their currents and extraordinary rates of evaporation; the biosphere, with its trees and their transpiration; and, in terms of human activities, the minerals mined from the lithosphere, the rock crust. Millions of years ago the sun encouraged the growth of the primeval forests, which became our coal, and the plant growth of the seas, which became our oil. Those fossil fuels, locked away for aeons of time, are extracted by man and put back into the atmosphere from the chimney stacks and the exhaust pipes of modern engineering. About 6 billion tons of carbon are mixed with the atmosphere annually. During the past century, in the process of industrialization, with its release of carbon by the burning of fossil fuels, more than 400 billion tons of carbon have been artificially introduced into the atmosphere. The concentration in the air we breathe has been increased by approximately 10 percent, and if all the known reserves of coal and oil were burnt at once, the concentration would be ten times greater.

This is something more than a public health problem, more than a question of what goes into the lungs of an individual, more than a question of smog. The carbon cycle in nature is a self-adjusting mechanism. Carbon dioxide is, of course, indispensable for plants and is, therefore, a source of life, but there is a balance which is maintained by excess carbon being absorbed by the seas. The excess is now taxing this absorption because of what is known as the "greenhouse effect." A greenhouse lets in the sun's rays but retains the heat. Carbon dioxide, as a transparent diffusion, does likewise. It keeps the heat at the surface of the earth and in excess modifies the climate.

It has been estimated that, at the present rate of increase, the mean annual temperature all over the world might increase by 3.6 degrees centigrade in the next forty to fifty years. The experts may argue about the time factor and even about the effects, but certain things are apparent, not only in the industrialized Northern Hemisphere but in the Southern Hemisphere also. The North-polar icecap is thinning and shrinking. The seas, with their blanket of carbon dioxide, are changing their temperature, with the result that marine plant life is increasing and is transpiring more carbon dioxide. As a result of the combination, fish are migrating, changing even their latitudes. On land the snow line is retreating and glaciers are melting. In Scandinavia, land which was perennially under snow and ice is thawing, and arrowheads of over 1,000 years ago, when the black soils were last exposed, have been found. The melting of sea ice will not affect the sea level, because the volume of floating ice is the same as the water it displaces, but the melting of icecaps or glaciers, in which the water is locked up, will introduce additional water to the sea and raise the level. Rivers originating in glaciers and permanent snow fields will increase their flow; and if ice dams, such as those in the Himalayas, break, the results in flooding may be catastrophic. In this process the patterns of rainfall will change, with increased precipitation in some areas and the possibility of aridity in now fertile regions. One would be well advised not to take ninety-nine year leases on properties at present sea level.

IV

At that same conference, there was a sobering reminder of mistakes which can be writ large, from the very best intentions. In the Indus Valley in West Pakistan, the population is increasing at the rate of ten more mouths to be fed every five minutes. In that same five minutes in that same place, an acre of land is being lost through water-logging and salinity. This is the largest irrigated region in the world. Twenty-three million acres are artificially watered by canals. The Indus and its tributaries, the Jhelum, the Chenab, the Ravi, the Beas and the Sutlej, created the alluvial plains of the Punjab and the Sind. In the nineteenth century, the British began a big program of farm development in lands which were fertile but had low rainfall. Barrages and distribution canals were constructed. One thing which, for economy's sake, was not done was to line the canals. In the early days, this genuinely did not matter. The water was being spread from the Indus into a thirsty plain and if it soaked in so much the better. The system also depended on what is called "inland delta drainage," that is to say, the water spreads out like a delta and then drains itself back into the river. After independence, Pakistan, with external aid, started vigorously to extend the Indus irrigation. The experts all said the soil was good and would produce abundantly once it got the distributed water. There were plenty of experts, but they all overlooked one thing—the hydrological imperatives. The incline from Lahore to the Rann of Kutch—700 miles—is a foot a mile, a quite inadequate drainage gradient. So as more and more barrages and more and more lateral canals were built, the water was not draining back into the Indus. Some 40 percent of the water in the unlined canals seeped underground, and in a network of 40,000 miles of canals that is a lot of water. The result was that the watertable rose. Low-lying areas became waterlogged, drowning the roots of the crops. In other areas the water crept upwards, leaching salts which accumulated in the surface layers, poisoning the crops. At the same time the irrigation régime, which used just 1-1/2 inches of water a year in the fields, did not sluice out those salts but added, through evaporation, its own salts. The result was tragically spectacular. In flying over large tracts of this area one would imagine that it was an Arctic landscape because the white crust of salt glistens like snow.

The situation was deteriorating so rapidly that President Ayub appealed in person to President Kennedy, who sent out a high-powered mission which encompassed twenty disciplines. This was backed by the computers at Harvard. The answers were pretty grim. It would take twenty years and $2 billion to repair the damage—more than it cost to create the installations that did the damage. It would mean using vertical drainage to bring up the water and use it for irrigation, and also to sluice out the salt in the surface soil. If those twenty scientific disciplines had been brought together in the first instance it would not have happened.

One more instance of the far-flung consequences of men's localized mistakes: No insecticides or pesticides have ever been allowed into the continent of Antarctica. Yet they have been found in the fauna along the northern coasts. They have come almost certainly from the Northern Hemisphere, carried from the rivers of the farm-states into the currents sweeping south. In November 1969, the U.S. Government decided to "phase out" the use of DDT.

Pollution is a crime compounded of ignorance and avarice. The great achievements of *Homo sapiens* become the disaster-ridden blunders of

Unthinking Man—poisoned rivers and dead lakes, polluted with the effluents of industries which give something called "prosperity" at the expense of posterity. Rivers are treated like sewers and lakes like cesspools. These natural systems—and they are living systems—have struggled hard. The benevolent microorganisms which cope with reasonable amounts of organic matter have been destroyed by mineral detergents. Witness our foaming streams. Lake Erie did its best to provide the oxygen to neutralize the pickling acids of the great steel works. But it could not contend. It lost its oxygen in the battle. Its once rich commercial fishing industry died and its revitalizing microorganic life gave place to anaerobic organisms which do not need oxygen but give off foul smells, the mortuary smells of dead water. As one Erie industrialist retorted, "It's not our effluent; its those damned dead fish."

We have had the Freedom from Hunger Campaign; presently we shall need a Freedom from Thirst Campaign. If the International Hydrological Decade does not bring us to our senses we will face a desperate situation. Of course it is bound up with the increasing population but also with the extravagances of the technologies which claim that they are serving that population. There is a competition between the water needs of the land which has to feed the increasing population and the domestic and industrial needs of that population. The theoretical minimum to sustain living standards is about 300 gallons a day per person. This is the approximate amount of water needed to produce grain for 2-1/2 pounds of bread, but a diet of 2 pounds of bread and 1 pound of beef would require about 2,500 gallons. And that is nothing compared with the gluttonous requirements of steel-making, paper-making and the chemical industry.

Water—just H_2O—is as indispensable as food. To die of hunger one needs more than fifteen days. To die of thirst one needs only three. Yet we are squandering, polluting and destroying water. In Los Angeles and neighboring Southern California, a thousand times more water is being consumed than is being precipitated in the locality. They have preempted the water of neighboring states. They are piping it from Northern California and there is a plan to pipe it all the way from Canada's North-West Territories, from the Mackenzie and the Liard which flow northwards to the Arctic Ocean, to turn them back into deserts.

V

Always and everywhere we come back to the problem of population—more people to make more mistakes, more people to be the victims of the mistakes of others, more people to suffer Hell upon Earth. It is appalling to hear people complacently talking about the population explosion as though it belonged to the future, or world hunger as though it were threatening, when hundreds of millions can testify that it is already here—swear it with panting breath.

We know to the exact countdown second when the nuclear explosion took place—5:30 A.M., July 16, 1945, when the first device went off in the desert of Alamogordo, New Mexico. The fuse of the population explosion had been lit ten years earlier—February 1935. On that day a girl called Hildegarde was dying of generalized septicaemia. She had pricked her finger with a sewing needle and the infection had run amok. The doctors could not save her. Her desperate father injected a red dye into her body. Her father was Gerhard Domagk. The red dye was prontosil which he, a pharmaceutical chemist, had produced and had successfully used on mice lethally infected with streptococci, but never before on a human. Prontosil was the first of the sulfa drugs—chemotherapeutics, which could attack the germ within the living body. Thus was prepared the way for the rediscovery of penicillin—rediscovery because although Fleming had discovered it in 1928, it had been ignored because neither he nor anybody else had seen its supreme virtue of attacking germs within the living body. That is the operative phrase, for while medical science and the medical profession had used antiseptics for surface wounds and sores, they were always labeled "Poison, not to be taken internally." The sulfa drugs had shown that it was possible to attack specific germs within the living body and had changed this attitude. So when Chain and Florey looked again at Fleming's penicillin in 1938, they were seeing it in the light of the experience of the sulfas.

A new era of disease-fighting had begun—the sulfas, the antibiotics, DDT insecticides. Doctors could now attack a whole range of invisible enemies. They could master the old killer diseases. They proved it during the war, and when the war ended there were not only stockpiles of the drugs, there were tooled up factories to produce them. So to prevent the spread of deadly epidemics which follow wars, the supplies were made available to the war-ravaged countries with their displaced persons, and then to the developing countries. Their indigenous infections and contagions and insect-borne diseases were checked.

Almost symbolically, the first great clinical use of prontosil had been in dealing with puerperal sepsis, childbed fever. It had spectacularly saved mothers' lives in Queen Charlotte's Hospital, London. Now its successors took up the story. Fewer mothers died in childbirth, to live and have more babies. Fewer infants died, fewer toddlers, fewer adolescents. They lived to marry and have children. Older people were not killed off by, for instance, malaria. The average life-span increased.

Professor Kingsley Davis of the University of California at Berkeley, the authority on urban development, has presented a hair-raising picture from his survey of the world's cities. He has shown that 38 percent of the world's population is already living in what are defined as urban places. Over one-fifth of the world's population is living in cities of 100,000 or more. And over one-tenth of the world's population is now living in cities of a million or more inhabitants. In 1968, 375 million people were living in million-and-over cities. The proportions are changing so quickly that on present trends it would take only 16 years for half the world's population to be living in cities and only 55 years for it to reach 100 percent.

Within the lifetime of a child born today, Kingsley Davis foresees, on present trends of population-increase, 15 billion people to be fed and housed—nearly five times as many as now. The whole human species would be living in cities of a million-and-over inhabitants, and—wait for it!—the biggest city would have 1.3 billion inhabitants. That means 186 times as many as there are in Greater London.

For years the Greek architect Doxiadis has been warning us about such prospects. In his Ecumenopolis—World City—one urban area like confluent ulcers would ooze into the next. The East Side of World City would have as its High Street the Eurasian Highway stretching from Glasgow to Bangkok, with the Channel Tunnel as its subway and a built-up area all the way. On the West Side of World City, divided not by the tracks but by the Atlantic, the pattern is already emerging, or rather, merging. Americans already talk about Boswash, the urban development of a built-up area stretching from Boston to Washington; and on the West Coast, apart from Los Angeles, sprawling into the desert, the realtors are already slurring one city into another all along the Pacific Coast from the Mexican Border to San Francisco. We don't need a crystal ball to foresee what Davis and Doxiadis are predicting; we can already see it through smog-covered spectacles; a blind man can smell what is coming.

The danger of prediction is that experts and men of affairs are likely to plan for the predicted trends and confirm these trends. "Prognosis" is something different from "prediction." An intelligent doctor having diagnosed your symptoms and examined your condition does not say (except in novelettes), "You have six months to live." An intelligent doctor says, "Frankly, your condition is serious. Unless you do so-and-so, and I do so-and-so, it is bound to deteriorate." The operative phrase is "do so-and-so." We don't have to plan for trends; if they are socially undesirable our duty is to plan away from them; to treat the symptoms before they become malignant.

We have to do this on the local, the national and the international scale, through intergovernmental action, because there are no frontiers in present-day pollution and destruction of the biosphere. Mankind shares a common habitat. We have mortgaged the old homestead and nature is liable to foreclose.

Human ecology

RENÉ DUBOS

I should first like to thank you, Mr. Chairman, for having invited me to deliver the first Jacques Parisot lecture before such a distinguished international audience. I am particularly sensible to this honor because I have endeavored throughout my professional life to take as my guide a medical philosophy which Parisot taught and practiced with outstanding success—a philosophy based on a synthesis of scientific knowledge and social conscience.

Nowadays there is a tendency to believe that modern medicine consists exclusively of a few sensational recent discoveries—miracle drugs, spectacular surgical techniques, sophisticated immunization methods. This tendency is dangerous, for it deflects attention from another aspect of modern medicine which is just as remarkable and perhaps of greater practical importance. If the health of the public has improved in many regions during recent decades, the improvement is due not only to certain specialized medical procedures but also—and probably to a greater extent—to a better understanding of the effects of man's environment and way of life on his physiological and mental state. Our health is better than that of our ancestors to the extent that our lives are more in accord with what I would choose to call biological wisdom. The scientific expression of that biological wisdom is human ecology, i.e., knowledge of the relationships between man and the innumerable factors of his environment.

It would be easy and pleasant for me to devote this entire lecture to an inventory of the progress of modern medical science. But I feel that it will be more productive to consider in what respects that science is inadequate, particularly when it comes to coping with the new ecological crisis that at the present time is threatening almost every country in the world.

The word "environment" has in our day acquired an ever more tragic connotation, both in primitive agrarian societies and in industrial urban

HUMAN ECOLOGY From *World Health Organization Chronicle*, Vol. 23, No. 11, November 1969. Reprinted by permission of the author.

societies. It connotes, for example, malnutrition and infection in most of the poor countries, chemical pollution and mechanization of life in all the prosperous countries. The ecological crisis is everywhere so menacing and takes such varied forms that the term "human ecology" has come to be used only for certain situations that might lead to biological or mental disaster. Yet human ecology embraces far more than this tragic view of the relationships between man and his environment. Ecology teaches us that all the physical, biological, and social forces acting upon man impart a direction to his development and thus mold his nature. The body and the mind are constantly being modified, and hence shaped, by the stimuli that induce formative reactions. It is to be hoped that a time will come when human ecology will be able to pay greater attention to the positive and beneficial effects of the environment than to its pathogenic effects.

The social mechanisms whereby society tries to create a more or less artificial environment better adapted to man's needs and desires constitute an extremely important aspect of human ecology which I shall not attempt to discuss here. The other aspect of human ecology consists of the biological processes whereby the organism as a whole tries to adapt itself to environmental forces. The importance of these adaptive phenomena for health has frequently been demonstrated in the course of history. I shall mention a few examples of this.

In the narrative of his travels, Christopher Columbus speaks with admiration of the magnificent physical condition of the natives he discovered in Central America. In the eighteenth century, Cook, Bougainville, and the other navigators who ranged over the Pacific also wondered at the excellent health of the island populations of Oceania. Many other explorers were similarly impressed on their first contact with the Indians, the Africans, and, later, the Eskimos. The legend of the noble savage, healthy and happy, thus has its origin in the descriptions published by the explorers who observed certain native populations when they were still undeveloped and almost completely isolated from the rest of the world.

There was certainly a lot of false romanticism in the illusion that the noble savage was free from disease and social restrictions because he lived in a state of nature. But all the same this romantic and over-simple view of man's estate has been partly justified by the studies in physical and social anthropology conducted on what contemporary anthropologists call man the hunter. These studies were recently the subject of a symposium under that title, in the course of which descriptions were given of the characteristics of populations that live without agriculture and even without tools, except for a few primitive objects they employ to derive their sustenance from wild plants and animals. It appears that this way of life, though so close to nature and therefore lacking any medical assistance, is compatible with a good state of health. But I should like to emphasize the fact that primitive populations undergo rapid physical and mental deterioration as soon as they come into close contact with the modern world and thus lose their ancestral manners and customs. The noble savage who seemed so healthy and happy in the eighteenth century had often become a human wreck by the nineteenth.

The epidemiological facts suggest that the good health of primitive peoples, like that of wild animals, is a manifestation of a biological equilibrium between the living creature and its environment. This equilibrium persists as long as the conditions of human ecology remain stable, but is broken as soon as the conditions change. The enormous problems of malnutrition, alcoholism, and infectious disease, which caused such a rapid physical deterioration among the primitive populations in the seventeenth, eighteenth, and nineteenth centuries, recurred in all the Western countries at the outset of the Industrial Revolution, when their working classes, originating largely from agricultural regions, underwent massive and sudden exposure to conditions of life that were then new to them.

Adaptation to industrial society is now far advanced in the prosperous countries, but this is only a temporary phase. New problems arc arising from the fact that the second Industrial Revolution is causing sudden and far-reaching changes in the physical environment and in everyday living, thus creating a new and as yet unstable ecological situation. The changes naturally bring their own specific dangers, which undoubtedly underlie what we nowadays call the diseases of civilization.

Indeed, we might say that in our day human ecology is undergoing an almost universal crisis because man is not yet adapted, and probably never will become adapted, either to the biological impoverishment of the very poor countries or to certain environmental influences that the second Industrial Revolution has introduced into the rich countries. It might be supposed that man, since he still has the same genetic make-up as in the past, could once again use the biological mechanisms that enabled him in the Stone Age to colonize a large part of the globe, and so could adapt himself to the conditions of physiological impoverishment or industrial intoxication of present-day life. But this is neither certain nor even probable, because the present changes are of a kind almost without precedent in human history.

Up till now, changes in the pattern of living have generally been so slow that it took several generations before they affected all classes of society. This slowness enabled the entire range of adaptive forces to be brought into play: physiological and even anatomical characteristics, as well as mental reactions and particularly social organization, little by little changed. Nowadays, on the contrary, everything changes so quickly that the processes of biological and social adaptation do not have time to come into play. Whether from the biological or the social point of view, the father's experience is now of practically no value to the son.

It is also a known fact that the human faculty of adaptation, great as it is, is not unlimited. It is quite possible that the stresses of present-day living are taking it near its extreme limits.

In the course of his evolution, man has constantly been exposed to inclement weather, fatigue, periodic famine, and infection. So as to survive these dangers, he has had to develop in his genetic code hereditary mechanisms that have facilitated certain processes of adaptation. But man now has to face dangers of another kind, without any precedent in the biological past of the human species. He probably does not possess adaptive mechanisms for all the new situations to which he is exposed. Moreover, the evolution of biological mechanisms is far too slow to keep up with the accelerated pace of technological and social change in the modern world.

It is certain, for example, that there is no possible means of adaptation to nutritional deficiencies that persist for long periods. Many children in their growth phase succumb to them. If they survive, they cannot satisfactorily realize the potentialities of their genetic endowment; they are condemned for the rest of their lives to anatomical, physiological, and mental atrophy. A population continuously subjected to nutritional deficiency cannot but degenerate.

Industrial technology has introduced into modern life a range of substances and situations that man has never known in his biological past. It is probable that he will never be able to adapt himself to the toxic effects of chemical pollution and of certain synthetic products; to the physiological and mental difficulties caused by lack of physical effort; to the mechanization of life; and to the presence of a wide variety of artificial stimulants. We should probably add to this list the disturbances to natural body rhythms arising from the almost complete divorce of modern life from cosmic cycles.

There are no grounds for the fear that all deviations from the natural order that result from technological change will be dangerous to health. Far from it. It remains true, however, that the more a population is exposed to modern technology the more it appears to be subject to certain forms of chronic and degenerative disease—conditions called for precisely that reason the diseases of civilization. Premature death caused by these diseases is not due to the lack of medical care. In the U.S.A., for example, scientists and especially physicians have, paradoxically enough, a shorter life expectancy than other groups, although they belong to an economically privileged class. Certain demographic studies show that the life expectancy beyond the age of 35 may have decreased somewhat during the last few years in the big cities of the U.S.A.

Everyday life seems to give the lie to the anxieties expressed in the previous pages, since modern man appears to be just as adaptable as Stone Age man. An extraordinary number of people have survived the terrible ordeals of modern war and the concentration camps. Throughout the world it is the most crowded and polluted cities, those in which life is at its most ruthless, that attract most people, and it is their population that is increasing at the greatest rate. Men and women are working all the time in the midst of the infernal noise of machines and telephones, in an atmosphere polluted with chemical fumes and tobacco smoke.

This remarkable tolerance of man towards conditions so different from those in which he has evolved has given rise to the myth that, through technological and social progress, he can modify his way of life and his environment indefinitely and without risk. That is simply not true. As I stated earlier, modern man can only adapt himself in so far as the mechanisms of adaptation are potentially present in his genetic code. Furthermore, it is certain that in many cases the apparent ease with which man adapts himself biologically, socially, and culturally to new or unfavorable conditions constitutes, paradoxically, a threat to individual well-being and even to the future of the human race.

This paradox arises from the fact that the word "adaptation" cannot be applied unreservedly to the adjustments that enable human beings to survive and function under modern conditions. Indeed, in man sociocultural forces distort the effects of the kind of adaptive mechanisms that operate in the animal kingdom.

For the biologist, the expression "Darwinian adaptation" implies harmony between a species and a given environment, a harmony that enables it to multiply and, at the appropriate moment, to invade new territory. In the terms of this definition, man would appear to be remarkably well adapted to the conditions of life that exist both in highly industrialized societies and in developing countries, since the world's population is continuing to increase and to occupy an ever greater proportion of the land surface of the globe. However, what would constitute a biological success for another species is a serious social threat to the human species. The dangers arising from the increase in world population show clearly that the Darwinian concept of adaptation cannot be used if the well-being of humanity is taken as a criterion of its biological success.

For the physiologist, a reaction to environmental stress is adaptive when it neutralizes the disturbing effects of such stress on the body and mind. In general, physiological and psychological adaptive responses are a factor tending towards the well-being of the organism at the time when they occur. In man, however, they may in the long term have detrimental effects. Man is capable of acquiring some degree of tolerance towards environmental pollution, excessive stimuli, a harassing social life in a competitive atmosphere, a rhythm completely foreign to natural biological cycles, and all the other consequences of his living in the world of cities and technology. This tolerance enables him to resist successfully exposure to influences which, at the outset, are unpleasant or traumatic. However, in many cases such tolerance is only acquired through a set of organic and mental processes that risk giving rise to degenerative manifestations.

Man can also learn to put up with the ugliness of the environment in which he lives, with its smoky skies and polluted streams. He can live without the scent of flowers, the song of birds, the life-enhancing spectacle of nature, and the other biological stimuli of the physical world. The suppression of a number of the pleasurable aspects of life and the stimuli that have conditioned his biological and mental evolution may have no manifest deleterious effect on his physical appearance or on his efficiency as a cog in the economic or technological machine, but there is a risk that, in the long run, it may impoverish his life and lead to the gradual loss of the qualities we associate with the idea of a human being.

Air, water, soil, fire, and the natural rhythms and diversity of living species are important not only as chemical combinations, physical forces, or biological phenomena but also because it is under their influence that human life has been fashioned. They have created in man deep-rooted needs that will not change in any near future. The pathetic weekend exodus towards the countryside or the beaches, the fireplaces that are still built in overheated urban apartments, the sentimental attachments formed for animals or even plants all bear witness to the survival deep down in man of biological and emotional urges acquired in the course of his evolution, of which he cannot rid himself.

Like the giant Antaeus in the Greek legend, man loses his strength as soon as he loses contact with the earth.

Human ecology therefore requires a scientific and intellectual attitude differing from that which would be adequate in general biology and even in the other biomedical sciences, because it has to deal with the indirect and long-term effects exercised by the environment and way of life, even if those factors have no apparent immediate influence. It would be easy to illustrate the importance of those indirect and long-term effects by discussing, for example, the part played by the abundance or scarcity of food, the various forms of chemical and microbial pollution, the effects of noise or other stimuli, the density of and especially the rapid changes in the population; in brief, all the environmental forces that act on man in every social class and in every country. Here, however, I shall confine myself to pointing out that the most important effects of the environment and way of life are often difficult to recognize because they only show themselves indirectly and after a lapse of time.

The early stages of life are of exceptional importance because to a large extent they determine what the adult will become. The young organism never forgets anything. All the factors that act upon it therefore contribute to the psychosomatic formation of the individual. The younger the person, the more malleable he is and the more easily affected by environmental influences. Hence the importance of the first stages of life, including those within the womb. These long-term and indirect manifestations of the environment are still poorly understood, but it is fortunately possible and even easy to study them experimentally since in animals, as in man, perinatal conditions have a profound and often irreversible effect, bearing on the anatomical features of the adult as well as on metabolism and behavior. Animal experiments will therefore make it possible to see what is not easily seen in man, to understand what is not obvious to our minds and, consequently, to take action with a view to alleviating certain untoward or even disastrous consequences of the influences to which man is exposed at the beginning of his life.

Of course the environment continues unceasingly to transform the organism. However, the first years of life have effects so profound and irreversible that they are the most important part of human ecology. I am emphasizing this fact because it seems to me that it should influence the general policy of WHO and encourage scientists to devote more effort to the problems of childhood. It is beyond doubt that the establishment of an atmosphere favorable to the biological and mental development of the child is the most economical way of improving world health.

A better understanding of the effect of environment at the beginning of life on growth and development gives a deeper sense to the definition of health made famous by the preamble to the WHO Constitution: "Health is a state of complete physical, mental and social well-being and not merely an absence of disease or infirmity." This "positive health" advocated by WHO implies that a person should be able to express as completely as possible the potentialities of his genetic heritage. That heritage, however, can only find true expression to the extent that the environment transforms genetic potentialities into phenotypic realities. It is in this way that human ecology might finally become identified, as I expressed the hope that it could at the beginning of this lecture, with the positive and beneficial effects of the environment.

The word "health" in the sense that I have chosen to give it describes not a state but a potentiality—the ability of an individual or a social group to modify himself or itself continually not only in order to function better in the present but also to prepare for the future. Ideal health will, however, always remain a mirage, because everything in our life will continue to change. The doctor and the public health expert are in the same position as the gardener or farmer faced with insects, molds, and weeds. Their work is never done. Man quickly grows tired of conditions of life that had originally seemed attractive. Individually and collectively he will look for adventure, and this forces him to live under constantly new conditions, with all the unforeseen occurrences and threats to health involved in change.

There is no question, however, of turning back. A society that does not move forward quickly deteriorates. Indeed, it cannot even survive in a world where everything is in a state of flux. Civilizations can only succeed and survive by exploring the unknown and accepting the risks involved in plunging ahead into the future. Technology would soon cease to develop if a certificate of absolute safety were required for every technical innovation and every new product.

It is therefore inevitable that economic and social progress should always be accompanied by hazards to health, whatever the advances made by medicine and hygiene.

This fact gives the doctor and the hygienist a still more important social role than they have at the present moment. It consists in recognizing as swiftly as possible, and even in anticipating, the medical problems that will arise increasingly as a result of the accelerated rate of technological and economic innovation. For this purpose it is becoming urgent to set up what might be called listening posts to record the first signs of pathological disorders that might threaten to spread to society as a whole. For example, the effects of atmospheric pollution, changes in food habits, the almost universal and constant use of new drugs, and automation in industry and in every aspect of life are still unforeseeable but could doubtless be detected before health disasters become widespread. It is a matter of satisfaction that this social responsibility is already recognized in certain sectors of the public service. Thus, thorough studies of the biological effects of ionizing radiation have been undertaken with a view to developing in advance practical methods of protection against the probable consequences of the industrial use of radiation. There would be no point in quoting here studies of the same kind already undertaken by WHO on the effect of drugs and insecticides. This farsighted attitude will have to be generally adopted. In the future the development of technological innovations should always include parallel scientific studies on the long-term effects of these innovations on human ecology.

As Jacques Parisot wrote, "To cure is good but to prevent is better." Humanity will only be able to avoid the hazards of the future by extending its scientific knowledge and showing greater social conscience.

Where will we put all that garbage?

TOM ALEXANDER

Just about any schoolboy can figure out that roughly as much material must be taken out of a community as is brought in if something altogether desperate isn't to happen eventually. But whereas goods are brought into communities via elaborate networks of transportation, organization, and management, the equally voluminous wastes are taken out and disposed of almost in afterthought. Up till now, Mother Nature has pretty well covered for these casual attitudes toward waste handling. The natural sinks of water, air, and land and nature's destructive processes have usually made it possible for urban, rural, and industrial man to manage, with a modicum of effort, to place his wastes far enough out of sight and smell to keep them out of mind. But urban man is finding out that this approach isn't good enough any more. Despite spending some $3 billion annually on municipal refuse disposal, most U.S. cities have fallen behind, and most face genuine solid-waste crises within two to fifteen years. Such cities as San Francisco, Washington, D.C., Chicago, and New York are at the crisis point already. Curiously, the agricultural community, too, finds itself with its manures and other wastes piling up faster than farmers can get rid of them.

Both the city's and the farm's problems come about for related reasons—shortage of disposal sites, changes of process and materials, plus the newly awakened concern over the health hazards of some of the traditional modes of waste disposal. And behind all of these is the relentless concentration of population. An analogy could be made with living organisms: simple one-celled animals need only primitive processes for handling wastes, such as exudation through their cell walls. But all large organisms have complex organs for excretion, often more elaborate than the organs for nourishment.

In belated recognition of the waste problem, considerable effort is now going into improving our technology of waste handling. The main spur was the federal Solid Waste Disposal Act of 1965, which exists only because of the recent alarm over air pollution. Solid-waste disposal was recognized

WHERE WILL WE PUT ALL THAT GARBAGE? Reprinted from the October 1967 issue of *Fortune* Magazine by special permission; © 1967 Time Inc. Tom Alexander is an Associate Editor of *Fortune*.

as a prime source of air pollutants, and to make federal funds available, a solid-waste act was passed as Title 2 of the 1965 air-pollution bill. The bait of federal funds attracted scientists into the notoriously uninspiring field of solid-waste research. What they found there provoked a shudder of alarm and a massive diversion of attention to solid-waste technology.

It now seems clear that technology alone is not the answer, and perhaps even that too many brains are now engaged in redundant investigations of the few conceivable engineering approaches. Before much long-term progress can be made in meeting the solid-waste crisis, new patterns of cooperation will have to emerge among federal, state, municipal, and county agencies. New systems of incentives may have to be legislated to encourage an economics of disposal to complement the orthodox economics of production, supply, and demand. New kinds of authorities or corporations may have to come into being to plan, capitalize, and manage new kinds of disposal systems—systems more versatile and flexible than a missile warning network or a telephone company, and just as important.

"Pollute thy neighbor"

The social metabolism of the urban U.S. currently appears to generate some six to eight pounds per person per day of waste products—garbage, paper, grass clippings, old autos, dead cats, demolition materials—or about double the weight of forty years ago. The U.S. Public Health Service expects this to double again in about twenty years. Most of the increase is attributable to the tremendous growth in use of paper products and packaging of various kinds. Nearly all foods and goods the housewife buys come in some kind of preprocessed packaged form. Furthermore, the *volume* of household waste is increasing far more rapidly than the weight. This reflects not only the shift toward paper but also the trend toward thinner grades of paper that, pound for pound, take up far more space when crumpled as refuse.

In the majority of U.S. cities and towns, the preferred solid-waste handling techniques entail gathering the trash noisily and expensively into trucks, carrying it outside the city limits, and dumping it upon a neighboring political jurisdiction. Sometimes when a dump becomes too large or too much of a nuisance, fires are started so as to permit obliging winds to carry off the dry and burnable fractions of paper, autos, and cats in the form of an oily, rich-smelling smoke.

But as surrounding communities have become either built up or fed up with this policy of "pollute thy neighbor," and as people have begun speaking badly of black, oily smoke, most cities appear about to run out of garbage room. In Washington, D.C., the citizenry has raised a barrage of organized protest over the city's famous evil-smoking Kenilworth Dump, located only five miles from the White House. Sixty percent of the refuse from the nine counties surrounding lovely San Francisco Bay is dumped along the bay shore. Now a state commission has ruled out the use of additional bay shore for dumping.

37

The most sophisticated techniques in common usage are the so-called "sanitary" landfill and municipal incineration. The principle of the sanitary landfill is to cover over each day's production of refuse with a layer of dirt to contain the odors and emerging fly pupae and to exclude rats and moisture. Unfortunately, landfilling takes a lot of dirt and a lot of space—an acre of ground piled seven feet high for every ten thousand people every year. New York annually uses up some 150 acres on the southern end of Staten Island even though the city first reduces the volume of part of its wastes through incineration. City officials estimate that New York will use up its supply of landfill space in about ten years. Meanwhile, it costs nearly $30 a ton to collect, transport, and dispose of New York's refuse—or three times the cost of a ton of West Virginia coal, mined and delivered in New York.

Theoretically, high-temperature incinerators should be able to reduce the total volume of municipal wastes by 75 to 90 percent, thereby cutting the demand for landfill. But almost none of the incinerators currently in operation in the U.S. meet the standards for air-pollution emissions that most experts recommend. Some have been shut down for this reason. New incinerators have been designed with elaborate electrostatic precipitators and gas scrubbers that can meet these standards, but both capital and operating costs are extremely high—totaling five or six times as much as the cost of sanitary landfill. Furthermore, such incinerators are usually designed for more or less specific refuse components, and such specifics are hard to predict over the next decades. Paper dresses, for example, are purposely made nonflammable, so that it takes higher-temperature incinerators to make them burn.

How to fertilize rhode island

Down on the farm, if anything, things are in some ways worse than in the city. It has recently been calculated, for instance, that one cow produces more waste material than 16.4 mid-twentieth-century Americans—some six to twenty-five pounds of manure for every pound of weight gained, three pounds for every pound of milk. In fact, total agricultural wastes of all kinds, including manures and food-processing residues, far outweigh the wastes produced by humans and their nonagricultural industries. Reports Professor Samuel Hart of the University of California at Davis, "If all the animal manure produced by the nation's livestock each year were spread evenly over the state of Rhode Island, forty-nine other states would have no agricultural sanitation problems and it would be several inches deep in Rhode Island."

Through the ages, most of the agricultural wastes were cycled back to the land and helped enrich its yield, but the economic urge to produce near the big markets is changing all that. Now most beef cattle and poultry spend all or much of their lives in the confines of a feedlot or poultry house, often on the outskirts of a large metropolis. Because of the transportation and labor costs of using manure, farmers now prefer the cheap, concentrated, and easy-to-apply artificial fertilizers. The upshot is that the far reaches of a number of big cities are marked by growing piles of manure, with attendant flies and severe drainage problems. For instance, rain runoff from feedlots has polluted nearly all the rivers and streams in Kansas. A complicating effect is that much of the soluble artificial fertilizer is leached from the fields during rains and finds its way into watercourses and lakes. There it stimulates the growth of aquatic plants that die eventually and in decaying deplete the dissolved oxygen in the water. This, in turn, lessens the water's ability to degrade sewage and, of course, the rain runoff from manure piles.

In both city and country, nature is increasingly being presented with a battery of wastes that she simply can't degrade. Nonreturnable glass bottles, aluminum cans, and junked autos litter the landscape and are virtually indestructible by natural processes. Bacterial cleanup agents are unable to break down many synthetic chemical products, including plastics and detergents. Industrial wastes such as steel-pickling and metal-plating baths are often discharged to persist with scarcely diminished toxicity for the entire length of a river. In other cases, toxic chemicals are impounded on land but percolate downward to pollute permanently groundwater sources. One alternative is to dry and burn some of the substances, but then they usually produce intolerable smogs, odors, or health hazards.

Several moves are afoot in federal and state agencies to ban or tax nonreturnable bottles and such nondegradable packaging materials as aluminum and plastics. (Sixteen states have introduced legislation against nonreturnable bottles.) The container and packaging industries are trying to come up with some kind of constructive measure to head off legislation. Two months ago, at the instigation of Chairman William F. May of the American Can Co., the trade associations from the container, paper, steel, aluminum, glass, and plastics industries formed a Materials Disposal Research Council to do something about the growing waste contribution from the packaging revolution. Whether this will turn into anything more than a public-relations gesture is still unclear, but May is suggesting that the council pursue a three-pronged approach: further attempts at antilitter education, studies of systems for collecting and reducing the volume of wastes, and research into container and packaging materials that either are not so durable or can be more easily processed for reuse. On and off for several years now various companies, notably the Adolph Coors brewery, National Brewing, Continental Oil, and Reynolds Metals, have experimented with paying the public to return empty aluminum cans, even though the salvage was uneconomical. Some of the tests have run into opposition from the retail outlets that were given the responsibility for collecting and sorting the salvaged items.

Many long-range thinkers cling to the view that somehow we must find ways of recycling waste materials back into useful form. Unfortunately the current economic trends seem to be against such a practice. Rising labor costs and the use of synthetic materials have virtually brought an end to most of the old picking and sorting of rags from municipal refuse. Large office buildings used to be paid for their wastepaper, which was then repulped and remade into paper. Today it can cost $37 a ton in New York to get it carried away. New industrial processes such as the oxygen steel-smelting process use less scrap iron, and as a consequence the derelict automobile is often not worth picking up and hauling to a processing yard.

Attempting to circumvent such economics, Dr. Athelstan Spilhaus, chairman of a recent blue-ribbon waste-management committee of the National Academy of Science–National Research Council, argues that potentially valuable wastes should be "banked" so they may easily be recovered at some later date when economics or technology has changed. Spilhaus points to the huge quantities of tailings from the gold mines in his native South Africa. As technology has developed, some of these tailing piles have been profitably reworked as many as three separate times, not only for gold but for uranium. Spilhaus suggests that all the junked autos, for instance, ought to be piled into landscaped dirt-covered hills, hills that might be mined when some future shortage of high-yield ores made scrap iron more valuable.

The goal of many of the ninety-two research and pilot demonstration projects funded under the federal Solid Waste Disposal Act is to find ways to salvage some kind of benefit from wastes. Notable among these is a project at Virginia Beach, Virginia, to use the sanitary-landfill technique to create a sixty-foot-high hill of municipal refuse. When finished, the hill will become a combination amphitheatre, soapbox-derby ramp, and landscaped park. University of Maryland scientists have a federal grant to develop foods and food additives for humans and animals from the wastes produced by the food-processing industries. They suggest, for example, that the U.S.'s annual ten million tons of tomato wastes—vines, leaves, and green and overripe tomatoes—could provide protein concentrates for undernourished parts of the world. Other federally supported research efforts are aimed at extracting waste heat from incinerators or methane gas and useful chemicals from waste materials. Europeans, in particular, have long put incinerator heat to work. West Berlin's huge new municipal incinerating complex provides steam for both electricity and central heating, while the residual clinkers are used as ersatz gravel. In the U.S., the town of Hempstead, Long Island, operates an imaginative refuse incinerator that drives both a 2,500-kilowatt electric power plant and a 420,000-gallon-a-day water-desalting plant.

The farmers' sense of humus

By conventional reckoning, the value added to waste through whatever processing is employed will usually be less than the cost of the processing. Take for example the efforts by a host of companies to turn municipal refuse into an organic compost that could be sold to farmers. Garbage and the paper components of refuse can be put through an accelerated bacterial process that in a few days or weeks turns them into a dark brown, odorless, soil-like material that is valuable as a soil conditioner. Such compost has long been used in Europe. But of the thirteen compost plants that have been set up in the U.S. by private firms or cities, nine have already closed down because of a lack of market. In most cases, transportation costs have forced the price of the compost up to the point where it could not compete with artificial fertilizers, especially since it needed a fertilizer supplement anyway.

Soil scientists agree that heavily farmed land should have some sort of organic humus added periodically. In the land-rich U.S. this is usually supplied by letting land lie fallow for a year and then plowing in a cover crop. But as the world's population grows, fallow land will become more and more of a luxury. Now it is being suggested that the city should pay the cost of making the compost and perhaps even of plowing it into the farmers' land and be thankful that it has a place to put its refuse. Chicago already helps defray the high cost of disposing of the semi-solid, nutrient-rich "sludge" residue from its sewage treatment plants by drying and barging it to Florida and selling it for use on citrus groves. Now Chicago is investigating piping the sludge some ninety miles for use on farmed-out lands in Kankakee County, Illinois. If this sludge could be mixed with refuse compost, it would make the compost considerably more valuable as a soil conditioner and nutrient.

Much of our helplessness in this area arises because most governmental units cannot cope with the problems. Political leaders don't find much glamour in solid waste. "You don't see a governor putting his gold plaque on a landfill," comments Dr. P. H. McGauhey, director of the University of California's Sanitary Engineering Research Laboratory at Richmond. In matters of waste handling, city does not speak to city, nor city to county. For instance, Leonard S. Wegman, an engineering consulting firm for solid wastes, recently worked out a cooperative disposal system for the three Connecticut towns of East Hartford, Glastonbury, and Manchester. The Wegman plan proposed modernizing East Hartford's air-polluting, inadequate incinerator for use by all three towns with the cost to be shared by all. But East Hartford citizens objected to the idea of handling the other towns' refuse and defeated the plan.

Individual towns often spend large sums on their own land-filling equipment, and it stands idle most of the day. Meanwhile the town can't afford to clean up the sewage discharge or the air pollution that is the bane of the neighboring town downstream or downwind. Air-pollution controllers end up cleaning up the air and discharging the wastes to rivers, while water-pollution controllers put theirs on land. The solid-waste controller pollutes all three.

The cost of curing an eyesore

Our accustomed totting up of benefits versus costs is difficult to apply in the instance of pollution. It is hard even to list all the direct and indirect costs of air, water, and land pollution to society—the shirts that must be changed twice a day, the funneling of vital soil nutrients and trace elements to the city and thence to irretrievability, the commuter's long, expensive haul to a cleaner suburb, the rat and fly eradication efforts, the foot cut on the beer-can tab. And how could anyone even attempt to put a price on an eyesore? But even if such calculations could be made, it is even more diffi- cult to devise economic incentives for recognizing the long-run needs of large regions. How do you persuade city dwellers to dispose of their wastes in such a way as to lessen the long-term drain on agricultural or industrial resources?

There are hopeful signs that some of the compartmentalization is van- ishing. At several places, such as Northwestern University and the uni- versities of Florida, West Virginia, and Cincinnati, the air, water, and land pollution experts are drawing together into "environmental engineering" groups, where "waste management" is the byword and "systems engineer- ing" the approach. And in those areas of the country where even minimal efforts have been made toward cooperation among political jurisdictions, the results have often been impressive. One of the best refuse-disposal sys- tems in the country serves seventy separate municipalities within Los Angeles County, including part of the city of Los Angeles itself. There col- lection and disposal costs—even with high land prices and long hauls—are among the lowest in the country. In the city of Los Angeles they average $12 a ton. The municipalities achieve this mostly through sharing landfill sites and through economies of scale. Some natural advantages, plus imag- inative area-wide planning and careful salesmanship, appear to be the main reasons why the county is already fairly well assured on its waste-disposal needs through the year 2005. And, through their pooling of resources, the Los Angeles County Sanitation Districts can afford a staff of engineers re- searching various advanced schemes for waste transportation and disposal for the periods after that.

Oddly, the spirit of cooperation in Los Angeles County stems from the joint need to provide a system of drains to carry off torrential rainfalls. Formed in the early 1900's, this Drainage District system later inspired a unique Sanitation District system that built a huge network of sewerage lines and treatment plants to serve a large section of the county. Finally, after World War II, the county woke up to its now famous smog problem. In 1957 the county banned the thousands of individual back-yard incin- erators and closed down the large municipal and industrial incinerators as well. It was left to the Sanitation Districts to find something to do with the 4,500 extra tons of refuse that would be piling up each day.

The districts' first move was to attempt to buy a huge abandoned quarry in Palos Verdes, ideally suited as a site for a sanitary landfill. Residents in that prosperous neighborhood fought the proposed purchase, being all too familiar with the smokes, odors, pests, and general unsightliness that characterized the privately operated refuse dumps then prevalent through- out the area. The Sanitation Districts nevertheless persisted, promising that not only would they cover each day's production of refuse in a nuisance- free way, but also that in the end the gaping quarry would become a land- scaped community asset for Palos Verdes. Sure enough, five years later a section of the scar had been quietly and painlessly converted into a public arboretum. With this and other similar triumphs skillfully publicized, the typical Los Angeles homebuyers' objections to having a "garbage dump" nearby were so well allayed that real-estate agents have little trouble selling $100,000 homes overlooking a working landfill with the bulldozers nudging up alongside the terrace. Often the houses overlooking the fill command the highest prices because of the promise of a park.

Envious officials from other cities point out that Los Angeles is exceptional in having natural canyons where refuse can be piled up to 600 feet deep. The districts' chief engineer, John Parkhurst, counters that ample landfill area can usually be found wihin easy-haul distance of most municipalities if (1) they can only overcome their mutual distrust long enough to cooperate, and (2) they can allay the legitimate doubts in the minds of nearby landholders that they will operate a nuisance-free landfill. Frank Bowerman, formerly Los Angeles County Sanitation Districts engineer, who did much of the planning for the landfills, has offered the New York area a free suggestion as to how it might solve *its* refuse problems. Bowerman, who is now working on Aerojet-General's waste-management research, recommends that the trash be barged out into lower New York Harbor and used to construct an artificial island for New York's much-needed new jetport. He estimates that enough material would be available to build at least one 12,000-foot runway per year.

The systems approach to garbage

Whatever the disposal method, the prerequisite to solving the waste-management dilemma is certainly some sort of regional approach. The regions might be small or very large—several villages or several states—but in each case they should be formed as geo-economic entities, rather than along political boundary lines. Moving in this direction, Sweden recently established a new central agency called Statens Naturvårdsverk—or "Nature Management Board"—that will attempt eventually to coordinate the handling of all waste products for the entire country.

Beginning in 1964, the state of California hired Aerojet-General to make a systematic series of studies of waste management on a statewide basis. Though Aerojet got off to a less than impressive start in its first reports, the company has by now developed some convincing adaptations of the defense industry's techniques of systems analysis and cost-benefit studies for the over-all waste management of large regions. In one study Aerojet is attempting to assess the relative seriousness of all the "bad effects" from wastes in Fresno County, California—rats from garbage dumps, odors from manure piles, air pollution from burning agricultural wastes, and so on. Once the sources and relative disagreeableness of all possible pollutants are established, Aerojet will be in a position to compute how the county can spend a limited amount of money to the greatest advantage. Such cost-benefit studies can also prevent uneconomic overkill; Professor H. B. Gotaas, Dean of Northwestern University's Technological Institute as well as head of the institute's Environmental Engineering Group, believes that many areas are proposing to make rivers and streams cleaner

43

than is economically justified. The money might better be spent on solid-waste or air-pollution technology, says Gotaas.

Ways to beat the freight rate

The major cost in any solid-waste disposal scheme, whether conducted on a regional basis or not, will be collection and transportation. As things stand now, from 75 to 90 percent of municipal refuse expenditures are absorbed by the armies of men and fleets of trucks that make the collections from individual households. The members of New York City's 14,000-man sanitation department make an average of $3 an hour, while the 1,800 garbage trucks contribute substantially to the noise, traffic congestion, and general nuisance of the city. New York's annual expenditure of nearly $130 million might better go for building some sort of automated, nuisance-free collection system. If long-haul transportation costs could be reduced, cities might find ample place for their residue in abandoned quarries, strip mines, swamps, or mountain canyons.

New York City and Philadelphia have studies under way with the New York Central and Reading railways, respectively, to see whether long-haul railroad transportation of wastes to the abandoned strip mines of Pennsylvania or West Virginia would be feasible. Spilhaus has suggested that since most freight cars enter a city full and leave empty, it might be possible to load the deadheading cars with bales of refuse. This recalls the laws of some medieval German towns that required every farm wagon bringing a load of produce to town to carry a load of municipal refuse out and dump it or plow it into the soil. With computers keeping track of railway cars, it is conceivable that even very long hauls might be possible, simply by taking advantage of the random movement of empty cars across the country.

The most sensible-sounding scheme for transporting wastes is simply to pump it out of town. Already Sweden and Britain have fitted several of their large scattered apartment complexes with tubes that transport bulk household refuse pneumatically to central incinerators as much as a mile and a half away. At the University of Pennsylvania, Professor Iraj Zandi has a federally supported project looking into the feasibility of collecting and pumping wastes in a liquid slurry form. Zandi has performed experiments that appear to show that if all ordinary municipal refuse—paper, tin cans, bottles, garbage, and so on—could be ground up in powerful household grinders or larger municipal grinders, it could be mixed with a small amount of water from the city sewer system and pumped out of town, perhaps more cheaply than it could be trucked out. Zandi's experiments show that the pipes could be surprisingly small—one only two inches in diameter could easily carry the wastes of a town of 10,000 or 15,000. And to save the costs of tearing up streets and buildings, most of these small solid-waste lines might be laid inside existing sewer lines, which are usually built outsize to accommodate storm runoff. The pipes could lead to far-off places where landfill is genuinely needed—perhaps to abandoned strip mines or low-lying swamplands. As for cost, Zandi points to the experience with pipelines used for transporting slurried coal. When the first 100-mile stretch of coal pipeline was laid in eastern Ohio, it had the effect of reducing the local rate for transporting coal by railroad. And rail transportation is cheaper than the truck transportation now used for hauling wastes.

Going even further, Zandi envisions the possibility of magnetic and centrifugal sorting devices to separate metals, glass, and perhaps the undecomposable plastics for possible salvage. The remaining organic material then might be mixed with the semisolid sludge residues from sewage treatment plants and manure from feedlots and the whole degraded biologically into compost, perhaps within the pipelines themselves.

A comsat for garbage

Though much needs to be learned about the costs and practicality of long-distance refuse pipelines, one could envision networks of such pipelines carrying compost and sewage from many sources to marginal agricultural areas. Even though the initial capital costs of such a system might be high, they would probably be offset by low operating costs. More important, there would be little noise, odor, unsightliness, and inconvenience. Furthermore, the network would double as an irrigation and fertilization system. It seems likely that some sort of utility company—wholly private like A.T. & T. or quasi-public like Comsat—would be best suited to plan, build, and operate such a regional network. The corporation could be paid a regulated price per ton or per household to get rid of all wastes. (Some items, such as bedsprings or large granite blocks from demolition, would probably still have to be hauled off specially, just as they are now.) Then such a profit-oriented company would try to make what extra money it could through cost cutting, salvage, irrigation charges, composting, or heat recovery.

But garbage network or no, one thing is clear: waste disposal will have to be done differently—and soon. The present approaches to waste handling are inadequate, expensive, and wasteful of natural resources. It appears to be only a matter of time before the congested areas of the U.S. will wake up to find garbage on their doorstep unless they reach out to avail themselves of the systems approach to waste disposal.

It's time to turn down all that noise

JOHN M. MECKLIN

In the Bronx borough of New York City one evening last spring, four boys were at play, shouting and racing in and out of an apartment building. Suddenly, from a second-floor window, came the crack of a pistol. One of the boys sprawled dead on the pavement. The victim happened to be Roy Innis Jr., thirteen, son of a prominent Negro leader, but there was no political implication in the tragedy. The killer, also a Negro, confessed to police that he was a nightworker who had lost control of himself because the noise from the boys prevented him from sleeping.

The incident was an extreme but valid example of a grim, and worsening, human problem. In communities all over the world, the daily harassment of needless noise provokes unknown millions to the verge of violence or emotional breakdown. There is growing evidence that it contributes to such physical ailments as heart trouble. Noise has become a scourge of our land, a form of environmental pollution no less dangerous and degrading than the poisons we dump into our air and water; it is one of the main causes of the exodus from our cities.

In many ways, noise is the most difficult form of pollution to combat. It has been recognized only recently as a major evil. It works so subtly on the human mind that it has gained a form of acceptance. Shouting over the din of an air compressor in New York recently, a newsman asked a construction foreman what he thought about the noise problem. "What are you," the foreman shouted back, "some kind of a Communist?"

Noise pollution is hardly a new evil. The word itself derives from the same Latin root as nausea. Noise bothered Julius Caesar so much that he banned chariot driving at night. In 1851, Arthur Schopenhauer wrote about the "disgraceful . . . truly infernal" cracking of whips in German streets. In a study published in October, 1955, *Fortune* reported "a rising tide of

IT'S TIME TO TURN DOWN ALL THAT NOISE From the October 1969 issue of *Fortune* Magazine. This article has appeared in a book, *The Environment: A National Mission for the Seventies*, published by Harper & Row, Inc. John M. Mecklin is a member of the Board of Editors of *Fortune*.

noise [in] U.S. streets, factories, homes, and skies" and asserted that Americans "have decided that noise should be abated." The optimism was unwarranted. Today the level of everyday noise to which the average urban American is exposed is more than *twice* what it was in 1955, and the cacophony continues to mount: the crash of jackhammers, whirring air conditioners, snarling lawn mowers, family arguments penetrating the paper-thin walls of homes and apartment houses, and the blast of traffic on freeways. Everyday noise is assaulting American ears at an intensity approaching the level of permanent hearing damage, if indeed the danger point has not already been passed.

A zone of "unacceptable annoyance"

As often happens with a slowly encroaching evil, it has taken a major outrage to stir up public concern. This is being provided spectacularly by the jet aircraft now bombarding some 20 million Americans every few minutes with a thunderous roar around our major airports. In the area of New York's John F. Kennedy Airport alone about one million people (including the students in about ninety schools) live within a zone of "unacceptable annoyance," as an official of the Federal Aviation Administration describes it. At Shea Stadium baseball games, the racket regularly drowns out not only the national anthem but also the players calling for fly balls. In Washington, jet noise so disrupted a ceremony attended by President Johnson at the Lincoln Memorial in 1967 that he ordered an aide to call the airport and stop it. In Los Angeles, concerts at the Hollywood Bowl have become virtually inaudible, and residents of nearby Inglewood have filed lawsuits that could total as much as $3 billion against the city.

The federal government is beginning belatedly to recognize that it has a problem—an awakening that may be partly due to the fact that approach paths to Washington National Airport pass directly over the homes of numerous top government officials. Congress last year voted to give the Federal Aviation Administration authority for the first time to fix aircraft noise limits, and the agency's initial order is expected momentarily. Though the effort may result in higher fares for air travelers, there is reason to hope that jet noise may be rolled back almost to the level of propeller planes within a few years.

But the same cannot be said for noise pollution in general. With a few exceptions, the steps taken so far have been palliatives. Memphis, for example, has enforced a ban on automobile horn blowing (instigated by an angry newspaper editor) since the 1930's. In New York in 1948 a landmark court decision upheld for the first time an award of compensation to an industrial worker who had suffered gradual hearing loss without losing work time. This type of claim is now recognized in some thirty states. Studies indicate, however, that only a small percentage of workers with legitimate claims have gone to court.

In Washington, at least a dozen federal agencies have become involved in the noise problem, and there has been one action of significance. That was the promulgation of a series of new regulations last spring under the Walsh-Healey Public Contracts Act of 1938, which limit industrial noise levels in most plants doing business with the government. The new regulations were initiated by the Johnson Administration, however, and were watered down by the Nixon Administration. Elsewhere a handful of unofficial organizations are agitating for noise abatement, notably in New York City.

Multitudes of special interests are arrayed against anti-noise measures whenever they are contemplated. When a state law was proposed to ban playing transistor radios in public vehicles, Buffalo radio-TV station WGR editorialized against such "inanities." Of about 125 industry representatives who testified last winter at Labor Department hearings leading to the new industrial noise standards, more than 90 percent were opposed to regulation. Sample argument: "It is unrealistic and literally impossible to comply with." The cause of noise abatement wasn't helped any when the *Journal of the American Medical Association* argued in an editorial earlier this year that "some noise must be tolerated as an unavoidable concomitant of the blessings of civilization."

Quiet doesn't cost much

To permit this kind of thinking to prevail is the true inanity. Virtually all man-made noise, whatever its source, can be suppressed. While some major problems, such as thin apartment walls and the roar of New York City's subway, would cost large sums of money to correct, many of the most irritating noises could be reduced at negligible cost. The screech of truck tires on pavement, for example, can be reduced at no extra cost or efficiency loss by redesigning the tread, and a quiet home lawn mower costs only about $15 more than the usual ear-jarring model. Some other examples of added costs: a garbage truck $2,400 (on top of original cost of $15,600), a small air compressor $500 ($5,300), and on most machinery an additional 5 percent atop the original cost. In some cases there is also a relatively small cost in reduced efficiency. Mass production of silenced equipment would lower costs still more.

The expense becomes even less formidable when measured against the savings from noise suppression. The World Health Organization estimates that industrial noise alone costs the U.S. today more than $4 billion annually—in accidents, absenteeism, inefficiency, and compensation claims. The human costs in sleepless nights, family squabbles, and mental illness are beyond measure, but they surely must be enormous.

In the cases of air and water pollution, one of the main obstacles to corrective action is the large governmental outlay required—e.g., for non-polluting municipal incinerators and sewage-treatment plants. But society's noise-makers are predominantly privately owned machines, many of which wear out and must be replaced within a few years anyway. Moreover, noise is not a uniquely big-city problem of little interest to suburban or rural taxpayers who are not exposed to it. Modern technology, its root cause, is everywhere, from grinding dishwashing machines in farm kitchens to outlying airports and thundering throughways that can be heard for miles.

The first and perhaps the most important course of action is to generate all possible public pressure on governments. It is no coincidence that one of the world's most effective anti-noise programs emerged in West Germany after the leading political parties there began including it in their election platforms. Once it becomes clear to Americans that noise is not an inescapable fact of life, that something *can* be done about it, and at manageable cost, the support for real action could be overwhelming. Says Judge Theodore Kupferman, a former Congressman from Manhattan and long-time anti-noise crusader: "In addition to the merits of the anti-noise cause, I don't see why more politicians don't take up the cudgel. Who's going to be in favor of noise?"

The most effective approach to governmental action probably lies in *federal* regulation. The legal authority already exists in the laws providing federal regulation of interstate commerce, health protection, and such specific functions as federal guarantees of housing loans, and there is a precedent for federal regulation of noise in the 1965 legislation empowering the Department of Health, Education, and Welfare to set limits on air pollutants emitted by motor vehicles. At the same time, state and local governmental action against noise, as well as support from enlightened businessmen, could go a long way toward reducing the problem, and perhaps in setting a trend—as a few localities have already demonstrated.

No lids to close

Noise—commonly defined as "unwanted sound"—works on humans in two ways. One, of course, is to cause deafness through deterioration of the microscopic hair cells that transmit sound from the ear to the brain. A single very loud blast, as from a cannon, can destroy the cells by the thousands and they never recover. (The Veterans Administration is spending about $8 million a year on the claims of some 5,000 servicemen whose hearing has been damaged by gunfire in training or combat.) Constant exposure to noises commonplace in our society can cause slower deterioration as the hair cells gradually rupture. There is a glimpse of the remarkable "redundancy" of the human body—in this case in spare hair cells—in the fact that all of us in modern communities have lost a substantial portion of our hearing mechanism without ever missing it. An experiment conducted by Dr. Samuel Rosen, a leading Manhattan otologist, has shown that aborigines living in the stillness of isolated African villages can easily hear each other talking in low conversational tones at distances as great as 100 yards, and that their hearing acuity diminishes little with age.

The second effect of noise upon humans is psychological and intensely personal. It relates not only to a lifetime of experience, but also to mood. Thus the scream of a siren at night may bring fright and anger to a thousand neighbors, but it means hope to a desperate accident victim. The human ear, unlike the eye, has no lids and cannot be turned off, not even in sleep. Nature's initial purpose in providing animals with hearing presumably was to alert them to enemies, with its function in communication coming at a later stage. Thus the instinctive human reaction to noise, especially unexpected noise, is fear and an impulse to flee. Children play games with this "startle effect," as psychologists call it. But to older people, just home from a hard day's work, for example, a sudden noise like the slam of a door or an automobile backfire or even the bell of an ice-cream vendor often can tip the balance of self-control and lead to an emotional eruption. Studies of sleep patterns have shown that people never "get used" to noise; on the contrary, the annoyance, and loss of sleep, worsen as the interruptions persist. This is the main reason why there is, rightly, such strong opposition to the use over populated areas of supersonic airliners whose sonic booms would cause psychic havoc among millions.

Hypertension and hallucinations

Clinical evidence has established conclusively that excessive exposure to noise constricts the arteries, increases the heartbeat, and dilates the pupils of the eye. Sigmund Freud wrote that noise could create an anxiety neurosis "undoubtedly explicable on the basis of the close inborn connection between auditory impressions and fright." One recent French study goes so far as to suggest that noise is the cause of 70 percent of the neuroses in the Paris area, compared with only 50 percent four years ago, and it blames noise for three recent premeditated murders. John M. Handley, a New York authority on industrial acoustics, recently wrote that "symptoms of hypertension, vertigo, hallucination, paranoia and, on occasion, suicidal and homicidal impulses, have been blamed on excessive noise... 'Noise pollution' may be one of the reasons why the incidence of heart disease and mental illness is so high in the United States." Other authorities have suggested that noise may be related to stomach ulcers, allergies, enuresis (involuntary urination), spinal meningitis, excessive cholesterol in the arteries, indigestion, loss of equilibrium, and impaired vision.

Tests of the effects of noise upon animals have produced dramatic results. Prolonged exposure has made rats lose their fertility, turn homosexual, and eat their young. If the noise is continued still longer, it eventually kills them through heart failure. There is clearly a limit to the amount of noise that any animal, including humans, can tolerate. But at what point does the noise in our daily lives begin to be dangerous? Dr. Vern O. Knudsen, former chancellor of the University of California at Los Angeles and a leading authority on noise pollution, believes we have already reached it. "Noise, like smog," he says, "is a slow agent of death."

Death by decibels

There is no single universally accepted criterion of what constitutes excessive noise. The most common noise yardstick is the decibel (db) scale, which is an expression of the sound pressure that moves the ear. The scale begins at zero db, which is the weakest sound that can be picked up by the healthy ear. Thereafter, because of physical laws, the scale increases as the square of the change. Thus so soft a sound as human breathing is about ten times greater than zero db, while an artillery blast is one thousand trillion (1,000,000,000,000,000) times greater. To simplify things, the scale is in logarithmic form so that ten times the minimum is 10 db and one thousand trillion times the minimum is 150 db. The db scale does not, however, take account of the tones in the sound being registered—i.e., the frequencies of the sound waves being propagated. Scientists' attempts over the years to work out techniques to weight such factors for accurate registration of the ways that noise sounds to humans have led to a plethora of measuring scales.

There is agreement that high-pitched tones are more annoying and thus should be given more weight than low tones, but there the agreement ends. The most common weighting system is the "A" scale, written dbA, which gives less weight to low tones and thus more nearly matches the effect of sound on people. Beyond that the variations are myriad. For example: dbC ("C" scale), PNdb ("perceived noise"), EPNdb ("effective perceived noise"), SIL ("speech interference level"), and the "sone" and "phon" scales.

Some sample noise readings in the dbA scale at distances at which people are commonly exposed:

Rustling leaves	20 dbA
Window air conditioner	55
Conversational speech	60
(Beginning of hearing damage if prolonged	85)
Heavy city traffic	90
Home lawn mower	98
150-cubic-foot air compressor	100
Jet airliner (500 feet overhead)	115
(Human pain threshold	120)

In the case of the laboratory rats mentioned earlier, death occurred after prolonged exposure at 150 dbA, or the equivalent of continuous artillery fire at close range. The take-off blast of the Saturn V moon rocket, measured at the launching pad, is about 180 dbA.

Very roughly, the noise level in busy sections of American communities is doubling every ten years. It has reached the point today where it is often greater than industrial noise levels. The main cause of the trend is the constant growth of the use of power. To cite one of the main new offenders, air conditioners are now in use in some 32 million homes. The giant machines on the top of large buildings often spew out more than 100 dbA and bother people for blocks around. No fewer than 89 million cars (up to 70 dbA) and about 18 million trucks and buses (up to 95 dbA) are cluttering our roads and streets. Millions of them are operating with defective mufflers, which always wear out faster than the vehicle. The beauty of our winters has been defiled by the din of some 700,000 snowmobiles, and our buses, trains, parks, and streets by millions of transistor radios. The racket in a modern American kitchen rises as high as 90 dbA midst an ever expanding profusion of dishwashers, mixers, grinders, exhaust fans, disposers, and the like. The National Institute of Mental Health is considering a proposal to wire up a typical housewife with telemetry like a spacecraft to try to study the effects of the pandemonium on her nervous system.

On top of all that, architects, engineers, and contractors in the $90-billion U.S. construction industry behave, says one acoustical expert, "as though they were born without ears." Thousands of new apartment buildings and homes are being thrown together like cardboard dollhouses, creating multimillion-dollar "noise slums," as one occupant puts it. Privacy, so badly needed by city dwellers, vanishes among the sounds of flushing toilets, electric razors, and family intimacies penetrating the walls, inhibiting conversation, and worsening tensions. Air-conditioning, heating, and ventilation ducts are made smaller and smaller to save space and weight, with the result that machinery must be faster, and therefore noisier, to move the same amount of air. Outside, meanwhile, some three million construction workers all over the U.S. create daily bedlam with jackhammers, air compressors, earth-moving equipment, riveters, and similar mechanical monsters.

Americans often seem to react to noise as if it were a narcotic, as though nature were compelling us to accept it, even savor it, rather than engage in a hopeless struggle. Researchers have found, for example, that workers in noisy jobs often refuse to wear ear plugs because they are proud of their ability to "take it." In truth, this kind of tough-guy syndrome seems to be a subconscious device for sublimating discomfort. Psychologists think a similar narcotic effect may help explain why teen-agers sit for hours in rock joints, overwhelmed by "music" (as high as 130 dbA) that blots out all else in the world and, like marijuana, enables them to escape temporarily from reality.

Muffling the jumbo jets

The first real test of the nation's capability to roll back the engulfing tide of noise will be the FAA regulations on aircraft. At this writing, the FAA is about to announce its plans. The agency reportedly will begin by fixing noise limits on the new generation of planes soon to go into service—such as the huge 325-passenger Boeing 747 due to begin operating early next year. The ruling probably will stipulate that such planes must generate the equivalent of no more than about 95 dbA at a point about four miles beyond the start of the take-off roll; today's big planes register as much as 105 dbA. An improvement of that magnitude is already being built into the 747's by Boeing engineers.

To supplement the new regulations, the National Aeronautics and Space Administration has launched a $50-million program to subsidize development of still another generation of even quieter engines through design and engineering innovations to slow engine fan-blade tips below supersonic speeds and thereby lessen the noise-making air turbulence. The agency hopes this will permit it a few years hence to begin further reducing the limit for new planes, perhaps to the equivalent of heavy city-traffic noise.

A third move, tentatively expected early in 1970, will apply noise limits to the 2,000 airliners now in service on the nation's airways. The problem is much tougher in this case and no decisions have yet been reached. There is a good chance, however, that there will be a dramatic program, to cost about $2 billion, to "retrofit" the whole airline fleet with engine silencers. How such a program would be financed remains to be worked out, but it seems likely that the government would require passengers to share in the added costs; a general fare increase of 5 percent has been suggested. A "retrofit" program might be accompanied by a change in flying procedures. Instead of gradual three-degree approach to airports, aircraft would make a two-segment approach, first at six degrees, then at three degrees for the final segment. That would permit them to stay longer at higher, and thus quieter, altitudes than is possible today. Such changes in procedure would also involve design changes in the aircraft.

A nixon compromise

In the area of general noise pollution other than aircraft, the one step that Washington has taken—new regulations under the Walsh-Healey Act—has been a disappointment to anti-noise advocates. The regulations benefit some 27 million workers in about 70,000 plants, but exclude millions of others in plants with fewer than twenty workers and less than $10,000 in government contracts, thus omitting small businesses where abuses are no less deplorable. The Johnson Administration, which initiated the action, originally proposed to fix a noise limit of 85 dbA, with higher levels permitted for short periods. The proposal was so hotly opposed, however, especially by high-noise industries like textiles, that the Nixon Administration compromised on a maximum of 90 dbA—or 5 dbA more than the experts regard as safe. Even at 90 dbA, however, the new regulations will have a notable, indeed historic, impact, if they are enforced. At least half of American industry today permits noise levels above 90 dbA. The American Petroleum Institute estimates the cost of compliance to the oil industry alone at $40 million to $50 million to modify its existing equipment.

Meanwhile, the federal government is acquiring a great deal of valuable expertise in studies ranging from apartment-house noise insulation to a computerized analysis of transportation noise. By far the most significant of the studies is an exhaustive document called "Noise—Sound Without Value," published last fall by a special ten-agency committee. The report asserted: "Increasing severity of the noise problem in our environment has reached a level of national importance and public concern." With notable political courage, it added that the solution "frequently will require actions that transcend political boundaries within the nation." i.e., it should not be left to the states. Not long afterward, the Johnson Administration, which had promoted the study, went out of business.

Which points directly to a central unknown today: what will the Nixon

Administration do about noise? The top authority is the newly created Environmental Quality Council, headed by Nixon himself, which to date has made no decisions on noise. There is fear among anti-noise advocates that Nixon's strong feelings about state responsibilities may lead him to stay out of noise control except perhaps for voluntary—and therefore ineffective—guidelines. Such concern is one reason why the Senate recently passed a bill proposed by Washington's Democratic Senator Henry Jackson to create a prestigious, independent council to recommend policy on all forms of environmental control, including noise. A similar bill is pending in the House.

If the Administration should leave non-aircraft noise pollution to the states, the outlook could be gloomy; few states have taken actions of any consequence. California has a law limiting the vehicle noise on freeways to 88 dbA, and a noise abatement commission will soon begin hearings aimed at producing recommendations by 1971. The law is so loosely enforced, however, that a Los Angeles police official confessed he did not know it existed. In New York State, indignant citizens along the roaring New England Thruway, where some 10,000 trucks create a steady din around the clock, persuaded the state legislature to fix a limit of 88 dbA on each vehicle. There have been only sixty-three arrests since 1965—and the maximum fine is only $10 anyway. Connecticut also plans to introduce a noise-abatement program soon.

In the long-suffering core cities, where noise works its greatest evil, the record is spotty. Several cities have anti-noise ordinances, e.g., Dayton, Dallas, Chicago, and Minneapolis. In San Francisco the Bay Area Rapid Transit System now under construction is spending $1,250,000 (only one tenth of 1 percent of the total cost) on noise suppression; it is expected to be the quietest subway in the country—85 dbA on the platform versus New York's numbing average of 102 dbA. Milwaukee attempted to reduce truck noise by a city ordinance, only to have it overturned by the courts on grounds that it invaded state jurisdiction; the effort was laughed into obscurity anyway when a newsman discovered that the city's own vehicles were violating the ordinance.

The man who moved a city

Despite its multitudes of other problems, New York City probably has tried harder than any other big community to mount a really effective anti-noise campaign. Much of the initiative came from a group of volunteers called Citizens for a Quieter City, Inc., headed by Robert Alex Baron, forty-nine, who was so incensed by the din of a construction project outside his Manhattan apartment that he quit his career as a Broadway play manager in 1966 to do something about it. His efforts helped coax Mayor John V. Lindsay to appoint, in 1967, a special anti-noise task force of technical experts and public-spirited citizens. These and other pressures combined to persuade the city council last year to pass the first building code of any major U.S. city with an anti-noise provision. It requires that new residential buildings must be constructed to cut noise penetration by about 45 dbA, which is appreciably less strict than the codes of several European countries but nevertheless a major stride forward.

To prove that Americans do not have to live with noise, Baron arranged for a public demonstration of silenced machinery in New York's Lincoln Center one day in 1967.

Among other items, he displayed a quiet air compressor imported from Britain. Within a few months, at least one major American manufacturer, Ingersoll-Rand, began actively promoting a similar machine. The city is running a test of the feasibility of using paper bags for garbage instead of cans, and it has contracted with General Motors to develop quiet garbage trucks to replace the present fleet of "mechanized cockroaches," as Baron calls them.

In a report to be published this month, the New York task force has also recommended an extraordinarily ambitious program for further steps, ranging from new zoning rules to creation of a corps of noise inspectors, with the objective of reducing the noise level in busy areas to 85 dbA and the residential level to 40 dbA in daytime and 30 dbA at night. The New York initiative is attracting considerable local attention. On N.B.C.'s Johnny Carson TV show recently, Baron appealed for people annoyed by noise to write him; the result was some 2,500 letters, most of them venting long-pent-up anger and frustration.

But the effort has a very long way to go. The anti-noise forces to date have failed even to persuade the New York Police Department to try to enforce the ordinance against needless horn blowing. The problem is compounded by the fact that the city has no direct authority to act against noisy vehicle engines (which are the state's responsibility), or noisy aircraft (the FAA's), or even the New York subway system (the Transit Authority's).

Even the french don't blow their horns

There is no mystery about how to control noise. At least sixteen European countries have building codes with anti-noise provisions, many of them tougher than anything even contemplated in the U.S. The Soviet Union, which began a "struggle against noise" in 1960, says it has banned factory noise above 85 dbA and limited the level in residential areas to 30 dbA. The West Germans, among other actions, have set up no fewer than eight categories of noise limits; they offer tax concessions and easy credit to manufacturers willing to silence machinery acquired before the limits were established; and they stamp the maximum noise permitted each vehicle on the owner's driver's license. In France, needless horn blowing has been successfully outlawed—much to the surprise of the French themselves—and other noise regulations are so well enforced that a peasant recently was fined $50 for a noisy cowbell.

Unlike other forms of pollution, noise comes from an infinite number of sources and cannot be cut off simply by cleaning up a few big operations such as garbage dumps. The answer, however, does not lie in brave new proclamations. Ways must be found to get at the problem through appeals to the self-interest of business and community leaders and through governmental regulations that are realistic and easily policed.

Two further federal moves are needed now to provide a legal framework for minimum national standards. One is to broaden the recent anti-noise regulations to protect workers in all factories engaged in interstate commerce. The second is to invoke the interstate commerce principle to permit the fixing of limitations on the noise created by the machines that industry produces. The objective of such a move would be to oblige manufacturers to design noise suppression right into their goods, and its national application would guarantee that no company would be hurt competitively. Says Leo L. Beranek of Cambridge, Massachusetts, chief scientist for the nation's largest acoustical consulting firm: "We have got to have noise regulation at the federal level. Controls in only a few scattered cities won't work; quiet products must have a national market."

A proposal for federal action on such a broad scale obviously invites innumerable problems. For one thing, it would require congressional action. It would compound the infighting already under way among the several federal agencies competing for anti-noise responsibility. Whatever the bureaucratic machinery, however, the approach probably should be to seek a broad mandate from Congress, and then to begin application of specific controls on a progressive basis, beginning with the most urgent problems— e.g., highway vehicle noise and outrageously noisy machines like air compressors.

The diverse opportunities

Federal laws, of course, are no panacea. At best they can be expected only to provide minimum standards that could then be reinforced through state and local action. In some cases such action can be carried out most easily through local regulation—e.g., anti-noise insulation of residential buildings, which can be enforced with relative ease through existing building inspectors. The mere existence of federal anti-noise laws would create strong psychological pressures on local governments and industry to act.

Apart from legislation, there are innumerable other opportunities for action. The federal government buys something like 35,000 vehicles annually. To require such vehicles, especially trucks, to be fitted with good mufflers, quiet tire treads, and other noise-suppressing equipment would go a long way toward encouraging manufacturers to make such items standard equipment. State and local governments could easily do the same. Procurement policy can be similarly useful across a broad spectrum of other items that are purchased by both consumers and government agencies —e.g., garbage cans, which can be quieted for about $1.50 apiece. The Federal Housing Authority and other national and local agencies have the power now to make compliance with noise standards a condition for publicly backed loans. The National Park Service has the same kind of authority now to bar noisy vehicles, transistors, and the like from our national parks. It should also be feasible for the federal and local governments to grant tax concessions to encourage industry to suppress noise. By relatively simple fiddling with electronic circuits, buses and trains could be fitted with jamming devices to discourage transistor addicts. And automobiles could be equipped with two horns, one for highways and a quieter beep for city streets, as is widely done in Europe. The Federal Highway Safety Bureau recently revealed that it is already considering a requirement of this sort.

Contrary to the view among some industrialists that noise control is an expensive luxury, it is in fact good business; the lack of effective noise control at the source, moreover, is bad for business. In the case of aircraft, anti-noise flight procedures—e.g., disuse of some runways—are further reducing the capacity of our congested airports, while popular reaction against aircraft noise is making it increasingly difficult to find sites for new airports. Cities like New York are losing tens of millions of dollars in traffic diverted elsewhere.

For industry in general, the mounting cost of hearing-loss compensation claims could easily become astronomic if workers began going to the courts in large numbers. In view of the growing evidence that noise is a significant health hazard, it would make eminent sense for insurance companies and labor unions to add their considerable weight to the battle. With a few exceptions, businessmen have been surprisingly slow to recognize that noise prevention can be marketed; for example, in advertising for quiet apartments or noiseless kitchen equipment. There is also a major public-relations consideration in the growing feeling among environmentalists that corporations have no more right to dump noise on communities than air and water pollutants.

"Let avoidable noise be avoided," said the late Pope Pius XII in a 1956 appeal from the Vatican. "Silence is beneficial not only to sanity, nervous equilibrium, and intellectual labor, but also helps man live a life that reaches to the depths and to the heights ... It is in silence that God's mysterious voice is best heard."

Secrecy and safety at rocky flats

ROGER RAPOPORT

The road from Denver northwest to Boulder, Colorado, is an enchanting, 20-mile drive, uncluttered by gas stations, hamburger stands or motels. At night, when traffic is light and fierce winds howl out of the 8,000-foot Flatirons, it can be a scary place to run out of gas or blow a tire. But more often than not, an angel of mercy will show up behind the wheel of a pickup truck, armed with a can of gas, the know-how to fix flats and plenty of Western hospitality.

The men in the pickups seem anxious to be good, unobtrusive neighbors to the 1.1 million people of metropolitan Denver. And in this way they have something in common with the people who run a plant at Rocky Flats nearby. But some of the reasons are different.

The Rocky Flats plant is operated by the Dow Chemical Company for the Atomic Energy Commission under a cost-plus contract. It employs 3,200 persons and its specialty is the fabrication and processing of plutonium, a radioactive grayish metal (worth $43 a gram) created as a by-product of nuclear reaction and the key ingredient in most atomic bombs. The plant also repairs and replaces defective bomb and warhead components which are sent back to it when spot checks of nuclear stockpiles turn up duds.

All this dangerous work so close to a metropolitan area has made the plant's management, certain union leaders and the AEC sensitive about the issue of safety, both for the general area and for the workers at the plant. How much of the safety is substantive and how much is empty reassurance has become a matter of bitter debate in recent years.

Plutonium is doubly hazardous to work with. Minute quantities of it inhaled or imbedded in the skin can be lethal. It has a radioactive half-life of 24,400 years (something that makes it imperative that any of it that gets away not be left to lie about). Its radiation, of course, can cause permanent damage to living cells leading to leukemia and other forms of cancer. It also oxidizes quickly, making it a serious fire threat.

From its side of the fence, Dow and the AEC emphasize super-safety precautions, and boast that the plant "ranks first in AEC facilities for safety and holds the fourth best all-time mark in American industry—2,122 consecutive days (24,295,542 man-hours) without a disabling injury."

Rocky Flats officials tell about the elaborate safety precautions taken in the final assembly area (buildings 776 and 777). All workers in the area were heavily shielded and the entire plutonium assembly line with its milling machines, furnaces and presses was enclosed in glove boxes (ventilated, shielded enclosures) connected by conveyors. Moreover, to guard against the accidental release of plutonium into the atmosphere, the entire production area was sealed off inside a self-contained unit with a special internal filtration system. An elaborate network of automatic heat and radiation sensors plus roving teams of safety monitors guarded against accidents.

But at 2:29 P.M. on Sunday, May 11, this fail-safe system fell through. A fire broke out in the final assembly area. Despite the efforts of the Rocky Flats fire department, the blaze spread through both buildings 776 and 777. Smoke billowed so thickly that some of the firemen (wearing air tanks to protect against radiation danger) had to crawl along exit lines painted on the floor to make their way out.

By 5:30 P.M., when the blaze was brought under control, it had caused more than $50 million worth of damage. The worst accident in AEC history, the fire put the final assembly area out of commission and forced a halt in American nuclear missile production for part of the year.

Potentially, the disaster was the biggest step the United States has ever taken toward nuclear disarmament. More than $20 million worth of plutonium burned in the fire—roughly enough to build 77 atom bombs like the one that incinerated Nagasaki.

But rather than signal Geneva, Congress quickly shelled out $45 million in supplemental funds to clean up the mess, a figure equal to the entire fiscal 1969 Rocky Flats budget. Now 240 Rocky Flats regulars and 60 summertime college students are sifting through charred debris to recover the burned plutonium. Meanwhile hundreds of railroad cars will ship 330,000 cubic feet of radioactive wastes to AEC for burial grounds in Idaho.

Anxious to understand how the AEC's safest plant could produce its worst disaster, I paid a visit to Rocky Flats recently. I learned that despite the vaunted precautions there have been over 200 small fires since the nuclear weapons facility opened in 1953. Recently, fires had been occurring about once a month in the buildings where the $50 million blaze took place. But on the Sunday afternoon the disaster started, only one ventilation system operator was in the building. Says Rocky Flats General Manager Dr. Lloyd M. Joshel: "I think we're going to have to review our monitoring procedures in this area."

All this has led local scientists to ask Rocky Flats officials if they shouldn't also review the possibility of moving their plant away from Denver. The Denver scientists are worried even though health surveys show that there was no release of plutonium from the plant site during the fire. Most of the smoke was trapped by the special filtration system.

Denver may not be so lucky next time.

Even the clean-up end of the May 11 fire is causing more trouble. On July 30 two plastic bags surrounding a can containing some of the plutonium recovered from the $50 million blaze caught fire. Two workmen in the area were contaminated.

Their names are only the latest addition to the roster of more than 325 workers who have experienced radioactive contamination at the plant. Officially, AEC spokesmen say there have been a mere 21 disabling injuries and one fatality since the plant opened. But they refuse to disclose the number of workers who have received their maximum permissable dose of radiation and been transferred to cold (non-radioactive) sections of the plant. The local union is not allowed to see medical files of contaminated workers or make an independent investigation of plant accidents.

Perhaps the biggest question looming over Rocky Flats is the number of workers who have cancer or have died from it. Dow public relations man Mike Carroll says "It would not be discreet to discuss this. I've got the figures but I won't give them to you."

One known cancer victim within the plant is 60-year-old Everett Holloway, an inspector with terminal leukemia: "I started checking into my medical records at the plant to see if I could establish some compensation. But I discovered that the company has lost some of my quarterly urine sample reports (which are taken to measure radioactive contamination). I was told that there was nothing the company could do for me until I become completely disabled. Supposedly they have switched me into a cold area but they're still machining a lot of radioactive material in my area and I don't know what effect it will have on my condition. I can't afford to quit because when a 60-year-old man like me comes asking for a job they look at you like you're poison."

Of course no one saw the plant as a liability when it came to Denver in 1953. Geographically, the rocky cow pasture 25 miles northwest of Denver was a smart choice because it was close by Colorado University in Boulder, skilled manpower in Denver and attractive recreational opportunities in the mountains. The plant soon grew into a crucial link in the AEC nuclear weapons complex.

In all, the bomb work was divided between eight AEC facilities. Design research and testing was done at New Mexico and California plants. Rocky Flats was responsible for plutonium components, the Kansas City plant made electro and electro-mechanical components, a Dayton, Ohio, plant made detonators and a plant in St. Petersburg, Fla., made neutron generators. These parts were assembled into nuclear weapons at plants in Burlington, Iowa, and Amarillo, Texas.

In the late 1950's, the plant mushroomed and radiation hazards grew with it. Between June 14, 1957, and October 28, 1958, there were 24 documented fires, explosions, plutonium spills, and contamination incidents at the plant. Testimony by Rocky Flats union leaders and government officials at AEC radiation hazards hearings in Washington during March, 1959, detailed many of the accidents; among them were serious fires in June and September of 1957.

Rocky Flats union leaders were particularly concerned about management's reluctance to bring in health physicists (who supervise worker health) after serious accidents took place. For example they testified that on October 28, 1957, a "chip fire in a production area occurred and as usual health physicists were not notified. No air samples were taken nor were any respirators worn to guard against inhaling dangerous plutonium. Health physicists learned of this operation after a worker involved in it coughed up black sputum at his home and became thus concerned with the method in which the incident had been handled by his supervisors."

The union leaders also pointed out that on September 4, 1958, supervisory personnel instructed workers to clean up a radioactive materials spill "using no respirators and without health physicists being informed of the situation." Subsequently, health physicists were notified, and recommended respirators and "area supervision gave in and allowed the workers to wear them on subsequent cleanup operations of the spill."

On October 3, 1958, another supervisor "stopped health physicists from allowing the men to know what the airborne contamination was in their production area on the grounds that it was his business only as to what the level was."

A variety of serious contamination incidents were also reportedly in supposedly cold areas. For example, on September 10, 1958, a "cafeteria survey showed 50 to 54 smears (taken to measure radiation) to be over allowable tolerance level." Ninety-seven of 99 smears in the locker room also showed contamination. Radioactivity was also found on drinking fountains, sinks, laundered caps, shoes, drums, flasks, carts, lifts and saws in cold areas.

As health hazards increased some workers were disappointed to see modification of some safety procedures. For example, prior to March, 1961, health physicists checked all employees out of hot areas with an alpha counter to make sure they were not carrying excessive radiation. But after March, 1961, workers were given more discretionary authority to monitor themselves out of hot areas.

Then and now, Rocky Flats officials felt that national defense precludes public discussion of these matters. But in the meantime they have been quietly documenting their problems in articles for the scientific community. For example, in 1964, Rocky Flats health physicists S. E. Hammond and E. A. Putzier had this to report in the sober international journal *Health Physics:*

The Rocky Flats wound counter was developed in 1957 to measure the amount of plutonium contamination present in wounds incurred in process areas. Since that time more than 900 wounds have been monitored of which more than 300 have indicated some degree of plutonium contamination.... The material is completely removed when possible. However, in cases where the plutonium is deeply imbedded or where physical impairment might result from complete excision, small amounts of plutonium may be left in the wound.

By 1965 union officials felt it was time to make a strong pitch for a new safety package in their contract negotiations with Dow. They asked for a joint "Radiation Safety Committee" with the company that would meet bimonthly "to discuss problems arising from radiation safety complaints from any employees." They also proposed adding three union members to the company's Executive Safety Council and making radiation records of all employees available to "the union at least once each year in writing." All the proposals were rejected by management.

By 1967 it was becoming clear to *Health Physics* readers that the situation at Rocky Flats was getting worse. In an article titled "Evaluation of Lung Burden Following Acute Inhalation Exposure to Highly Insoluble PuO_2 (plutonium oxide)," J. R. Mann and R. A. Kirchner of the Rocky Flats staff reported that

> On 15 October 1965, a fire in a plutonium fabrication plant resulted in a large-scale spread of plutonium oxide. The Rocky Flats body counter (a device that measures radioactivity in the body) was used to measure the plutonium in the lungs of all employees working in the area. Of approximately 400 employees counted, 25 were found to have enough plutonium in their lungs to deliver a dose of 15 rem/year. (In line with federal radiation standards Rocky Flats generally tries to keep worker exposure under 5 rem/year, although a complicated formula permits special exceptions.) On the average, 30 percent of the material initially deposited was cleared in 2 to 3 months. The remaining material is clearing very slowly with little or no measurable absorption into the bloodstream.

In another 1967 *Health Physics* article, C. R. Lagerquist, E. A. Putzier and C. W. Piltingsrud of the Rocky Flats staff described the gradual amputation of the thumb and second finger of a worker injured by the "explosive reaction between hot plutonium metal and carbon tetrachloride." They wrote that eleven months after the amputation "it was thought that there was a high concentration of plutonium in a small portion of the remaining thumb stump." But the operation was only a partial success and six months later "the remaining portion of thumb was removed."

Dissident members of Rocky Flats Local 15440 of the International Union of District 50 of the United Mine Workers finally got a little of the safety story out into the open in late 1967. At the time the coal-conscious international leadership of the United Mine Workers was conducting a vigorous campaign against a proposed nuclear power plant at Platteville, 30 miles north of Denver. Spearheading the campaign was the Ralph Nader of the atomic energy industry, a United Auto Workers official named Leo Goodman.

As Secretary of the Atomic Energy Technical Committee of the AFL-CIO, Goodman had served as a consultant to unions working in atomic energy and proved a nemesis to the AEC.

His files suggest about 6,000 Western states uranium miners are now dying of cancer. He also points out that there have been 1,400 known accidents in atomic plants and 200 known cases of cancer. Naturally these statistics are useful to the United Mine Workers in their fight to protect coal power and guard against the inherent dangers of nuclear power.

So in November, 1967, Goodman joined UMW leaders in a trip to Denver where they worked to block the proposed atomic power plant at Platteville.

After reading in a Denver paper that Goodman was in town, a group of Rocky Flats employees visited him at his motel room. They told the atomic hazards expert that safety was deteriorating rapidly in their plant, and reviewed case histories of workers who had contracted cancer and then been denied medical pensions. Reporters for the *United Mine Workers Journal* and *Cervi's Journal,* a muckraking Denver business weekly, were present and published accounts of the meeting. To the chagrin of Dow officials and leaders of Rocky Flats Local 15440 of District 50 of the UMW the stories pointed out that "Officials of District 50 of the UMW representing the Dow Chemical workers will not discuss the radiation dangers involved for workers at Rocky Flats. If they do, they face loss of their security clearance."

This story ignited a feud within the UMW. International Leaders of the UMW were already sore at District 50 (with a regional office in Denver) because it refused to join their fight against the proposed atomic plant at Platteville. After the stories on the meeting with Goodman were published, District 50 officials went out of their way to back the new atomic plant. In February, 1968, a delegation of Rocky Flats local 15440 leaders headed by President Jim Kelly traveled to Washington for a regional directors conference of District 50. Aided by their Denver regional director Sam Franklin, the Rocky Flats union leaders extolled the virtues of the safety program at their AEC plant. Using color slides provided by the Rocky Flats management they showed how "the Rocky Flats plant has achieved one of the world's best safety records ... through a highly effective program of industrial safety." They pointed out that "The design of Rocky Flats facilities insures that each worker's exposure to radiation is kept to a minimum. ... The average work-related exposure of a Rocky Flats employee for an entire year is barely above the radiation received during a chest x-ray ..." Gene DeCarlo, chairman of the union's radiation committee told how "all employees are particularly careful about cuts and scratches on their flesh as the radiation danger increases in an open flesh."

According to District 50's Denver Regional Director Sam Franklin, the assembled directors "were so impressed by the presentation that they subsequently passed a resolution calling for the expansion of District 50's role in the atomic power industry."

Back at Rocky Flats, workers soon received news of the meeting in the February 26, 1968, edition of *District 50 News.* In the lead story it was reported that District 50 International President Elwood Moffett declared that "District 50's future is 'clearly interwoven' with the progress and development of the atomic energy industry." Further, the International Executive Board of District 50 promised to "continue to represent and safeguard our membership employed in every phase of that industry ..."

The paper also carried the text of District 50's resolution endorsing atomic power plants "... contrary to the thinking of those who sporadically would remind us that progress in the field of nuclear energy represents a destructive force which could annihilate humanity. ... mounting scientific statistics amassed through the 2,000 man-years of experience in the Atomic Industry discount this pessimism."

Rep. Chet Holifield, chairman of the Joint Committee on Atomic Energy, inserted the District 50 resolution into the Congressional Record. Beneath the Holifield story in the March 11, 1968, *News* issue was a Freudian slip of a filler that did not amuse the Rocky Flats workers: "1.4 million Americans now alive have been cured of cancer. Early detection and prompt treatment saved their lives. The American Cancer Society urges you to become familiar with cancer's seven warning signals and to fight the disease with a checkup and a check," it read.

The international leadership of the United Mine Workers was also not amused by District 50's endorsement of atomic power at the expense of coal. In March, 1968, the UMW International expelled District 50 charging that it was "willing to risk the lives of every citizen of this country in potential nuclear reactor accidents for the sake of a few members they have in atomic plants."

Since the break, District 50 has been getting along better with Dow and worse with the UMW. In March, 1968, just after District 50 endorsed atomic power, one of its biggest locals, 12075 in Midland, Mich. set a "chemical industry precedent" by winning an 80-cent-plus, three-year package from Dow. This paved the way for a 60 cent-an-hour direct wage hike plus a wage reopener in the third year for Rocky Flats Local 15440. The latter contract was ratified in June, 1968. But Local 15440 again lost its demand for the safety package originally proposed in 1965.

The UMW, through Washington atomic consultant Leo Goodman, subsequently charged that "Because the workers revealed the real hazards in the *UMW Journal* and *Cervi's Journal* of Denver (in November, 1967) ...a sweetheart agreement was negotiated between District 50, Dow and the AEC (June, 1968) to foreclose any public discussion of the unsafe operating practices in the Rocky Flats plant. ... Thus, in order to cozy up to Dow Chemical, District 50 not only abandoned labor's traditional role in behalf of workers' safety in the plant but also collaborated with AEC–Dow Chemical in hiding from the people of the Denver community the great hazard which this plant brought to them."

Rocky Flats Local 15440 President Jim Kelly hotly denies these charges. The senior radiation monitor says that "If anyone told me to my face that we were playing sweetheart with management I'd knock him clear across the table. The real problem is that individual workers are afraid to turn their own plant health records (which they are eligible to see) over the union. They think they'll lose their job. These guys raise a lot of hell in the locker room but they don't have the courage to get involved."

But on July 24 Kelly suddenly found that 200 of his chicken-hearted men had turned into wildcats. They walked off their jobs in building No. 44 when a plant official sent a union vice-president home because he refused to stop investigating an alleged work violation on company time. The grievance was the use of an inadequately trained radiation monitor on the cleanup of the May 11 fire. It is now in arbitration. The union vice-president and 154 of the wildcats received temporary layoffs and were docked on pay.

Both President Kelly and District 50 Denver Regional Director Sam Franklin are reluctant to talk loudly in public about their problems. They refuse to give out their records on the number of workers who have picked up their maximum permissible body burden of radiation and been transferred out of hot areas of the plant. Explains Franklin: "I'd appreciate it if you wouldn't bring up anything about this radiation business and men getting cancer because it will scare a lot of people."

But quietly, Local 15440 is trying to arrange for some Washington-style publicity. Letters have been sent to Senator Edward Kennedy and to chairman Chet Holifield and vice chairman John Pastore asking for a meeting to discuss safety problems surrounding the fire on May 11 as well as discriminatory hiring practices. Chairman Holifield has already spoken with the union leaders by phone and they say Sen. Kennedy's staff is trying to set up a meeting in Washington for mid-September.

But even should the meeting come off, the Q clearance may well save the day for the AEC. For the Q clearance is the real barrier to the truth about Rocky Flats. Ostensibly invoked to protect the national defense, it is really used by plant security officials for self-defense. The Q clearance is the nation's highest security classification and explains why every Rocky Flats employee down to janitor is reluctant to discuss plant safety. For violating security can cost an employee his clearance, job, and pension as well as leave him open to federal prosecution. In the end, though, this silence may be shattered by disaster.

The May 11 fire has led the Colorado Committee for Environmental Information, a group of scientists from colleges and industries in the area to voice "real concern for the health and safety of Colorado citizens because of possible accidents involving large quantities of radioactive chemicals at Rocky Flats, located in the rapidly growing metropolitan area between Denver and Boulder."

Rocky Flats officials are not oblivious to this fear themselves. The AEC's Mike Sunderlind, who has been with the plant since it opened, keeps a thick civil defense manual nearby at all times: "If some plutonium smoke went up we'd call all the police agencies, tell them which way the smoke was going and ask them to move everybody out of the path. Afterwards decontamination teams would have to scrape all the plutonium off everyone's roofs—it would take months. Then we'd have to bring in all the people and put them through our one body counter (designed to measure radiation). It would be one hell of a mess."

The AEC is particularly anxious to minimize fears about atomic power, and with good reason. At this writing, there are 15 American atomic power plants in operation, 31 being built and 42 in the planning stage. Several have had serious accidents and two good new books *The Careless Atom*, and *Perils of the Peaceful Atom*, document the hazards. One accident in Michigan endangered the lives of 133,000 people. After a 1957 accident at the Windscale Works breeder reactor in England, authorities had to seize all milk and crops within 400 square miles of the plant. And a 1957 AEC survey shows that a reactor built 30 miles from the nearest city could kill 3,400 people, injure 43,000 and cause $7 billion damage in a bad accident. The risks of atomic power are so bad that insurance companies will not sell policies for these reactors. Only a special act of Congress provides $500 million worth of insurance for atomic power plants and absolves them for liability over that amount.

Thus a panic in Denver over Rocky Flats could jeopardize the future of the entire atomic energy industry. For if the public figures out that nuclear war is not inevitable and nuclear accidents are, the AEC is in trouble. Of course the AEC does its best to discourage this kind of thinking. When I first started work on this story, the AEC made a special effort to dissuade me from visiting Rocky Flats. After I insisted on taking a look, I was accompanied by three p.r. men (one flew in 400 miles from Albuquerque; another was an FBI agent) who shadowed me into toilets and wouldn't let me within 100 yards of the firesite. George Dennis, the AEC man who came in from Albuquerque (his office governs Rocky Flats) pleaded with me "not to give any of our secrets away to the Russians."

At a time when six nations have atom bombs and most high school physics students know the basics of atom bomb making, it seemed like he was really trying to invoke old-fashioned patriotism to keep AEC secrets from the Americans. After all, the AEC is spending a record $7,891,000 on Q clearance investigations of 17,300 personnel in fiscal 1970. Each investigation takes several months and one middle-aged Rocky Flats worker told me that "When they investigated me they went all the way back to my first grade teacher and she was 84."

Apparently the AEC is getting its money's worth. For security is a good way of keeping problems like leukemia, plutonium spills, and $50 million fires in the AEC family. Veteran Rocky Flats employees confess they still don't know what really happened on May 11: "Normally they have 8 to 10 guys patrolling those buildings for fires and radioactive contamination. Either they were playing around with something they don't want to admit to or they're guilty of the most incredible safety blunder I've ever heard of. If you had fires regularly in a building wouldn't you keep people on guard?"

In the end, the plant work force and the people of the Denver area are dependent on the AEC's good faith for their safety. Responding to public concern, Colorado Governor John Love arranged for a private briefing on the fire with Brig. Gen. Edward B. Giller, director of the AEC's military applications division. In an interview with *West*, Gov. Love indicated he found the AEC reassuring: "They seemed to be quite certain no radiation escaped from the plant site during the fire and will take precautions to make sure this kind of thing doesn't happen again. If you've got to have nuclear devices in the country I guess you might as well have the work done here as any place else."

But at a time when the United States has enough nuclear weaponry to wipe out the world several times over, one wonders what Rocky Flats is doing with enough plutonium to make at least 77 Nagasaki size atom bombs. While cleanup crews put the final production area back together

Rocky Flats is moving ahead with a $75 million dollar expansion program. Some critics feel this is the wrong direction in the wake of the AEC's worst disaster. Says UMW atomic consultant Leo Goodman: "Now's our chance to get together with the Russians and ban nuclear weapons together. It will save us a lot of money and be a lot safer."

But this is only wishful thinking. Clearly the AEC will continue running the plant, paying the salaries, regulating security, determining health standards, monitoring radioactive leaks and investigating accidents. Questions about deteriorating safety conditions, accidents and worker health will remain unanswered. For Dow officials are beholden only to the AEC.

As criticism has grown there has been a predictable reaction inside the plant. Rocky Flats General Manager Dr. Lloyd M. Joshel inserted a brief message in his house organ *Dow Newsline* to remind employees that silence is golden:

We are facing a difficult situation as a result of the fire May 11. Certain uninformed people have questioned the value of our presence here and have attacked the integrity of both the AEC and Dow. It is hard not to make an angry rebuttal, but I hope each of you will help our efforts to solve this problem by not commenting on the situation either by letters or by discussions off the plant site.

Medicine in the ghetto

JOHN C. NORMAN, M.D.

Any analysis of the evolution of the problems of medical care in the ghetto that ignores the issue of race is relatively meaningless. Reduced to essentials, the prototype ghetto today, urban or rural, is a Negro community with all the attendant social illnesses of economic, political, moral and medical exploitation.

This is not to say that other minority groups do not also suffer serious inequities.[1] However, it is primarily the Negro, 1,000,000 in Los Angeles and 1,000,000 in New York, with highly visible aggregates in nearly every area of the country between, that constitutes the major human element of the contemporary ghetto. It is reasonable, then, to focus on the evolution of the Negro, [2-6] the largest constituency of the ghetto, when one is considering its needs and how to meet them.

America, at large, has known for more than 300 years that its Negro minority has been a problem. At various times, society has attempted to suppress, ignore or evade these issues; yet the same society built an entire economic system on slavery and fought a war to determine whether or not that economic system should continue. At times, various "solutions" have been proposed ranging from total deportation to total segregation or total integration. Few of these proposals have been implemented, and none have gained majority acceptance. The Negro remains today an important majority in the ghetto population, an alien minority in his own country, exploited, dehumanized, oppressed and impinged upon by forces that are beyond contemplation, much less control.

The experience of the Negro is unique for he is a member of the only group among all those who have immigrated to this country who did not come of their own free will. To the English, the Dutch, the Germans, the

MEDICINE IN THE GHETTO From *New England Journal of Medicine*, December 4, 1969, Massachusetts Medical Society. Reprinted by permission of the *New England Journal of Medicine* and the author.

Italians, the Irish, the Poles and the Puerto Ricans, this nation represented a land of freedom and opportunity, a haven from oppression and a country where a man could shape his destiny free from the stultifying rigidities of established social and economic structures. Brought here in chains, the Negro had no such expectations and no hope that the American dream might come true. Physically, and subsequently psychologically, enslaved, the Negro was forcibly and systematically taught to be subservient, to endure endless indignities and to accept instant categorization by color. And, in spite of three centuries on these shores, most Negroes, contrary to the experience of others, have been prevented from joining the dominant culture and have been forced to exist in a bewildering limbo, neither slave nor free. That they have survived at all is remarkable. That some, if not all, carry a heavy baggage of profound suspicion, subliminal rage and covert hatred can hardly be surprising.[7-10]

Moreover, the American Negro, abruptly severed from his African ancestry and immediately unwelcome in America, has been effectively deprived of his own traditions. With few exceptions, historians, have patronized and all but ignored him, treating his evolution as an appendage rather than an integral part of the development of this country. How many, for example, are at all aware of any of the contributions to medicine of Dr. Daniel Hale Williams,[11-13] Dr. Louis P. Wright[74] or Dr. Charles Drew[11-15]? Until very recently, white Americans tended to view the Negro in terms of society as it existed at the time of the Civil War. Plantation life has been vividly represented in the literature of Joel Chandler Harris and in the music of Stephen Foster. Whites, however, are almost totally ignorant of any other aspects of Negro life and historical development. In these circumstances, is there any question why black students rebel against the stereotypes created by whites and insist on black studies in the universities, why they demand exposure to the "black experience" and raise the disturbing questions of "relevancy"?[7]

Nonetheless and perhaps not too late, society is being made aware that the Negro is a person and not a statistic and that he has problems. One of his major problems is ill-health, and that is linked inextricably to his problems of poverty, ignorance and racial prejudice. Society's usual reaction when faced with problems of great magnitude, is to form commissions or committees[16] to attempt definition, study, analysis and consultation. All these mechanisms are now being employed to understand and repair medical deficiencies in the ghetto. Doubtless they are necessary. However, in the preoccupation with theories, guidelines, solutions and programs, regardless of how well intentioned these efforts may be, it should be remembered that there are people in the ghetto to whom dignity and pride[17] are as important as they are to those who grandly assume the responsibility for ordering the lives and habits of others. However, theories, guidelines, solutions and programs imposed from without often lack relevance to the ills they are intended to alleviate and, if ill conceived, poorly executed or badly administered, frequently end by creating further hardship and perpetuating oppression. Bedford-Stuyvesant must know that it shares little in common with Sutton Place, but do Shaker Heights and Beverly Hills delude themselves into believing that they understand, or worse, can decide the better courses of action for Hough and Watts?

Patterns

To understand the medical problems of ghetto residents, one must recognize the differential patterns of treatment of the Negro and the white. These patterns have been woven into the fabric of our culture for 350 years. The first Negroes who came to Virginia in 1619 were indentured servants entitled to freedom by 1629. Nevertheless, when in 1640 three runaway servants, two white and one Negro, were recaptured, the courts ordered the white servants to serve their masters one additional year; the Negro was ordered "to serve his said master or his assigns for the time of his *natural life* here or elsewhere." and the pattern was initiated.

By 1700 Virginia and the other colonies had recognized and condoned slavery with all its debasement of humanity in laws that were as proscriptive as they were precise. In 1775 General George Washington issued an order forbidding recruiting officers to enlist "Negroes, Boys unable to bare Arms nor Old Men unfit to endure the Fatigues of the Campaign," and the pattern was reinforced.

The framers of the Constitution went another step, implicitly recognizing the institution of slavery by devising a formula whereby representation in the lower house was determined on the basis of equating five slaves to three white men. And the pattern was perpetuated.

Between 1767 and 1790 more than 80,000 slaves were brought here each year; by 1787 there were nearly 700,000, and the invention of the cotton gin in 1793 sent the outlook for slave labor soaring. The patterns of differential treatment of human beings were established. The outlawing of slave trading in 1808 did little more than challenge the ingenuity of those able to take advantage of America's unprotected coastline, and by 1830 the slave population had reached 2,000,000. When the Civil War began there were almost 4,000,000; when total emancipation became effective in 1865, one of every three Southerners and one of every nine Americans was a recently liberated slave. Emancipation had minor impact, however; the patterns had been set. Negroes were no longer property, but neither were they citizens. They could not vote, sit on juries or hold public office, and in both the North and the South they were subject to violence, abuse and legalized repression. In fact, little had changed; Negroes lived at a level of bare subsistence, worked on the plantations for their previous masters and were careful not to offend, for the lynch rope had replaced the lash as quick and convenient punishment.[2-6] But, tentatively at first and then with increasing urgency, Negroes began the bitter, frustrating struggle to rise above the traditional patterns of degradation and injustice to claim the equality and respect other Americans assumed as a birthright. Part of this struggle was manifested in migration.

From the rural south to the urban north and west

Every census from 1790 to 1900 revealed that at least 90 percent of the Negro population lived in the South. After the turn of the century, Negroes began to move from the South to the North and West, and from rural to urban areas.[18-20] The reasons for migration were and are many and include the search for economic and social improvement and better educational opportunities. Many fled from frustration and fear. It is difficult to ascertain the relative importance of any of these factors. However, 3,407 fatal lynchings of Negroes, mostly in the rural South, had been documented by World War II, and each was followed by a wave of local migration.

As recently as 1948, Governor Fielding L. Wright advised the Negroes of Mississippi that "if they contemplated eventual social equality and the sharing of school, hotel and restaurant facilities ... they should make their homes in some other state than Mississippi." Negroes migrated to the North and West, crowding into already teeming cities, and were forced into substandard and antiquated housing in areas of the central cities that were being abandoned by lower and middle class whites moving outward (and upward) to the suburbs. For example, in the 1930's Newark's population peaked at 500,000, 9 percent of whom were Negroes. By 1950, reflecting the influx of migrants from the South, the Negro population of Newark had risen to 17 percent and in 1960 to 34 percent. In 1969 as the middle class exodus continues, the city's population is 52 percent Negro, making it the nation's second municipality to have a Negro majority, the first being Washington, D.C. By 1975 demographers believe that Newark's population will be 75 percent Negro. Other major cities are experiencing similar trends and suffering from an accompanying escalation of welfare costs, shrinking tax bases, polarization of public opinion toward ethnic groups and deteriorating delivery of public services, of which medicine can be considered a prime example.

In the North and West the immigrant Negro hoped to find a freedom and opportunity denied him in the South. This has proved to be, more often than not, a miscalculation. Forced by economic limitations and social pressures into deteriorating inner-city ghettos, the newcomers found that they had exchanged one form of bondage for another, perhaps less blatant but more difficult to combat. They are told that they lack skills that "qualify" them for obtaining and keeping a job. Defeated and demoralized, they have little faith in the ability of the segregated ghetto school to lead the succeeding generation to prosperity and self-respect and little trust for the "outsider," the teacher, merchant, social worker, employer, government official or hospital-based physician who represents one more link in the endless chain of oppression and exploitation extending over centuries.

John C. Norman

Is racism relevant?

To raise the question of the relevancy of racism in considerations of the evolution of the problems of the ghetto is naive. [21-25] The United States Riot Commission Report of the National Advisory Commission on Civil Disorders (the Kerner Commission), written largely from ghetto analyses, summed up the situation in agonizingly clear terms: "America is, and has always been, a racist society. Bigotry penetrates every level and every region of the country, North and South, business, labor, journalism, education and medicine. The causes [of racism] are ignorance, apathy, poverty and above all a pervasive discrimination that has thwarted each and every American Negro in all avenues of his life." [9] The full meaning of this conclusion becomes more ominous when it is realized that the Negro census is younger and is increasing significantly more rapidly than the white population; the mean age of American Negroes is 21.1, and that of whites 29.1. One out of nine Americans in 1966 was Negro; by 1972 the proportion will be one out of eight. The great majority (70 percent) of Negroes now live in the decaying central cities.[19, 20] In general, and in ghetto areas particularly, Negroes with the same job skills and educational attainments as whites are paid far less in jobs with no possible upward mobility. For the same size substandard (10 to 15 percent deficient) housing units, Negroes pay an average 10 to 15 percent higher rent. In these areas more than 2,300,000 Negro children under 15 are living in circumstances below the poverty level ($3,335 per year for a family of four). The young people of the ghetto are increasingly conscious of a system that seems to offer rewards to those who exploit others (narcotics sellers, numbers runners and so forth) and failure to those who struggle under traditional responsibilities. Many adopt the former as a life style, and these patterns reinforce themselves from one generation to the next.[9]

No aspect of life within the ghetto is free from racism. Few chain stores operate in these areas, and, contrary to stereotypes, few ghetto residents own automobiles. As a result, inner-city residents are forced to shop at stores where prices are 10 to 15 percent higher and quality is 10 to 15 percent lower. In one northeastern metropolitan area, the Kerner Commission found that it took police four times as long to respond to a call from a predominantly ghetto district as compared to a call from white areas of the same city. In another metropolitan district, delays of six to eight hours in emergency services in municipal hospitals were recorded. Within the law-enforcement ranks the following patterns were found: one Negro on the 1,502-man Michigan State Police Force; five Negroes on the 1,224-man New Jersey State Police Force; seven on a 707-man force in Phoenix; and 49 on a 2,504-man force in Boston. In comparison, however, Negroes constituted 11 percent of the enlisted personnel in Vietnam in 1967. And in the first eleven months of that year Negro soldiers, the majority of whom now live in our urban ghettos, constituted 22.4 percent of all Army troops killed in action. It can be said, as previously, " 'the point' during the war, and the ghetto during peace."

72

The Kerner Commission decided that it is primarily racism, not poverty or cynicism, that is the basic cause of the current schism in American life. As one Commission staff member summed it up, "We've got to see it as a system and attack it as a system."

The "system"

The "system" has existed in America since the beginning. Our nation's educational facilities,[25] medical schools,[16] teaching hospitals [22] and health-care delivery systems [21, 23] are part of the system and equally guilty of complicity. Consider why, at a national level, a Negro's life expectancy is 64.1 years and a white's is 71 years, or why in urban areas in general Negro mothers die in childbirth four times as often as white mothers, or why Negro babies die in infancy three times as often as white babies.[26] Consider why further differentials pertain within the ghetto. Why, for instance, infant mortality in Chicago is 50 percent higher among recent Southern migrants than it is among other ghetto residents. Consider why the pharmacy dispenses food as prescription medicine to the 1,300 members of the Negro township of Mound Bayou, Mississippi, in 1969 or why the median weekly income of an employed Negro male household head in Boston's Columbia Point is $55.23.[1]

The "system" that permits and promotes these inequities is acquired, nurtured and promulgated from generation to generation, and it is uniquely American. The "system" created the urban ghetto by fostering migration of the Negro from the South and by applying intense social pressures in the North and West, with devastating ecologic impact. The "system" engenders a general inability of the citizenry to understand or deal with the problems of ghetto residents, their degradation, their misery and hopelessness. Under the guise of maintaining standards of quality or property values, the system repeatedly frustrates attempts to pursue any meaningful and profitable goals by ghetto residents. The "system" seems unable to grasp the concept that failure breeds failure and that an ingrained sense of inferiority leads to "unteachable" children, "unreachable" patients and escalating cycles of self-destructive behavior. The system has produced generations of Negro tradesmen, skilled workers, professional men and scholars who have been forced to lower aspirations, to compromise integrity and to accept in desperation whatever may have become available, ultimately achieving far less than their capabilities warrant simply because the "system" has been unwilling to give them opportunities and responsibilities commensurate with their training and ability. The "system" has produced a nation in which Negroes were excluded from "soup-kitchen" lines during the Depression, in which separate blood banks for white and Negro soldiers were maintained during World War II [11] and in which, in 1963, 84 percent of Southern and 43 percent of border state hospitals were permitted to segregate Negroes by race.[21] With public funds, the "system" has built a medical school in the State of West Virginia, whose population is 10 percent Negro, which has graduated 2,400 students, including 35 Puerto

Ricans, but only two Negroes.[27] The "system" has produced Southern medical societies that still bar Negroes from membership.[24] The "system" has permitted perhaps one but never more than two American Negroes to graduate from Harvard Medical School in any given year [14, 28, 30] and has allowed virtually none to train for specialization in any of its 18 affiliated teaching hospitals. None has remained to practice in Boston, where the ghetto population has now reached 85,000.

Insight into the problem

The plight of the ghetto resident cannot be fully appreciated by those who lack a heritage of perpetual disenchantment, disillusionment, alienation, frustration and apathy bordering on despair. Ghetto residents and their ancestors have been exposed to three and a half centuries of overt and covert oppression and exploitation, the perpetuation of which can be likened to a subtle and lingering, but effective, form of genocide. The strategies and tactics have included the removal of initiative and its replacement with patronage, the demand for subservience and the denial of responsibility, the creation of barriers and the questioning of innate capabilities, the focus on shortcomings and the ignoring of achievements, the alleging of inherent inferiority and the decrying of misdirected efforts, the postponement of ambitions and the attack, directly or by innuendo, of protests, the display of concern from afar, but the scrupulous avoidance of involvement, secure in the knowledge that moral responsibilities have been discharged by the mere "awareness" of the problems of the ghetto, and finally, the sudden demand for instant qualification and leadership.[31]

Any effort to improve the health of ghetto residents cannot be separated from equal and simultaneous efforts to remove the multiple social, political and economic constraints currently imposed on inner-city residents. Nor will medicine be successful without basic changes in attitudes so deeply embedded in the "system" that they are seldom questioned or even considered. Ideally, the ghetto should not exist. However, each ghetto resident at least should have a responsible physician whom he knows and trusts, who is unhurriedly attuned to his needs and aspirations and who understands and is concerned with his domestic and employment situations. Nonetheless, the collective apperceptive mass of ethnic experience of the ghetto resident dictates that he demand and accept far less than this along with far less than adequate political representation, employment, housing, public services and medical care. The ghetto resident offers, in the depersonalized language of the medical profession, excellent teaching "material," and many, if not most, physicians continue to be trained in institutions serving indigent populations in metropolitan areas. What better way to perpetuate the "system" of exploitation than to learn basic clinical medicine from ghetto residents and subsequently deliver that expertise to suburban patients? Cynically, one could present an excellent case that the ghetto is best suited for exploitation. For it is there that we obtain practical nurses but not supervisors, janitors but not hospital administrators, domestics but not executive secretaries, "disadvantaged" students but not national merit scholars, "neglected teaching cases" but not private patients, and the endless entourage of convenient political issues, case studies in violence and targets for countless federal programs. Without the ghetto, would there be the flight to the burgeoning suburbs on which so much of the economic growth of the country depends? And if ghettos did not exist, with what would they be replaced?

Despite these comparisons and conjectures in cynicism, the medical problems of the ghetto have evolved and exist as monuments to one of the most unjust aspects of our society. They will continue to exist and increase until we realize that the quest for dignity is universal and that adult ghetto residents should not be called by their first names on ward rounds. They will continue to exist and increase until we realize that outward appearances belie ambitions, motivations, aspirations, anxieties and capabilities. They will continue to exist and increase until all of us realize that each little yellow, white, red, black or brown baby represents the hopes and fears of generations, and that the future of each is predicated on equal measures of opportunity, challenge, empathy, understanding, compassion and dignity.

References

1. Sources, a Blue Cross Report on Health Problems of the Poor, Blue Cross Association, Chicago, Illinois, 1968.
2. G. Myrdal, *American Dilemma: The Negro Problem and Modern Democracy.* New York, McGraw-Hill Book Company, 1943.
3. *A Documentary History of the Negro People in The United States.* Edited by H. Aptheker. New York, International Publishers, 1951.
4. M. J. Butcher, *The Negro in American Culture.* New York, Alfred A. Knopf, 1956.
5. R. Bardolph, *The Negro Vanguard.* New York, Vintage Press, 1959.
6. J. H. Franklin, *From Slavery to Freedom: A History of Negro Americans.* Third edition. New York, Alfred A. Knopf, 1969.
7. D. E. Pentony, "The Case for Black Studies." *Atlantic Monthly* 223 (4):81–89, 1969.
8. W. H. Grier, P. M. Cobbs, *Black Rage.* New York, Basic Books, Inc., 1969.
9. *Report of the National Advisory Committee on Civil Disorders.* New York, Bantam Books, Inc., 1969.
10. Malcolm X, *The Autobiography of Malcolm X.* New York, Grove Press, 1966.
11. M. Stratton, *Negroes Who Helped Build America.* Boston, Ginn and Company, 1965.
12. H. Buckler, *Doctor Dan: Pioneer in American Surgery.* Boston, Little, Brown and Company, 1954.
13. S. Redding, *The Lonesome Road.* Garden City, New York, Doubleday and Company, 1958.

14. *Ebony* Magazine 3: Nov. 7, 16, 1948.
15. E. G. Sterne, *Blood Brothers: Four Men of Science.* New York, Alfred A. Knopf, 1959.
16. *Preliminary Report of the Commission on Relations with the Black Community.* Harvard Medical School, April, 1969.
17. I. F. Swan, "The Inner City Oriented Physician." *J Nat Med Ass* 58:139, 1967.
18. *The American Negro Reference Book.* Edited by J. P. Davies. Englewood Cliffs, New Jersey, Prentice-Hall, 1966.
19. P. M. Hauser, "Demographic Factors in the Integration of the Negro," *The Negro American.* Edited by T. Parsons, K. B. Clark. Boston, Houghton Mifflin, 1966, p. 79.
20. Senate Sub-committee on Government Research, *The Rural to Urban Population Shift: A National Problem,* Washington, D.C., Goverment Printing Office, 1968.
21. J. D. Snyder, "Race Bias in Hospitals: What the Civil Rights Commission Found." *Hosp Manage* 96:52–54, 1963.
22. M. Seham, "Discrimination Against Negroes in Hospitals." *New Eng J Med* 271:940–43, 1964.
23. M. S. Melton, "Health Manpower and Negro Health: The Negro Physician." *J Med Educ* 43:798–814, 1968.
24. M. Scheck, unpublished data.
25. Undergraduate enrollment by race. Chronicle of Higher Education, April 21, 1969.
26. United States Department of Health, Education, and Welfare, Public Health Service, Vital and Health Statistics, *Infant Mortality Trends: United States and Each State, 1930–1964.* Washington, D.C., Government Printing Office, 1965 (Publication No. 1000, Series 20, No. 1), pp. 1–70.
27. J. Rasmussen, "Medical Crisis in Black and White." Charleston, West Virginia *Gazette & Mail,* September 20 and October 5, 1968.
28. Harvard Medical School Archives, AA 1.20 Bx 3.
29. *Idem:* Harvard Medical School Faculty Minutes, 11/4/50, 12/26/50 and 11/16/53.
30. W. M. Cobb, "Medical History Column on Martin Robison Delany." *J Nat Med Ass* 44:232–37, 1952.
31. J. Z. Bowers, L. Cogan, E. L. Becker, "Negroes for Medicine, Report of a Conference." *JAMA* 202:213–14, 1967.

The health
of haight-ashbury

DAVID E. SMITH, JOHN LUCE,
and ERNEST A. DERNBURG

Conventional middle-class populations receive the best care our present conventional medical institutions can supply. Middle-class people pay their bills on time or have health insurance, which does it for them. They trust the doctor to do what is best for them. They have diseases that go with respectability, and the doctor who treats them need not feel tainted by associating with people whose medical problems arise from activities that are illegal or immoral.

People who do not measure up to middle-class standards pose a problem for organized medicine. They require medical care no less than others, but the profession does not do well in providing it. People who have no money or insurance, who mistrust doctors, who seem to the physician to be immoral criminals, find it difficult to get care. Doctors don't like them; they don't like the doctors. The profession, used to providing medical care in a style that suits it and supplied with plenty of middle-class patients who like that style, has never bothered to figure out how to deliver medical care in a way that suits other populations who live differently.

San Francisco's hippie invasion of 1967 created an acute problem of this kind. The city's officialdom made no adequate response to the medical and public health problems it produced, but a number of volunteers founded the Haight-Ashbury Free Medical Clinic, a unique experiment in providing medical care to a deviant population on terms it would accept. The story of the clinic—the problems of staffing, supplies, finances and the changing population needs it encountered—suggests some of the difficulties and some of the possibilities involved in such an innovation.

Three years ago *Time* magazine called San Francisco's Haight-Ashbury "the vibrant epicenter of America's hippie movement." Today the Haight-Ashbury District looks like a disaster area. Some of the frame Victorian houses, flats and apartment buildings lying between the Panhandle of Golden Gate Park and the slope of Mount Sutro have deteriorated beyond

THE HEALTH OF HAIGHT-ASHBURY From *trans*action, Vol. 7, No. 6, April 1970. Reprinted by permission of David E. Smith, M.D.

repair, and many property-owners have boarded over their windows or blocked their doorways with heavy iron bars. Hiding in their self-imposed internment, the original residents of the area seem emotionally exhausted and too terrified to leave their homes. "We're all frightened," says one 60-year-old member of the Haight-Ashbury Neighborhood Council. "The Haight has become a drug ghetto, a teen-age slum. The streets aren't safe; rats romp in the Panhandle; the neighborhood gets more run down every day. The only thing that'll save this place now is a massive dose of federal aid."

Nowhere is the aid more needed than on Haight Street, the strip of stores that runs east to west through the Flatlands. Once a prosperous shopping area, Haight Street has so degenerated by this time that the storefronts are covered with steel grates and sheets of plywood, while the sidewalks are littered with dog droppings, cigarette butts, garbage and broken glass. According to Henry Sands, the owner of a small realty agency on the corner of Haight and Stanyan streets, over 50 grocers, florists, druggists, haberdashers and other merchants have moved off the street since the 1967 Summer of Love; property values have fallen 20 percent in the same period, but none of the remaining businessmen can find buyers for their stores. The Safeway Supermarket at Haight and Schrader streets has closed, Sands reports, after being shoplifted out of $10,000 worth of merchandise in three months. The one shopowner to open since, stocks padlocks and shatterproof window glass. "The only people making money on Haight Street now sell dope or cheap wine," the realtor claims. "Our former customers are all gone. There's nothing left of the old community anymore."

Nothing is left of the Haight-Ashbury's new hippie community today either. There are no paisley-painted buses on Haight Street, no "flower children" parading the sidewalks, no tribal gatherings, no H.I.P. (Haight Independent Proprietor) stores. Almost all the long-haired proprietors have followed the original merchants out of the district; the Psychedelic Shop at Haight and Clayton stands vacant; the Print Mint across the street and the Straight Theatre down the block are both closed. Allen Ginsberg, Timothy Leary, Ken Kesey and their contemporaries no longer visit the communal mecca they helped establish here in the mid-1960s. Nor do the rock musicians, poster artists and spiritual gurus who brought it international fame. And although a few young people calling themselves Diggers still operate a free bakery and housing office out of the basement of All Saints' Episcopal Church on Waller Street, Father Leon Harris there considers them a small and insignificant minority. "For all intents and purposes," he says, "the peaceful hippies we once knew have disappeared."

They started disappearing almost three years ago, when worldwide publicity brought a different and more disturbed population to the Haight and the city escalated its undeclared war on the new community. Today, most of the long-haired adolescents the public considers hip have left Haight Street to hang out on Telegraph Avenue in Berkeley or on Grant Avenue in San Francisco's North Beach District. Some of the "active" or "summer" hippies who once played in the Haight-Ashbury have either returned home or reenrolled in school. Others have moved to the Mission District and other parts of the city, to Sausalito and Mill Valley in Marin

County, to Berkeley and Big Sur or to the rural communes operating throughout northern California.

A few are still trapped in the Haight, but they take mescaline, LSD and other hallucinogenic drugs indoors and stay as far away from Haight Street as possible. When they must go there, to cash welfare checks or to shop at the one remaining supermarket, they never go at night or walk alone. "It's too dangerous for me," says one 19-year-old unwed mother who ran away from a middle-class home in Detroit during the summer of 1967. "Haight Street used to be so groovy I could get high just being there. But I don't know anybody on the street today. Since I've been here, it's become the roughest part of town."

A new population has moved into the district and taken over Haight Street like an occupying army. Transient and diverse, its members now number several thousand persons. Included are a few tourists, weekend visitors and young runaways who still regard the Haight-Ashbury as a refuge for the alienated. There are also older white, Negro and Indian alcoholics from the city's Skid Row; black delinquents who live in the Flatlands or the Fillmore ghetto; Hell's Angels and other "bikers" who roar through the area on their Harley Davidsons. Finally there are the overly psychotic young people who abuse any and all kinds of drugs, and psychopathic white adolescents with criminal records in San Francisco and other cities who come from lower-class homes or no homes at all.

Uneducated and lacking any mystical or spiritual interest, many of these young people have traveled from across the country to find money, stimulation and easy sex in the Haight and to exploit the flower children they assume are still living here. Some have grown long hair and assimilated the hip jargon in the process, but they resemble true hippies in no real way. "Street wise" and relatively aggressive in spite of the passive longings which prompt their drug abuse, they have little love for one another and no respect for the law or for themselves. Instead of beads and bright costumes they wear leather jackets and coarse, heavy clothes. Instead of ornate buses they drive beat-up motorcycles and hot rods. Although they smoke marijuana incessantly and drop acid on occasion, they generally dismiss these chemicals as child's play and prefer to intoxicate themselves with opiates, barbiturates and amphetamines.

Their individual tastes may vary, but most of the adolescents share a dreary, drug-based life-style. Few have any legal means of support, and since many are addicted to heroin, they must peddle chemicals, steal groceries and hustle spare change to stay alive. Even this is difficult, for there is very little money on Haight Street and a great deal of fear. Indeed, the possibility of being "burned," raped or "ripped off" is so omnipresent that most of the young people stay by themselves and try to numb their anxiety and depression under a toxic fog. By day they sit and slouch separately against the boarded-up storefronts in a drug-induced somnolescence. At night they lock themselves indoors, inject heroin and plan what houses in the district they will subsequently rob.

Although the results of this living pattern are amply reflected in the statistics available from Park Police Station at Stanyan and Waller streets, the 106 patrolmen there are apparently unable to curb the Haight-Ashbury's crime. Their job has been made easier by the relative decrease in amphetamine consumption and the disappearance of many speed freaks from the district over the past few months, but the rate of robbery and other acts associated with heroin continues to rise. Making regular sweeps of Haight Street in patrol cars and paddy wagons, the police also threaten to plant drugs on known dealers if they will not voluntarily leave town. Yet these and other extreme measures seem only to act like a negative filter in the Haight, screening out the more cunning abusers and leaving their inept counterparts behind.

Furthermore, the narcotics agents responsible for the Haight-Ashbury cannot begin to regulate its drug flow. According to one agent of the State Narcotics Bureau, "The Haight is still the national spawning ground for multiple drug abuse. The adolescents there have caused one of the toughest law enforcement problems we've ever known."

Public health: a suicide license

They have also created one of the most serious health problems in all of San Francisco. Many of the young people who hang out on Haight Street are not only overtly or potentially psychotic, but also physically ravaged by one another as well. Although murder is not particularly popular with the new population, some of its members seem to spend their lives in plaster casts. Others frequently exhibit suppurating abrasions, knife and razor slashes, damaged genitalia and other types of traumatic injuries—injuries all caused by violence.

Even more visible is the violence they do to themselves. Continually stoned on drugs, the adolescents often overexert and fail to notice as they infect and mangle their feet by wading through the droppings and broken glass. Furthermore, although some of the heroin addicts lead a comparatively stabilized existence, others overlook the physiological deterioration which results from their self-destructive lives. The eating habits of these young people are so poor that they are often malnourished and inordinately susceptible to infectious disease. In fact, a few of them suffer from protein and vitamin deficiencies that are usually found only in chronic alcoholics three times their age.

With gums bleeding from pyorrhea and rotting teeth, some also have abscesses and a diffuse tissue infection called cellulitis, both caused by using dirty needles. Others miss their veins while shooting up or rupture them by injecting impure and undissolvable chemicals. And since most sleep, take drugs and have sex in unsanitary environments, they constantly expose themselves to upper respiratory tract infections, skin rashes, bronchitis, tonsillitis, influenza, dysentery, urinary and genital tract infections, hepatitis and venereal disease.

In addition to these and other chronic illnesses, the young people also suffer from a wide range of drug problems. Some have acute difficulties, such as those individuals who oversedate themselves with barbiturates or "overamp" with amphetamines. Others have chronic complaints, long-term "speed"-precipitated psychoses and paranoid, schizophrenic reactions. Many require physiological and psychological withdrawal from barbiturates and heroin. In fact, heroin addiction and its attendant symptoms have reached epidemic proportions in the Haight-Ashbury, and the few doctors at Park Emergency Hospital cannot check the spread of disease and drug abuse through the district any better than the police can control its crime.

To make matters worse, these physicians appear unwilling to attempt to solve the local health problems. Like many policemen, the public health representatives seem to look on young drug-abusers as subhuman. When adolescents come to Park Emergency for help the doctors frequently assault them with sermons, report them to the police or submit them to complicated and drawn-out referral procedures that only intensify their agony. The nurses sometimes tell prospective patients to take their problems elsewhere. The ambulance drivers simply "forget" calls for emergency assistance. They and the other staff members apparently believe that the best way to stamp out sickness in the Haight is to let its younger residents destroy themselves.

Given this attitude, it is hardly surprising that the adolescents are as frightened of public health officials as they are of policemen. Some would sooner risk death than seek aid at Park Emergency and are equally unwilling to got to San Francisco General Hospital, the city's central receiving unit, two miles away. Many merely live with their symptoms, doctor themselves with home remedies or narcotize themselves to relieve their pain. These young people do not trust "straight" private physicians, who they assume will overcharge them and hand them over to the law. Uneducated about medical matters, they too often listen only to the "witch doctors" and drug-dealers who prowl the Haight-Ashbury, prescribing their own products for practically every physiological and psychological ill.

A few are receptive to responsible opinion and anxious to be properly treated, particularly those individuals who want to kick heroin and those younger adolescents who have just made the Haight their home. Unfortunately, however, they have nowhere to go for help. Huckleberry's for Runaways and almost all the other service agencies created to assist the hippies in 1967 have suspended operations in the area. Although Father Harris and several other neighborhood ministers offer free advice at their respective churches, they can hardly deal with all the young people who come their way. Indeed, the only major organization that can reach the new population is the Haight-Ashbury Free Medical Clinic. But today, the first privately operated facility in America to employ community volunteers in providing free and nonpunitive treatment of adolescent drug and health difficulties has serious problems of its own.

The clinic: an alternative

This is ironic, for although it is still somewhat at odds with the local medical Establishment, the clinic is better staffed and funded than at any point in its 2-1/2-year history. It is also more decentralized, with several facilities in and outside of the Haight-Ashbury. Its oldest operation, a Medical Section located on the second floor of a faded yellow building at the corner of Haight and Clayton streets, is now open from six until ten five evenings a week. Over 40 dedicated volunteers are on hand in the 14-room former dentist's office, so that 558 Clayton Street can accommodate more than 50 patients a day.

Of the young people who use the facility, only half live in the immediate area. The rest are hippies, beats and older people who come with their children from as far away as southern California. Accepting the clinic because it accepts them, the patients are treated by a staff of over 20 volunteer nurses and physicians in an atmosphere brightened by poster art and psychedelic paraphernalia. Some of these health professionals are general practitioners committed to community medicine. Others are specialists hoping to broaden their medical understanding. Many are interns and residents looking for experience or studying the Medical Section as a philosophic alternative to the practices of the Public Health Department and the American Medical Association.

Whatever their motivation, the doctors' primary objectives are diagnosis and detoxification. After examining their patients, they attempt to treat some with donated drugs which are kept under lock and key in the clinic pharmacy. Others require blood, urine and vaginal smear tests that can be performed in the laboratory on equipment furnished by the Medical Logistics Company of San Francisco and its 35-year-old president, Donald Reddick, who serves as the clinic's administrative director. Most of the patients have chronic problems, however, and cannot be treated adequately on the premises. They must therefore be referred and/or physically transported to other facilities, such as Planned Parenthood, the Society for Humane Abortions, the Pediatrics Clinic at the University of California Medical Center on Parnassus Street six blocks south, Children's Hospital, San Francisco General Hospital and the Public Health Department Clinic for VD. The Medical Section maintains a close working relationship with these institutions and can therefore act as a buffer between its hip patients and the straight world.

Although the physicians and nurses contribute to this mediating process, much of the referring, chauffeuring and patient-contacting at 558 Clayton Street is carried out by its staff of clerks, administrative aides and paramedical volunteers. Twenty such young people donate their time and energy to the Medical Section at present, most of them student activists, conscientious objectors fulfilling alternative service requirements and former members of the Haight-Ashbury's new community. Emotionally equipped to handle the demands and the depressing climate of ghetto medicine, several core members of the paramedical staff live together in the Haight as a communal family.

Supervising the volunteers is Dr. Alan Matzger, a 37-year-old general surgeon from San Francisco who developed an interest in community medicine after working at 558 Clayton Street for over a year. The clinic's first full-time resident physician, Dr. Matzger is actually employed by the United

States Public Health Service, which has asked him to conduct a long-range investigation of health needs in the Haight-Ashbury. He is now nearing completion of this study and will soon develop an objective and comprehensive plan for community medical care.

Since heroin addiction is such a pressing current problem, Dr. Matzger and an anesthesiologist named Dr. George Gay have recently launched a heroin withdrawal program at the Medical Section. Working there five afternoons a week for the past four months, the two physicians have treated over 200 patients, less than 50 percent of whom consider the Haight their home. "The remainder are adolescents from so-called good families," Dr. Matzger reports, "most of them students at local colleges and high schools. Significantly, they follow the same evolutionary pattern as young people have in this district, progressing from hallucinogenic drug abuse to abuse of amphetamines and then to abuse of barbiturates and opiates. The 'Year of the Middle-Class Junkie' in San Francisco may well be 1970. If it is, we hope to expand our program as addiction problems mount throughout the entire Bay area."

Another expansion being considered at the clinic is a dentistry service. Organized by Dr. Ira Handelsman, a dentist from the University of the Pacific who is paid by a Public Health Service grant to study periodontal disease, this would be the first free program of dentistry in the city outside of the oral surgery unit at San Francisco General Hospital. As such, the service is under fire from the local dental society, which is opposed to this form of free dental care. Nevertheless, Dr. Handelsman is committed to his effort and has recently secured three donated dental chairs.

Although this and other programs at 558 Clayton Street are intended to operate somewhat autonomously, they are closely coordinated with those operated out of the clinic's second center in the Haight-Ashbury. Known as "409 House," it is located in a pale blue Victorian residence at the corner of Clayton and Oak streets, across from the Panhandle. On the first floor of this building is a reading and meditation room supervised by Reverend Lyle Grosjean of the Episcopal Peace Fellowship who counsels some adolescents about spiritual, marital, draft and welfare problems and offers shelter for others coming in from the cold.

On the third floor at 409 Clayton Street is the clinic publications office, staffed by volunteers who oversee the preparation of *The Journal of Psychedelic Drugs*, a semi-annual compilation of articles and papers presented at the drug symposia sponsored by the clinic and the University of California Medical Center Psychopharmacology Study Group. Aided by several health professionals, the volunteers also answer requests for medical information and administer the affairs of the National Free Clinics Council, an organization created in 1968 for the dozens of free facilities in Berkeley, Boston and other cities that modeled their efforts after those of the Haight-Ashbury Free Medical Clinic programs.

Sandwiched in between the Publications Office and Reverend Grosjean's sanctuary is the Psychiatric Section. This service, which is supervised by Stuart Loomis, a 47-year-old associate professor of education at San Francisco State College, provides free counseling and psychiatric aid for over 150 individuals. Roughly one-half of these patients are hippies and "active hippies" who either live in the district or commute from rural and urban communes where physicians from the Medical Section make house calls. The remaining 50 percent is made up of young people who suffer from the chronic anxiety and depression common in heroin addicts.

Loomis and the other 30 staff psychologists, psychiatrists and psychiatric social workers at 409 Clayton Street are able to counsel some of these patients in the Psychiatric Section. They usually refer the more disturbed multiple drug-abusers and ambulatory schizophrenics now common to the Haight either to such facilities as the drug program at Mendocino State Hospital or to the Immediate Psychiatric Aid and Referral Service at San Francisco General, whose director, Dr. Arthur Carfagni, is on the clinic's executive committee. When intensive psychiatric intervention is not called for, however, they frequently send the patients to the clinic's own Drug Treatment Program in the basement downstairs.

Project "free fuse"

This project, nicknamed the Free Fuse, is led by a Lutheran minister in his mid-thirties named John Frykman. Financed by personal gifts and by grants from such private foundations as the Merrill Trust, its goal is to wean drug-abusers away from their destructive life-style. Using methods developed by Synanon and the Esalen Institute, Frykman and the other Free Fuse counselors have attempted to create a close and productive social unit out of alienated adolescents living together as the clinic's second communal family. They have also provided educational and employment opportunities for more than 500 young people in the past 1-1/2 years.

Since many Free Fuse graduates are still involved in his project, Frykman has also found it possible to expand. Having recently opened an annex in the drug-ridden North Beach District under the supervision of a psychiatric nurse, he has allowed the Drug Treatment Program to geographically qualify for inclusion in the Northeast Mental Health Center, a cachement area encompassing one-quarter of San Francisco. Because of this, the Free Fuse will participate in a substantial grant from the National Institute of Mental Health being administered by Dr. Carfagni. Frykman's Drug Treatment Program has already received some of these funds, and he is therefore making arrangements with the downtown YMCA to open a similar center in the city's Tenderloin area. "We've never gotten a penny from any public agency before," he says, "but the future looks bright from here."

This optimism certainly seems justified, and Frykman is not the only staff member who insists that the clinic is in better shape than at any other point in its history. Yet, as indicated earlier, the facility has problems all the same. In the first place, although the volunteers working at 409 and 558 Clayton Street can point to their share of therapeutic successes, they cannot really help most of the individuals who now live in the Haight-Ashbury. Many of the volunteers are actually former patients; some of them can keep off drugs only if they are kept on the staff.

Second, and most important, is the fact that the Haight continues to deteriorate in spite of the clinic's efforts. Thus, the relatively healthy adolescents tend to abandon the district, leaving behind their more disturbed counterparts, as well as the older individuals who preceded them in the area. Because of this, some staff members at the Medical and Psychological Sections believe that the clinic has outlived its usefulness in its present form. Others argue that the facility should address itself to the problems not only of the new population but of the old community as well. Dr. Matzger will probably have an important voice in this matter, and although his study might prompt the United States Public Health service to support the work at 409 and 558 Clayton Street, it may mean a radical transformation in these centers as they now stand. This is a distinct possibility, for the clinic's future, like its past, is intimately connected with the district it serves.

Haight-ashbury history

To fully appreciate this it is necessary to visualize the Haight in 1960, before its present population arrived. In that year, rising rents, police harassment and the throngs of tourists and thrill-seekers on Grant Avenue squeezed many beatniks out of the North Beach District three miles away. They started looking for space in the Haight-Ashbury, and landlords here saw they could make more money renting their property to young people willing to put up with poor conditions than to black families. For this reason, a small, beat subculture took root in the Flatlands and spread slowly up the slope of Mount Sutro. By 1962 the Haight was the center of a significant but relatively unpublicized bohemian colony.

Although fed by beats and students from San Francisco State, this colony remained unnoticed for several years. One reason was its members' preference for sedating themselves with alcohol and marijuana instead of using drugs that attract more attention. Another was their preoccupation with art and their habit of living as couples or alone. This living pattern was drastically altered in 1964, however, with the popular acceptance of mescaline, LSD and other hallucinogens and the advent of the Ginsberg-Leary-Kesey nomadic, passive, communal electric and acid-oriented life-style. The beats were particularly vulnerable to psychoactive chemicals that they thought enhanced their aesthetic powers and alleviated their isolation. Because of this, hallucinogenic drugs swept the Haight-Ashbury, as rock groups began preparing in the Flatlands what would soon be known as the "San Francisco Sound." On 1 January 1966 the world's first Psychedelic Shop was opened on Haight Street. Two weeks later, Ken Kesey hosted a Trips Festival at Longshoreman's Hall. Fifteen thousand individuals attended, and the word "hippie" was born. A year later, after Diggers and H.I.P. had come to the Haight, the new community held a tribal gathering for 20,000 white Indians on the polo fields of Golden Gate Park. At this first Human Be-In, it showed its collective strength to the world.

The community grew immeasurably in size and stature as a result of this venture, but the ensuing publicity brought it problems for which its founders were ill prepared. In particular, the immigration of more young people to the Haight-Ashbury after the Be-In caused a shortage in sleeping space and precipitated the emergence of a new living unit, the crash pad. Adolescents forced to reside in these temporary and overcrowded structures started to experience adverse hallucinogenic drug reactions and psychological problems. The new community began to resemble a gypsy encampment, whose members were exposing themselves to an extreme amount of infectious disease.

Theoretically, the San Francisco Public Health Department should have responded positively to the situation. But instead of trying to educate and treat the hippies, it attempted to isolate and thereby destroy their community. Still convinced that theirs was a therapeutic alternative, the young people packed together in the Haight grew suicidally self-reliant, bought their medications on the black market and stocked cases of the antipsychotic agent Thorazine in their crash pads. Meanwhile, the Diggers announced that 100,000 adolescents dropping acid in Des Moines and Sioux Falls would flock to the Haight-Ashbury when school was out. They then tried to blackmail the city into giving them the food, shelter and medical supplies necessary to care for the summer invasion.

Although the Public Health Department remained unmoved by the Diggers' forecast, a number of physicians and other persons associated with the University of California Psychopharmacology Study Group did react to the grisly promise of the Summer of Love. Among them were Robert Conrich, a former private investigator-turned-bohemian; Charles Fischer, a dental student; Dr. Frederick Meyers, internationally respected professor of pharmacology at the Medical Center; and Dr. David Smith, a toxicologist who was then serving as chief of the Alcohol and Drug Abuse Screening Unit at General Hospital. Several of these men lived in or were loyal to the Haight-Ashbury. Many had experience in treating bad LSD trips and felt that a rash of them would soon occur in the district. All had contacts among the new community and were impressed by the hippies' dreams of new social forms. But they also knew that the hippies did not number health among their primary concerns, although they might if they were afforded a free and accepting facility. In April then they decided to organize a volunteer-staffed crisis center which might answer the growing medical emergency in the area.

As they expected, the organizers had little difficulty in gathering a number of hip and straight persons for their staff. However, they did face several problems in implementing their plans. First, they were unable to find space in the Haight until Robert Conrich located an abandoned dentist's office and obtained a lease for one-half of its 14 rooms. Paying the rent then became problematical, but Stuart Loomis and an English professor from State College, Leonard Wolf, offered funds if they could use half the facility for an educational project called Happening House. Finally, the organizers learned that local zoning regulations prohibited the charity operation they envisioned. This obstacle was overcome only after a sympathetic city Supervisor, Jack Morrison, suggested that Dr. Smith establish the clinic as his private office so that his personal malpractice insurance could cover its volunteers.

Once this was accomplished, the organizers dredged up an odd assortment of medical equipment from the basements of several local hospitals. Utilizing the University of California Pharmacology Department, they also contacted the "detail men" representing most of America's large pharmaceutical houses and came up with a storeroom full of donated medications, including some vitally needed Thorazine. They then furnished a calm center for treating adverse LSD reactions at the facility.

Next, the organizers told the Public Health Department of their efforts. Its director, Dr. Ellis Sox, indicated that he might reimburse the organizers or open his own medical center if it was required in the Haight-Ashbury. Encouraged by this, the organizers alerted the new community that they would soon be in business. On the morning of 7 June 1967 the door to 558 Clayton Street was painted with the clinic's logo, a blue dove of peace over a white cross. Underneath this was written its slogan, Love Needs Care. The need itself was demonstrated that afternoon when the door was opened and 200 patients pushed their way inside.

Sickness and drugs

Although the organizers anticipated the need for a regional health center in the Haight, they never dreamed that so many adolescents would seek help at the Medical Section. Nor did they suspect that the Diggers would be so close in their estimate of the number of individuals coming to the district that summer. Not all 100,000 showed up at once, but at least that many visitors did pass through the Haight-Ashbury during the next three months, over 20,000 of them stopping off at 558 Clayton Street along the way. A quarter of these persons were found to be beats, hippies and other early residents of the area. A half were "active" or "summer" hippies, comparatively healthy young people who experimented with drugs and might have done so at Fort Lauderdale and other locations had not the media told them to go West. The final quarter were bikers, psychotics and psychopaths of all ages who came to exploit the psychedelic scene.

Most of these individuals differed psychologically, but sickness and drugs were two things they all had in common. Some picked up measles, influenza, streptococcal pharyngitis, hepatitis, urinary and genital tract infections and venereal disease over the summer. Uncontrolled drug experimentation was rampant so others had bad trips from the black-market acid flooding the area. Many also suffered adverse reactions from other drugs, for the presence of psychopaths and multiple abusers brought changes in psychoactive chemical consumption on the street. This first became obvious at the Summer Solstice Festival, where 5,000 tablets were distributed containing the psychomimetic amphetamine STP. Over 150 adolescents were treated for STP intoxication at the clinic, and after an educational program was launched, the substance waned in popularity in the district. But many of its younger residents had sampled intensive central nervous system stimulation for the first time during the STP episode. As a result, many were tempted to experiment next with "speed."

Such experimentation increased over the summer, until the Haight became the home of two separate subcultures, the first made up of "acid heads" who preferred hallucinogens, the second consisting of "speed freaks" partial to amphetamines. At the same time, the district saw the emergence of two different life-styles, the first characterized by milder adolescent illnesses, the second marked by malnutrition, cellulitis, tachycardia, overstimulation and the paranoid-schizophrenic reactions associated with "speed." This naturally affected the calm center, where student volunteers were treating more than 50 adverse drug reactions every 24 hours. It also made extreme demands on the doctors in the Medical Section, who were dealing with more than 250 patients a day. Discouraged and exhausted by their efforts, the physicians pleaded with the Public Health Department for assistance. Yet the department refused to help the facility and never attempted to open a crisis center of its own.

Fortunately, this refusal did not pass unnoticed by the local press, and 558 Clayton Street received a great deal of community aid. Shortly after the clinic's plight was reported, the facility was flooded with doctors disappointed by the Public Health Department and with medical students who came from as far as Indiana to volunteer. Several Neighborhood Council members dropped by with food for the workers, while contributions began arriving through the mail. One of us (Dernburg) and more than 30 other psychiatrists arrived at 558 Clayton Street and established a temporary Psychiatric Section on the premises. They were followed by Donald Reddick and his partners in Medical Logistics, who donated over $20,000 worth of equipment and organized the staff procedures along more efficient lines. The second set of seven rooms was leased; a laboratory, pharmacy and expanded calm center were installed. Then, Dr. William Nesbitt, a general practitioner, invited the organizers to join Youth Projects, an agency he headed, and to use its non-profit status to accept donations. When all was completed, the clinic was the best-equipped neighborhood center in town.

It was also the most chaotic, of course, a fact that was causing increased friction with the psychiatric staff. Once a Psychiatric Section was furnished at 409 Clayton Street, however, the doctors were able to counsel young people in relative privacy, to segregate the more violent amphetamine-abusers and to reduce the traffic in the Medical Section to a more manageable flow.

While this was going on, the clinic was also involving itself in the crumbling new community. *Time* and other publications somehow assumed that the Haight was still full of hippies at this point, but the physicians at 558 Clayton Street knew otherwise. Realizing that the district was becoming even more disorganized, they created an informal council with Huckleberry's for Runaways, All Saints', the Haight-Ashbury Switchboard and other groups trying to prevent its total collapse. They then launched *The Journal of Psychedelic Drugs* to disseminate pharmacological information and started to participate more actively in community town hall meetings at the Straight Theatre. These several activities greatly enhanced the clinic's reputation in and outside of the Haight-Ashbury.

Although this publicity proved helpful to the facility in certain respects, it also caused several new crises. The first occurred two days after the publication of a *Look* magazine article on the clinic, when Dr. Smith was notified that his malpractice insurance was to be cancelled because he was "working with those weirdos in the Haight." This crisis was resolved when Dr. Robert Morris, a pathologist who was then chairman of the executive committee, suggested that he apply for group coverage under the auspices of the San Francisco Medical Society. Dr. Smith doubted that this organization would ever support his advocacy of free medical care. He was therefore delighted when the Medical Society not only granted him membership but also endorsed the programs at 558 and 409 Clayton Street.

"Where has all the love gone?"

His delight did not last long, however, for shortly after the endorsement the clinic had to contend with a number of persons who tried to capitalize on its good name. First were a number of bogus doctors, most of whom worked under stolen or forged medical licenses in the Haight-Ashbury. Then came the Diggers, who resented the facility's influence in the community. Finally, the Medical Section was besieged by several older psychopaths, one of whom, a drug-dealer named Al Graham, hoped to turn it into his base of operations in the Haight. "Papa Al" was ultimately exposed and run out of the clinic, but shortly after he left, Robert Conrich, who was close to collapse after serving for two months as administrator, retired.

Although a severe blow in itself, Conrich's departure was also an ill omen. In fact, less than a week after he tendered his resignation, the Medical Section ran out of funds. The volunteers rallied to meet this new crisis; phone calls were made to potential contributors; and several paramedical staff members begged for money on Haight Street. Two dance-concert benefits with local rock groups that used the facility were also held, but only one was successful. In desperation, Peter Schubart called Joan Baez, who helped take patient histories and sang to entertain the lonely youngsters as they sat quietly in the waiting room. Yet even she could not save the clinic. On 22 September the door was locked at 558 Clayton Street. Two weeks later, what was left of the new community held a "Death of Hip" ceremony to bury the term "hippie" and remove the media from its back. "Haight used to be love," a participant wrote on the steps of the Medical Section after the event. "Now, where has all the love gone?"

This question could be easily answered, for by the end of the Summer of Love almost all of the original hippies had moved to urban and rural communes outside of the Haight. Many summer hippies had also left the district, and those who remained either fended for themselves or were assimilated into the new population. Staying in the Haight-Ashbury, they quickly changed from experimental drug-users into multiple abusers and needed even more help. For this reason, the clinic organizers were determined to open the Medical Section again.

At the same time, they had another good reason to renew their efforts in the Haight. With the hippie movement spread across the United States by this point, other cities—Seattle, Boston, Berkeley, Cambridge, even Honolulu—were being swept by drug problems. New clinics were being created in the face of this onslaught, all of them looking to the Haight-Ashbury for guidance. Although always a confused and crisis-oriented center, the Haight-Ashbury Free Medical Clinic had become the national symbol of a new and successful approach in reaching a deviant population of alienated adolescents. Thus, its organizers had not only their medical practice but also their position of leadership to resume.

However, not all of them could still work in the Haight, a few were turning to other projects, others went back to prior commitments such as teaching.

The money game

But in spite of the losses the organizers looked to what was left of the new community for support. Another dance-concert benefit was held, this one under the guidance of Fillmore Auditorium owner Bill Graham, and several thousand dollars were raised. Smaller events were hosted at the Straight Theatre and at the John Bolles Gallery. In addition, a wealthy local artist named Norman Stone stepped forward to finance a substantial part of the Medical Section program. The clinic had still received no private or public grants, but by the end of October it had the funds necessary to open again.

When operations were resumed, however, the staff had a great deal more speed and more violence to contend with. In late February of 1968 a tourist ran over a dog, prompting a large crowd of adolescents to assemble on Haight Street. This in turn allowed Mayor Joseph Alioto to unleash his latest weapon for crime control, the 38-man Tactical Squad. After cleaning the street with tear gas and billies that afternoon, the squad vowed to return and enforce its own type of law and order. It did so four months later, when the district was ripped by three nights of rioting, rock-throwing and fires.

After the flames died down, it became apparent that the disturbance had marked yet another turning point in the history of the clinic. Many of its nurses, doctors and paramedical volunteers interpreted the riot as a sign that the Haight was now hopeless; mail contributions also ceased; and several psychiatrists who felt they could do little with or for the new population resigned from their positions. Low on money at this point, the clinic's business manager decided to host a three-day fund-raising benefit over the Labor Day weekend at the Palace of Fine Arts. The Affair was sabotaged by Mayor Alioto, who denied the cooperation of his Park and Recreation Commission. When the benefit, Festival of Performing Arts, was finally over, the organizers had lost $20,000. Two days later, the Medical Section was once again closed.

But, in spite of these obstacles, some progress was made. First, one of us (Smith) was awarded a grant to study adverse marijuana reactions which could be run in conjunction with the clinic. Stuart Loomis was installed as chief of the Psychiatric Section; Roger Smith raised more money for the Drug Treatment Program. In December the clinic received financial pledges from Norman Stone, the San Francisco Foundation and the Mary Crocker Trust. By 7 January 1969, 558 Clayton Street was in business again.

In contrast to previous years, its business went relatively smoothly in 1969. The amphetamines gradually ran their course in the district, and many of the multiple drug-abusers here switched to opiates, barbiturates and other "downers" after becoming too "strung out" on "speed." This change in chemical consumption naturally affected treatment practices, as heroin addiction increased tenfold and young people suffered even more types of chronic illness as a result of their drug abuse. Yet, in spite of the new population's problems, the year was a productive one for the clinic. Over 20,000 patients were treated at the Medical and Psychiatric Sections; research programs were initiated; efforts were made to reach the hippies in their communes; the volunteers became more experienced, although fewer in number; and several ex–staff members became involved in treatment programs of their own.

This year has also been a period of growth. More grants have been secured, and the inclusion of the Drug Treatment Program in the Northeast Mental Health Center, which provides for 14 new paid staff positions, has meant the facility's first official recognition by a public agency. In sum, the Haight-Ashbury Free Medical Clinic has finally become established—and, some say, part of the Establishment. From its third opening until the present, it has enjoyed a time of expansion, improvement and relative peace.

Whether these conditions continue depends, as always, on the Haight-Ashbury. This is particularly true today because its resident population seems to be changing once again. As some of the drug-abusers drift out of the area, their places are apparently being taken by adventurous college students. More black delinquents from the Fillmore ghetto are also frequenting the district, contributing to its heroin problem, though participating in the Drug Treatment Program for the first time. The Neighborhood Council and Merchants' Association still function, but both are demoralized and at a political impasse. In addition, the area is seeing an increased influx of older Negro families. Because of this, some staff members are urging changes at Medical and Psychiatric Sections. One faction sees the clinic evolving into a health center for the entire neighborhood and wants to purchase one of the abandoned buildings on Haight Street so that all future programs can be consolidated under one roof. Another argues for more decentralization, de-emphasis of certain activities and/or increased expansion within and without the Haight.

Dr. Matzger, who knows the district intimately, has not yet decided what policy changes will stem from his United States Public Health Service study. However, he does not feel that both 409 and 558 Clayton Street will be different tomorrow from what they are today. "The clinic is at a cross-roads," he says. "It may continue as a screening, diagnosis, detoxification and referral unit. It may become an expanded Drug Treatment Program. It may evolve into a large neighborhood health facility, particularly if we get the required dose of federal aid. On the other hand, it may have to cut back on some of the present programs. But whatever happens, it will continue to be an amalgam of individual efforts and an inspiration to people who seek new approaches in community medicine. Furthermore, no matter how the Haight-Ashbury changes, we are certain that the clinic will never close again."

The world of the haight-ashbury speed freak

ROGER C. SMITH

Very little is currently known about the kinds of experiences which individuals have who are compulsively injecting large doses of methamphetamine or "speed." This is particularly due to the fact that the "speed freak" as we know him today is a relative newcomer to the drug scene. Perhaps most important, however, is the frantic and violent life style which make on-the-street observation both difficult and dangerous. The researcher or observer, regardless of his intentions, is suspect and not likely to be drawn into the life of a group using speed.

The Amphetamine Research Project is in a unique position in San Francisco's Haight-Ashbury community, however. Since its inception, in June of 1968, the project has served dual roles of treatment and research. The staff has been of assistance in matters of obtaining housing, food, and legal services and obtaining help did not require that the patient subject himself to the questions of the researcher. In short, the staff was represented to the community as both helpful and interested in the problems of "speed" abuse.

This paper is concerned with the kinds of experiences with which individuals enmeshed in the speed scene have to deal, how they interpret these experiences, and how this shapes the direction they may take within the speed scene. It is by no means a complete picture. The research is currently in progress, and there are many gaping holes in our information. The data to be presented represents both formal taped interviews with speed users as well as observations made during informal contacts both in the research offices and on the street. Much of what will be said is frankly speculation, based on some of the hunches we have about the typical career of the "speed freak."

No attempt is made to analyze the many social or psychological variables which pre-date involvement in the speed scene, since these factors appear to be less important in determining what happens to an individual who

THE WORLD OF THE HAIGHT-ASHBURY SPEED FREAK From *Journal of Psychedelic Drugs*, Vol. II, 1969, Haight-Ashbury Medical Clinic, 1969. Reprinted by permission of David E. Smith, M.D.

involves himself in speed use than such factors as drug availability, subjective interpretations of the drug experience, the quality of social interactions, the sanctions which the community imposes on certain types of behavior, and the crucial problems which the speed freak is forced to confront as a result of his particular pattern of drug use.

Turning on to speed is almost always accomplished within a group setting, where the majority of individuals present are using speed. There are great pressures to use for the newcomer. He may be completely overwhelmed by the compulsive talking, the frantic activity, and the apparent euphoria and friendliness of the drug using members of the group. It is also true that the individual in such a group who is not "high" is unable to communicate with others in the group, for talk and the activity seem to have little meaning or relevance for him.

Since most of the young people we have seen come from middle class backgrounds, the notion of sticking a needle in their arm may initially be repugnant to them. For many, the presence of outfits and spoons is reminiscent of the "horror movies" they remember from high school hygiene classes, where such activities were associated exclusively with heroin addicts. Rarely can an individual fix himself the first time, and for many users, fixing is an impossibility and must be handled by a friend. Initially there is the fear that some permanent harm may result from missing a vein, others are fearful of the possibility of overdosing or contracting hepatitis from the needle.

Although most of the individuals with whom we talked had used other drugs in the past, primarily marijuana, the psychedelics and occasionally oral amphetamines or barbiturates, few could conceive of using a needle. How then were they turned on? A Berkeley student's experience seems fairly typical:

> I'd always heard about people shooting drugs, but I'd always looked down on it pretty thoroughly, but when it was actually presented to me it took less than an hour to talk me into it. Mainly because I was at the level where I would have tried anything.

Another young speed user recalls his first experience this way:

> If you're around someone that would do it and like you see them doing it around you, pretty soon you'll do it yourself. I'm pretty sure it doesn't take a particular kind of person, it doesn't take an irresponsible person.

The majority of users seem to have been turned on either by close friends who recommended it, or were turned on by a group with whom they were staying. This has particular significance in the Haight-Ashbury district, which, despite the reputation it has acquired locally for violence and misery, still attracts large numbers of youngsters from outside the Bay Area. It is quite conceivable that these same youngsters, had they appeared on the scene during the 1967 Summer of Love, would have found a "crash pad" with those who used marijuana socially and the psychedelics for religious or philosophical reasons, and who were unalterably opposed to the use of speed, which is generally regarded by this group as an "ego trip." It is quite clear that the peer sanctions against the use of speed and other injectable drugs have broken down with the mass exodus of the "Flower Children," and that speed is now the drug of choice in this youthful subculture.

For some, the first experience with speed is quite frightening. We have seen numerous young people in the Amphetamine Research Project who were acutely anxious following their first experience with speed. It is probable that the acute anxiety reaction is the most common clinical pattern presented at the Haight-Ashbury Medical Clinic or other medical facilities for this reason. For many the rapid heartbeat, excessive sweating, compulsive talking or physical agitation are unbearable, and some fear that they will never be able to return to a normal state. For others, the adverse effects are perceived during the come-down, with the feeling of extreme physical fatigue and mental depression, a feeling which can be immediately alleviated by repeating the process.

Those who have adverse reactions to speed following the initial experience are in a decided minority. For most, it is a gratifying physical experience. As one Berkeley user put it:

I was pretty stoned on grass at the time, and all of a sudden
I just felt elated, you get a feeling of elation, at least I do. I
feel wonderful, like my whole body is just doing a physiological
flip-flop.

Part of the sought after effect is the "rush" or "flash" which the user experiences immediately after fixing, a feeling which may last from five to fifteen minutes. Although many young speed freaks make no distinction between the rush and the flash, there are those connoisseurs of speed who do. The speed manufactured by street chemists of cooks generally contains ether, used to dry the liquid methamphetamine. It is the ether, or any additive, which makes for the "flash," often described as a total body orgasm. Street speed is also cut with a variety of substances, the most common being "Accent" a meat flavorizer which contains monosodium glutamate. Almost any substance which resembles the white crystal is used to cut street speed, although sometimes a "burn artist," or one who sells a substance like Accent for speed, may be more vicious. A 24-year-old dealer, specializing in "rush" speed describes an incident of this sort:

I had an old lady last year that did about a dime (ten dollar bag)
hit cut with rat poison. She turned purple and started gasping
for breath and fell on the floor and damn near croaked.

Fearing the "burn artists," many "speeders" will use only amphetamines which they think are commercially manufactured. A young dealer who is typical of this group will use only Desoxyn tablets, boiled down and injected, or what he labels "white floaty," which he claims is part of a shipment of methamphetamine phosphate stolen from an interstate shipment. Contemptuous of street speed, which he labels garbage, and fit only for "flash freaks," he prefers the less violent "rush," which he describes as a more "mellow" feeling, without the gagging in the throat which accompanies the injection of street speed that contains ether.

Although the physical pleasure of the rush or flash is sometimes mentioned as the reason for continued use of speed, most users are attracted to the feeling which they experience within a group setting. Most are able to relate to others in a very open and confident fashion. This experience is described by a 21-year-old female user as follows:

> When your friends get off you feel so good, you get so close and the vibrations are just wider on speed, everybody's feeling so groovy. Like my girl friend got off. She was kind of up tight, and Joe got her off and she sat there and didn't move and she said "Wow, I just don't believe it, this is too much." We just sat and drew all night, like she drew pictures of me and I drew pictures of her and back and forth. And we rapped just furiously to our innermost soul, but it was really fun.

For some, the initial speed experience seems to enable them to talk out all of their problems to others, even though no one else may be interested or even listening. Whether people are listening or not seems to make little difference. One user describes it this way:

> Like, when you're talking constantly, you always think that people will be glad to listen and you're sure that you know everything. If you listen, it's out of a sort of deference, it's because you're brilliant, but you're humble too.

The first few speed experiences tend to produce an optimism and sense of well-being that can lead to actions which may later be regretted. One user described a letter which he had written to his family in the East while stimulated, in which he gushed about his love for them, how he had found religion, and how well he was doing. Others may decide that a casual acquaintance is the finest person he has ever met or profess undying love for a member of the opposite sex.

As the effect of the amphetamine wears off, the user will begin to feel depressed and physically fatigued. He may either conteract this by again shooting up, or by crashing. In some cases, crashing occurs after a prolonged run, regardless of how stimulated the individual is. In most instances, however, the come-down is hastened by the use of depressants or "downers," commonly barbiturates or heroin.

Novices who happen to be turned on by users who are protective of them are generally instructed as to proper methods of self-protection. A 24-year-old male, deeply involved in the speed scene offered the following pointers for staying alive and sane when using speed:

1. Use clean hypodermic paraphernalia, and do not circulate your outfit (syringe, or eyedropper and needle) among anyone. Procure it new if possible, and keep it clean, if not sterile. One good system is using permanent stainless steel needles, and a glass syringe and sterilizing them in a pressure after each day of use.
2. Take plenty of vitamins, nutritional supplements and drink plenty of liquids. Vitamin C, ascorbic acid, is a must, as are multivitamins and as much good food as possible. I recommend taking dessicated liver, so as to strengthen the vital organ, and protect it from becoming weakened and receptive to hepatitis.
3. The last thing of great importance is that one should never, no matter what the reason, stay awake for longer than 72 hours, as any longer than three days awake causes irreversible brain damage. If necessary in order to avoid this, a person is better off taking barbiturates or tranquilizers.

Although it is possible to be a "weekender" with speed, the chances are good that a young person living in an area such as the Haight-Ashbury will tend to repeat the speed experience if he finds it a pleasurable one, and, as a consequence, more and more of his life will center around obtaining and using drugs. If the newly initiated speed user fails to heed the above advice, he may quickly experience his first adverse reaction to the drug. With some it comes about with the appearance of "crank bugs," imaginary bugs under the skin. It is common to see speed freaks with open running sores or scabs on their faces or arms as a result of picking or cutting out these hallucinated crank bugs. An experienced 24-year-old speed freak described crank bugs as follows:

It's just that when you're shooting speed constantly you start to feel like there's bugs going around under your skin and you know that they're not there, but you pick at them anyway. You go through all these changes scratching. Once in a while you'll see a little black spot and you'll watch it for 10 minutes to see if it moves. If it doesn't move it isn't alive. You can feel them on your skin. I'm always trying to pick them out of my eyebrows.

Extended runs on speed, sometimes as long as two or three weeks inevitably lead to feelings of paranoia or even a full blown psychotic reaction. A common feeling, one which is usually reinforced by others within the individual's social group, is that the police are about to make a massive sweep into the house or apartment for the purpose of confiscating whatever speed one has and arresting the user. One begins to see himself as the focus of attention, and every comment or every occurrence, no matter how far removed it may be from the user, somehow takes on new importance for him. Thus, every police car he sees becomes the lead car in a task force dedicated to tracking him down, while strangers or even friends who make comments that are seemingly innocent become plotters against him, or undercover narcotic agents. This reaction has been observed in love relationships where one partner is suddenly seen as a conspirator against the other. We have observed groups of as many as 10 individuals where each felt that others in the group were plotting against him. In some instances, one person within the group will be singled out for no apparent reason, and the wrath of the entire group vented on him.

The paranoid speed freak is highly prone to violent behavior, but more than this, he begins to expose himself to arrest because of highly erratic and irrational behavior. Threats of mayhem and murder are common within speed groups, and many begin to collect guns and knives to make the threats more convincing. Although there is the possibility that direct assaults may take place within such a group, the impression we have is that more often direct assaults come about as a result of the individual's relationship to the speed marketplace.

As the user becomes more deeply involved in the world of speed, he must necessarily make certain commitments to that life, and must reject or is rejected by other members of the conventional community and even members of the "grass and acid" culture. As mentioned previously, a meaningful relationship between a user and a non-user is virtually impossible, both because of the speed freak's suspicions that anyone who is not using may be an undercover agent, and because few non-users are willing to put up with the constant talking, and fever pitch of activity, and the generally irresponsible behavior that the freak exhibits. In some instances, the threatened disruption of a meaningful love relationship at this point will cause the speed freak to break away from this pattern of drug use. In other cases, former friends or relatives will force the individual into a treatment situation, either by persuading him to voluntarily present himself for help, or by obtaining court authority for commitment as one who is potentially a danger to himself or others.

One cannot expect to be treated to speed by friends for long, thus he must begin to score for himself. Dealing speed on the street is a relatively easy way to obtain the drug, with little outlay of money. The most common pattern is to begin dealing in small quantities, generally nickel or dime bags (five or ten dollar bags). This is the lowest level of dealing and is generally engaged in by people who are heavy users. It also is the most dangerous form of dealing, both in terms of the possibility of arrest and the more certain probability that he will be "ripped off" or robbed of either his money or his speed by others within the scene. There is very little profit by further cutting the speed to be sold, or by "burning" the customer by selling any substance which resembles speed. This is perhaps the most dangerous form of activity the street dealer can involve himself in, for it is common for those who have been burned to seek revenge, either by "snitching," or shooting or beating him. In some instances the "burn artist" will be injected with his own product in large doses, particularly if his customers have suffered adverse effects from his "burn speed."

The novice dealer is perhaps the most vulnerable individual in the speed scene. Learning to protect oneself on the street is an art which takes time to learn. For instance, an experienced dealer will never have the speed on him when he makes the initial contact, if he is dealing in quantities of a quarter ounce or under on the street. The exchange of speed for money should take place in a setting where the dealer will have some assurance that the customer intends to pay him for the drug. The more successful dealers seem to be those who have a reputation for fairness; where the customer is reasonably assured that the drug is what the dealer says it is, and that if the dealer himself has been burned by his connection, he will replace the bad speed. If the dealer is compulsively using the drug, it is important that he have numerous contacts and be able to get rid of the speed quickly. Not being able to "turn over" speed quickly has proven disastrous to many dealers as in this example:

When you are dealing speed and doing it both at the same time it gets fantastically involved. You're sitting with ounces all around you, and you are saying . . . hey, wow . . . I can do a whole spoon. That's what's happening to my connection right now. He brought up two ounces the other night and did one and a quarter before we got any of it sold. You've got to learn to maintain with it a little.

To the speed freak who has learned to "maintain," it would be unthinkable to buy speed from a "nickel or dime" dealer on the street. He prefers to deal with a known and trusted connection who deals in quantities from one eighth ounce to pounds. In such a situation, the customer is allowed to "taste" prior to making a purchase, which allows him to determine the quality before buying.

The lowest status in the speed world is assigned to the individual who has not learned to "maintain." He is the speed freak that "snivels over used cottons," that is, pleads with other users for the use of cottons which have been used to strain out impurities when drawing speed from the spoon. He also is unable to "get his bread together," or save enough money to make a purchase larger than five or ten dollars. Such an individual would never be "fronted" speed, or given speed on consignment, since the connection knows from experience that he is not likely to get his money back. Although "fronting" speed is uncommon, it is still done occasionally if the user is not seen as "strung out" and if he appears to be responsible and rational. Occasionally a usually reliable user will begin to get "strung out" and the connection will balk at "fronting" to him. In response to the question "What would happen if the guy who is fronting you speed noticed that you were getting freaky and paranoid?" a 21-year-old dealer-user replied:

He would cut me off, just like he did my partner. He would say, I'm sorry man, friendship is friendship, business is business. We can still be friends and do hits together and get loaded, but I can't front you no more because you're not coming back with my money.

Another source of money for drugs is hustling, although there are few hustlers in the speed world to compare with those in the heroin world. Perhaps the most common hustle by heroin addicts is burglary, which requires a great deal of skill to avoid arrest, and a knowledge of the kinds of items which are most easily sold to a fence. This kind of an operation is run by professional fences who do not regard the speed freak as a reliable burglar, since his demeanor and irrational behavior may well call attention to himself and others involved in the operation. Usually the goods obtained by the freak in a burglary are simply traded for speed or money on an informal basis.

Another major source of speed and or income in this scene is the "rip off," or theft directly from a dealer who has large quantities of speed or money on his person. Because this is common practice, the more experienced dealers and users usually cover themselves, either by having a friend along for protection, or by carrying a weapon. Many cases have been reported where, following a highly confidential sale of speed, the dealer will leave an apartment or house and immediately be held up for his money by someone who has been tipped off by the group that made the purchase.

Our hypothesis is that it is this kind of activity related to the marketplace, coupled with the paranoia induced by long runs on speed which accounts for the excessive amount of violence which prevails in a speed using community. In some cases, a speed user who has been arrested will try to talk his way out of this situation by agreeing to give the police names of users and dealers within the community. The "snitch" or "dime dropper" as he is referred to, is the object of immediate and forceful retribution if his identity becomes known, or if one is suspected of being a "snitch" or "dime dropper." Said one user of a friend who had turned "snitch":

> A cat I knew fairly well, last time he got busted he gave up 42 names. He's up in County right now giving up every name he can think of. He got a lot of people some righteous time. If he does manage to get back out on the street, he's dead this time. If he goes to the joint, he is definitely dead, without any hesitation whatsoever. When people start copping out on everyone on the street, pretty quick they get turned off. Or else they get stomped out or shot out. It's becoming a very violent scene up there.

The snitch, dime dropper, burn artist, rip off and others are just some of the hazards with which the speed freak must contend if he is to survive in this scene, for the typical speed freak soon finds that he is unable to control the paranoia which inevitable overtakes him. It is at this point that he begins to use other drugs to counteract the effects of speed. Most common among the young persons we have talked with are barbiturates, generally Seconal, Tuinal and Nembutal. Few of the speed users will wait for the effect of the drug taken orally, and prefer to boil them down and shoot them for the immediate effect. Interestingly enough, most report that barbiturates also have a "heavy flash" similar to that experienced when shooting speed. Drug switching becomes a common practice, and few users or dealers are without an ample supply of both speed and "downers." Barbiturates have several advantages over other depressants, such as heroin or morphine, in that they are easily obtainable, cheap and don't carry felony penalties for possession. On the other hand, the heavy shooter of barbiturates is seen as a menace, even to the most violent and paranoid speed freak because of the aggressive and surly demeanor of most "barb freaks." In addition, barbiturates prepared for injection by the speed freak contain numerous impurities and are sometimes difficult to get through a needle. It is common for even the most expert "fixer" to miss a vein while doing barbiturates, resulting in cellulitis or abcesses, while others force the heavy solution through the needle with such pressure that they "blow" a vein.

In such a scene, the sanctions which most middle-class youngsters have against the use of heroin break down. Several bad experiences with the barbiturates may convince the user to try heroin as a downer. Most users report that heroin is a more "mellow" down, that one rarely develops or "blows" a vein, and that surly or aggressive behavior generally doesn't follow its use.

At one time heroin was most difficult to obtain, since the major source of supply was the East Coast. West Coast heroin has traditionally been of low quality and extremely expensive. Recently, however, a low-grade Mexican heroin, almost brown in color has appeared on the streets and is used extensively by speed freaks to come down. Although most users are aware of the addictive nature of heroin, they are also aware that barbiturate addiction is a far more serious problem to deal with on the streets. It is our opinion that this new source of supply will give rise to an increasing heroin problem in San Francisco, since it is now more freely available than ever before, according to most persons close to the heroin market.

There are many reasons why speed use may be terminated after a few months. There is always the obvious possibility of arrest and incarceration for possession or dealing drugs, or possession of an outfit. Some youngsters become anxious about their erratic behavior and may seek help during a period of extreme anxiety or paranoia, if they perceive the helpers as nonpunitive and understanding. There is a great fear among street speed freaks of conventional or "Establishment" agencies because of their possible relationship with the police, or the possibility that they may be involuntarily committed to a treatment institution. Many young speed freaks who have become addicted to heroin, and are therefore capable of more rational thinking will voluntarily seek help for their addiction.

Perhaps the most common contact with traditional agencies comes about as a result of contracting serum hepatitis from using an infected needle. This is a common health hazard in the speed scene, and interestingly enough, the reputation of the hepititis ward at S.F. General Hospital is a good one; that is, the staff is seen as "hip" and understanding, the food and medical care good, and the company of fellow patients enjoyable.

The long-term speed freak is a phenomenon which is difficult to understand. How can one find satisfaction in a social scene which offers a steady diet of violence, suspicion, disease and possible death? For the speed freak who is not able to "maintain," his stay within this world is limited. For those who remain, two major routes seem to develop. For the speed freak who knows his limits, has numerous contacts within the speed scene, and who has acquired a reputation as a shrewd but fair dealer, he may move into the higher levels of the marketplace, either as a higher level distributor of speed and other drugs, as a supplier of raw chemicals for the manufacture of speed, or into the actual manufacture of the drug itself. It is on this level that the possibility of arrest decreases, the quality of the drug is assured, and the relationship between members of his group are more congenial and trusted. In addition, he can make fairly large sums of money and can afford his own apartment as well as decent clothing and food, something of which the street level speed freak is generally deprived.

The second route is perhaps the most difficult to understand. It involves a total commitment to the use and procurement of drugs, and an identity as the "biggest freak on the street." Status for such an individual is derived from how much speed he can shoot, how bizarre his dress, demeanor or behavior is, and his knowledge of drugs in general. Even the names which they give themselves reflect this orientation, names such as "Mad Bruce," "Dr. Zoom," "Crazy Tom," "Mr. Clean," "Supercrank," "Nickidrene." In one instance, a group of individuals banded together, wore quasi-military uniforms, and labeled themselves the "Methedrine Marauders," or "Crank Commandos."

In a community such as the Haight-Ashbury, being the biggest freak in a community of speed freaks is not an easy task. Pride in one's ability to shoot massive doses is reflected in the following statement from such a speed freak:

> I know I scared an intern half to death once. He said that a person who took 500 milligrams would croak, so I shot a flat gram right in front of him, he turned every color of the rainbow just watching me. I fixed two spoons in Marin County, I'm a legend in Marin County now. They're always talking about the guy who shot two spoons.

The same individual recalled a speed shooting contest, which he frankly admitted was a self-destructive act:

> This was a down to the death dope shooting contest. One of the two of us was supposed to die when the thing was all over. He'd shoot a half a gram and I'd shoot a gram, and he'd shoot one and a half, and I'd shoot 2 grams, then he'd shoot 2 and a half and I'd have to shoot 3. Nobody would back out, we'd die before we'd back out.

Much of the attraction of this style of life is in the fantasies which the speed freak maintains. For example, if one freak asks another if he can score five pounds of speed within the hour, both are extremely flattered and gratified. For the one who makes the request, he imagines the other will see him as a big-time dope dealer, about to make the sale of the year, while the other is flattered that someone thinks he is capable of getting his hands on five pounds of speed.

The speed freak is constantly living in a fantasy world, making plans which will elevate him out of his misery into a position of power and great prestige within the criminal world. Perhaps the most articulate description of the kinds of plans which are made nightly in the speed world is this, by a 21-year-old male speed freak:

I make lots of plans, but I don't ever carry any of them out. I get into this megalomaniac bag about five days into it, and I'll build these mountainous castles in my mind, all the far out things I'm going to do, and all the money I'm going to make. I'll be driving a Rolls Royce and have 2 speed labs going at once, a heroin refining plant, my own private 2 engine plane, I'll be running the Mafia, and then when I start to come down I realize that none of this stuff is existing and that none of it is going to exist and it's like you pulled the bottom out of my brain. I feel empty and suicidal in about 4 or 5 hours.

Another describes the way in which he rationalizes his existence in the speed world:

I really enjoy the whole thing. When I'm out there hustling I haven't got a thing. I'm really up tight. Part of me is up tight, the rest of me is having a good time, I'm talking all this expansive shit to everybody else. I'm building my castles about a block ahead of me, and when I get there it's gone, so I build another one. But I do all right; I have my basic necessities of life and things like that. I stay a step above some of these other people who just turn into animals.

There is no way to determine how such an individual will react to you from day to day, as his life is a series of clashes with others in the scene, scheming to score or deal, trying to kick a barbiturate or heroin habit, freaking out after a long run on speed, or surprisingly calm and rational when mixing drugs to achieve a state of apparent normalcy.

Such a career terminates in one of three ways generally. The most common hazard is being arrested, usually after getting extremely loose or erratic because of the particular drug he is using at the time. Secondly, he may be involuntarily committed by relatives or by a court following arrest, and finally, death, either from an overdose of heroin or barbiturates or being murdered by others within the scene. If the latter possibility seems overly dramatic, one has only to look at the homicide rate involving speed dealers and users in the Haight-Ashbury during the last year.

Although many speed freaks will assure you that they have little desire to change their life style, and that they are quite happy with their lives, this concluding quote, from a young man deeply involved in the speed scene, reveals the hopelessness, despair and misery he feels:

> My life, though freaky, has assumed a sense of quasi-normality, at least compared to some of the righteous freaks and loose people on the street. But, in the last two years, I have attempted suicide three times, and have blown my mind at least two score and ten times. I will cop out to being freaked out, and generally loose. As to speed . . . they tell me it will kill me, but they don't say when.

The first probe

CHARLES C. BRAUNER

Rain and mystery opened and closed the pre-season workshop for students entering architecture at the University of British Columbia. Foul weather and wonder about what was to come provided the only obvious threads linking three weeks of activities that ran from foraging to feast, Spartanism to splendor, privation to saturation. Shrouded in rumors as thick as the clouds overhead, fifty-five students from all over Canada and several distant countries gathered together for the first time in mid-August on a dock opposite Vancouver's Stanley Park. As college graduates with a common interest in architecture they had no trouble combining into spontaneous conversation groups. When the six members of staff arrived a sense of relief rippled through the crowd as they quieted to hear where they were going. Disappointed at not being told, they managed to load their camping equipment on one of the boats and divide themselves into two parties for boarding. All the way out to Horseshoe Bay and up Howe Sound they speculated. After two hours of sailing through ever thickening fog they no longer knew whether they were traveling north or south. When the boats dropped anchor at a small island a few miles off Britannia Beach they had no way of knowing where they were. Small boats took them ashore on Defense Island in groups of six. Densely forested, and guarded by an Indian mask carved in a drift log at the landing, the island was deserted. Being no more than three-quarters of a mile long and a quarter of a mile wide, with a backbone of rock that ran its length, it seemed to offer a minimum challenge. By the time the last boat landed the two girls and the main party had a fire going in the opening on the crest. Since it was noon, everyone stood around waiting to be fed. Wet, having nothing but what they wore and carried in their pockets, but reassured by seeing the staff similarly unequipped, they did not take alarm when the boats sounded their horns and pulled away.

After a half hour of exploration, John Gaitanakis, a co-director, called the

THE FIRST PROBE From *Architectural Review*, Vol. CXLVI, No. 874, December 1969. Reprinted by permission of the publisher and the author.

students together and explained that the boat would return in forty-eight hours.

Meanwhile, there was no food, no shelter and no equipment. The time was theirs to use as they saw fit. The first reaction was disbelief. Having found an axe and some nails on their brief tour, a small group insisted other necessities only awaited discovery. The fact that two five-gallon coffee urns of water had been brought ashore from the boats convinced others that food was there for the finding. A general unwillingness to accept the likelihood of deprivation sent everyone on an hour of fruitless searching. Reassembling with nothing new to report, they conjured up their first fears of famine. They all knew that man could do quite well without food so long as he had water, and fresh water was plentiful both from rain and springs. Nevertheless, half-a-dozen individuals insisted they would succumb to nausea and disability at the very least. Those most fearful set about to forage for edibles. We warned them that a recent red tide had made the shellfish temporarily poisonous. This came as a blow. The gloom did not persist, however. Soon half the group was busy gathering salal berries and toasting sea kelp. No other edibles could be found. By mid-afternoon a dozen self-selected groups were busy building shelters and gathering wood for night fires.

Having coalesced into personality groups of three to five, the shelter parties remained intact as living units for the rest of the time on the island. Confronted with the basic choice of whether to improve and inhabit existing shelters from half-formed caves to semi-tunnels formed by overturned trees, or to cut and interweave cedar branches, the majority shied away from using the existing natural cover. However, their finished dwellings distinguished them far less than the characteristics that drew them into alliance. To the staff they became known as the hoarders, the sharers, the defilers, the isolaters, the raiders, the excluders, the worriers, the trusters and the grumblers. Those who found no common cause in personality, location, habitat or conversation remained around the fire on the crest.

Since this cluster-by-default was three times as large as any of the separate living units, their clearing served as a common ground. A more barren commons would be hard to imagine. Once fire and rude shelter were assured the group found it had absolutely nothing to do but pass time. No game of matchsticks or burning of twigs was too trivial. There was not even enough common concern for anyone to do more than note that one of the groups had made off with half the reserve water-supply. Efforts to open discussions on why they were there or what they might do proved so fruitless that the dozen who started the talks could not sustain them for half an hour. In the evening a longer chat on "What is architecture" was started. With the downpour and darkness punctuated only by massive tree-trunks and widely spaced fires, boredom dictated the effort at conversation.

Unable to develop a cohesive thread, the only thing that sparked interest was why the staff was made up of only two members of the architecture faculty, the rest being a visitor from Outward Bound, a specialist in contemporary dance, a sociologist and an educational philosopher. The thing that seemed to impress the students most was that the staff saw fit to share their discomfort on equal terms, though they had foreknowledge of what was to come. Again, all question about future events went unanswered. When it became clear no profitable discussion would develop, the staff withdrew to the semi-shelter of a huge cedar tree and bedded down around a fire.

Wetter and colder, only four things distinguished the second day: the end of the berries, the building of a raft, the appearance of a boat, and underground fires that threatened to burn the island down. What had been planned as minimal existence experience turned out to be no existence to speak of at all. The hope had been that by being freed of cooking, eating, preparation, clean up, and denied the opportunity to lavish time on such mindless occupations, the students might try to make something special of their stay. Instead they lavished all their time on the mindless activities left them: buttressing shelters, improving fireplaces, gathering wood. Beyond that, they were determined simply to sit out their time like convicts awaiting parole. Some spent hours just cleaning their fingernails. Even the making of the raft was undertaken with half an eye to floating somewhere to get food. When a boat came in a group tried to signal their need for supplies. Informed that just three weeks before the Provincial Department of Correction had put some hard cases ashore for survival training, those on the boat did not linger. Surviving their fast in good health but low spirits, the several groups greeted the last night with huge fires. These burned through the ground-cover of rotten needles and branches to ignite the dry mulch that coated the ground to a depth of twelve feet in places. A group in a cave on a rock ledge burned themselves out entirely when a covering tree went up in flames taking two more with it. Three other groups had runaway fires during the night, and the *Lord of the Flies* bunch who took the communal water-supply had to use more than forty buckets of the water to damp underground fires which they insisted that, as experienced woodsmen, they had under control at all times. When it was time to leave, the staff spent three hours doing nothing but uprooting underground fires that had been left as extinguished. If it had not been for heavy and continuous rain the island would have become an inferno.

By far the most interesting thing to be seen during the island experience was the students' behavior toward food when it arrived. Before taking us off, the captain of the Columbia landed oranges, apples, and bread. The "marooned" were told that there was enough for each to have a fruit and two slices of bread. The *Lord of the Flies* group was the first to the food, followed by several kindred parties. They raided the stores like seasoned pirates. Half the loaves of bread disappeared inside jackets, only because pockets were filled to bursting with fruit. Eight people got more than half the supplies for sixty-one people. The pattern of resentment among those who went without was remarkable. No one could be heard blaming the gluttons, though they were known to most. First the captain became the villain for landing so little. Secondly, there was general resentment that they had not been given a feast. Finally, annoyance focused on the staff for not anticipating the raiders and deterring them. This settled down to a criticism of a more general nature. Somehow the staff had failed to make the experience meaningful. What happened with the food became symbolic of that failure.

When the boat landed everyone at Britannia Beach, there was a station wagon waiting with enough bread, sliced meat, fruit, cookies and candy bars for all. Or so it seemed. But again the mighty eight plundered the stores. They made sandwiches with more than an inch of meat. Not one, but four and six apiece. Even so, the meat and the bread held out. Everyone, except one girl who could hardly eat, overate. The raiders took whole packages of ten chocolate bars or thirty-six cookies against future uncertainties. Again, nothing was said. Interesting in itself, what makes it significant is that, except for the girl, no one had suffered severe hunger past the slight pangs of the second day. There was a general feeling of having been physically cleansed. The unanimous overeating and the special greed of a few seemed more a ritual atonement for failure or a common urge to make up for the empty hours by stuffing their bodies. Overeating remained a characteristic of the group throughout, students and staff alike.

A mystery in itself, this hangover from the island cloaked an even deeper feeling. Before going, several students had known the forest on intimate working terms. Others from cities and foreign countries had heard of it in terms that mixed awe and grandeur. Yet the wood-wise had been as unable to face the challenge of the forest-island as the forest unfamiliars. Both had been equally helpless against what neither had expected to encounter—Time. Having brought almost nothing ashore they found themselves stranded with even less than they imagined. Had they been truly marooned, desperation would have given them common cause that would have filled every moment. Denied even that last resort, they encountered themselves as truly useless. Each one was, harrowingly, alone. Only for two days; but that mystery became the yeast that leavened all that followed. However slight, all had suffered a common adversity. However profound, all had faced a common humiliation. In just forty-eight hours the props of a quarter-century of customary daily activity had been knocked flat. They were ready for a new beginning. It was, as it turned out, a workshop of beginnings.

Dawn broke clear at 5,300 feet revealing snow-caps surrounding the camp in Garibaldi meadow. Warmed by cooked food and rations of rum, everyone slept half-dry in sleeping bags sheltered by stretches of plastic. Grouped in seven-man teams for the stay on the glacier, some bathed and shaved in mountain streams while others packed for the trip to the top. Rain settled in and efforts to keep dry failed. The question became "Will the weather break long enough for a helicopter to drop in and make eighteen lifts from the meadow to the broad back of the glacier?" By mid-afternoon the enveloping mist thinned. Heather, high up the hills, showed magenta against wet grass as if struggling to serve as tiny beacons. From over the ridge the beat of rotors chopped away at the remaining mist. As sky opened the turbo-jet copter swung in, trailing a fifty-five gallon drum of fuel at the end of a long line. It set the drum between two logs as neatly as a woman might place a vase. The lift was on.

In groups of four, and three, lifts of twenty backpacks hung in a cargo net beneath the machine, the base camp went to the glacier. The flight up became a personal experience from the moment of lift-off. Skimming off the meadow, the machine circled inside the basin and darted through a gap in the peaks. The lush Alpine meadow dropped away into rock canyon stripped of vegetation. With the five-hundred-foot face of the glacier coming up at a hundred and twenty miles an hour, the machine slipped between clouds and ice like a razor parting tissue. Racing across the frozen ridges of snow that spread like a still ocean all around brought the full fascination of speed up through the glass bubble. As if about to topple over a crest that dropped half a mile, the machine floated into a stall and touched to a stop. Set down at 6,500 feet, each new arrival looked from the rough crown of encircling peaks into the abyss. A mile across the valley trees disappeared into blue-black on the mountainside. Printed in a solid wash, the stone seemed a clear crystal darkened only by the blue air between. Some took running slides down steep slopes. Others raced away to the highest ledge they could find. Groups held brief skirmishes in the snow. Still others just sat and looked.

Andrew Gruft and two friends experienced in climbing took charge. Safety guidelines were set forth and the pre-arranged groups were set the task of building shelter. A third of the parties chose to use the snow to their advantage. The rest decided to build their camps on the clear outcropping of rock around the main field.

With cooking and shelter under way, half the company set out to use the remaining light to climb by. Curving past blue-green crevasses toward a crest two miles away and 2,000 ft. above, they strung out like ski-troops on maneuvers. Those who stayed behind drank, cooked, joked, built fires from mountain driftwood, improved shelters and attended to idle busywork. Though the rain came back, the mood was as opposite from the island as the surroundings. Cold, wet, getting hungry, tired, no one was bored. The new groupings jelled around work, chatter, pranks and meals. The real chance of a thunder-storm on the glacier, rumored to be capable of making experienced climbers panic, held no fear. The known difficulty of climbing down through fog that hid all bearings posed no concern beyond the challenge. The outside chance of severe cold at night worried no one. Where 48 hours on the island had seemed interminable, 36 hours on the glacier seemed no time at all.

Where the dense stand of evergreens reaching up out of sight had hemmed everyone in until each became trapped in some barren patch of self, the broad expanse with nothing on all sides and above became truly timeless. Drawn out from the cramped quarters of self, as vapor must expand in a vacuum, their spirits bubbled to the surface. For the first time there was singing. Who could but help but sing on the top of the world? There was play. Joy. Reborn on the glacier while chaffing under unexpected discipline, they surged back to life. The island, not the want of food, the gloom of the forest, not the rain, the self inflicted isolation, not the division into camps, had made them old. On the island they behaved like retired folks so old that all they had left was to await their final departure. On the glacier they became young again. But the growth they found, like the agedness they settled into when most lost, came from psychological depths none had ever plumbed. Indeed, on the glacier and all through the trip, only a few ever sensed that the territory covered during the workshop paralleled the topography of their spirit. Like animals in a maze they were much too busy reacting to stimuli to analyze, or even to formulate, their responses. That would come later.

The climb down the glacier and back to base camp was their first small test of physical endurance. Seven miles over the ice field, down the face, into the valley and up four thousand feet, confronted them with the task of covering in each hour what they had flown over in a minute. Sixty-pound backpacks and fog thick enough to limit vision to fifty feet made it a challenge. Divided into three teams of twenty joined by a long stretch of rope, they set out over waist-high ridges of soft snow. The experienced climbers lead each unit to the face of the glacier. In a running, tumbling, sliding, skidding, free-for-all, each person balanced his pack as best he could and slid down the forty-five degree slope. Once down in the valley on an unmistakable trail they were left to make their way up and back to the meadow like draft-horses free to find the barn. Those who faced it as a show of strength made it in less than three hours. Others who found it an enjoyable if demanding stroll took as long as five. Saddled with a pack and confronting an unavoidable two-and-a-half mile climb up a twenty-degree slope, each one had to balance energy against endurance, progress against tedium, interest against fatigue.

Eventually they had to settle down to some common denominator for completing the task. In a narrow, special, private and very physical way, each one had to work out his own "one best means." Some rushed and rested every hundred yards. Others plodded. Many forgot they were climbing at all for as much as a half-mile, caught by the change in perspective that rising above the valley brought. A few cursed almost every step. One by one they settled into what Jacques Ellul calls a "technique." They came up against what freedom was left them within the rigid limits of physiological ability and physical conditions. For that brief passage each one worked out his personal style under a special condition of stress. That style told those around him volumes. It was a story that did not take long to tell. Yet it was the style of others that remained most apparent. Even so, without knowing accurately, fully, or coherently *what* he had exposed, each one sensed *that* he had exposed himself in some important way. The climb back to the meadow made it clear why certain groups had grown spontaneously on the island, and why other combinations of people would not naturally occur. The return from the glacier marked the emergence of an awareness of individual techniques for achieving ends and styles-in-means previously unnoticed.

The new awareness came at the best possible time. Having first been plucked from society and comfort and held in contact with nature for five days, the students were plunged back into the system and surrounded with conveniences. Comfort was a modern motel that provided all facilities and good food and the freedom to roam Port Alberni every evening. Twice each day they would tour a different aspect of the lumber industry. Reborn as social beings, they noticed not only the emperor's nakedness but the alleged cut and fabric of his imaginary gown.

A satrapy of MacMillan Bloedel in the Middle of Vancouver Island, this company town, left over from an earlier century, enjoys polluted streams, hepatitis, noxious air, odors that would stun a horse, soot, fumes, loud traffic, periodic layoffs, alcoholism and treeless hills as side benefits of having but one major employer. Yet the effects of industrial technique on the life-style of the town were trivial compared to their influence on the men at work. In three days the students saw modern industrial technique at work in fire-fighting, paper manufacture, logging, cutting lumber, and plywood production. Everywhere the most modern equipment stood out as the only evidence of the twentieth century. The two surviving Martin Mars were kept ready as water bombers. The largest planes to see active service in World War II, they pick up 6,000 gallons of water in a twenty-two second sweep across the surface of a lake. The pulp and paper mill was as fully automated as possible. Gigantic vats collect, grind, soak, stew and feed a sticky juice into a block-long oven of drums that press, stretch, dry, bake and roll up finished newsprint. The nattering of powerful chain saws throughout the forest made it sound as though the whole mountain was host to a swarm of mechanical locusts that would eat it bare.

Where the crews had left, the mile-square stands made a cutover wheatfield look scraggly. Everything was down. At China Lake the water scooters cut logs from the dumping pools more efficiently than a trained quarterhorse culls a herd. In the sawmill, blades man-high made beams from trees in two cuts. The plywood factory had presses three storeys high. Everywhere one technique stood out: enlarge the machine. Each replacement was more gigantic than its predecessor. Gradually, the attendant technique became apparent; rationalize the internal steps of each separate process until that stage is automated. Only then did the discontinuity between gigantic machines begin to make sense. Specialists had automated isolated processes separately, and that separation set the tasks for human labor. Men did not work so much on, as between, machines. Whenever one complex of machinery finished a set of tasks, and another assemblage waited to take it another stage, there was a flurry of human activity. Men rushed pell-mell to fill the gap between two independent mechanical processes.

Unique, specialized, temperamental, costly and irreplaceable, the machines received irreproachable care. Indeed, the machinery was the only thing unique in any of the operations. The company could no more use a six-million-dollar paper dryer to put out forest fires than it could dry paper with the Hawaii Mars. Only the men were standardized, interchangeable, expendable and indistinguishable.

Posted everywhere, the signs announced the daily life-style for workers. Like front line troops they had learned to live in the company of constant danger. The numbers themselves gave a precise arithmetic index of danger, job by job. They announced that the machinery could not be made man-safe. "No matter what you do the machine will get you. It's just a matter of time"; "Look, so and so has escaped injury for 283 days." Yet when you are hurt, "It's your fault"; "Men *make* accidents." Whenever anyone was asked about the company's concern for the workers, the safety signs were pointed out. After the second day no one asked. Discussion with management pro-voked hostility. The very thought that unintended psychological and social contaminants might develop as side effects of company policy came as an unpardonable insult. The safety-game stood out as symbolic of a funda-mental absurdity. Practical businessmen regarding themselves as deeply involved in the basic struggle to provide necessary commodities were more prisoners of their own fantasies than the students had been on the island. Practical laborers committed to bread and butter wage earning were more lost than they would have been on the glacier when the fog closed in. Worse, both groups believed they were "communicating." Neither suggested its isolation from the other. A huge industrial complex had grown up between them and yet it remained invisible.

The result of this mutual blindness was Port Alberni, a peculiar but somehow typical wasteland. For all the devastation of physical resources for the production of commercial exports, they came to little by comparison to the degradation of human resources. The forests, the streams and the air could still replenish themselves. The people had been used beyond any point of return.

Having seen *how* industrial technique devastates a population, the students went on to follow up that human devastation in a more advanced stage. Their next stop was Skid Row in downtown Vancouver.

Arriving in the usual downpour, everyone checked into the West Hotel at Carrol and Pender Streets just off Chinatown. With two students to a room at $1.50 each per night, they had the next four days to explore eight square blocks. Before turning them loose, Bud Wood, the other co-dirctor, gave each one his five-dollar-a-day allotment of cash. Dressed in boots, camping clothes, beards and untrimmed hair growth, they had only manners, speech and curiosity to separate them from the native inhabitants. The hotel's bar served as base camp, refresher station, rest home, take off point, runway, rally ground and seminar room. Low slung, huge, noisy, pillared, blue, black ceilinged, gilded, mirrored, busy, threadbare and orderly, it catered to a cross section of the population two beers at a time. It came as a surprise that there was nothing especially bawdy, frantic, violent, boisterous or hostile about the patrons. A gravel-voiced citizen entertained each newcomer with the offer of a diamond from "the crown jewels of Czechoslovakia" smuggled on the last plane out of Prague. A few lads lent themselves to the embraces of an Indian girl happy to give them vivid details of her decline and fall. Others received fatherly advice from pensioners about keeping their cash in a side pocket and not flashing anything bigger than a two-dollar bill. They saw and heard drunks, but found the vast majority quite content to drink well within their budget and limit. After buying a few rounds they found themselves treated in return.

Even before they ventured out on the streets they knew a good deal about the community. Most of all, they knew it was a community. The people they had expected to find broken and in a continuous stupor had a spirit and individuality not to be found in Port Alberni. They reflected, without having heard, Camus' dictum in *The Myth of Sisyphus:* "There is no fate that cannot be surmounted by scorn." These survivors of industrial displacement had many battle scars. Yet herded together in a ghetto left over as an omission in city planning, they retained a certain small measure of independence from commercial-industrial technique. By working little, unsteadily, or not at all, they avoided having to stay in anyone's "good grace." They were, in a most limited way, being themselves. The limitation was that by the time they got there, not much of the "self" was left intact. Contrary to expectation, these people had not given up. They laughed, drank, hoped, fought occasionally, talked endlessly, listened, argued, smiled, dreamed, sang, cried, visited, made friends and worried. The notable difference was that they had no assigned places in which to do these things. They were "at home" on the street or in an alley, in a bar or a temporary room. They were at home in their bodies instead of in some set space; and it soon became clear that this was not a matter of choice but of necessity.

Being architecture students they soon noted how little space existed to serve Skid Row's inhabitants. By day and early evening businessmen came in to open shops for customers who came from outside. Only when the outsiders withdrew, and the stores and offices were dark and padlocked, did the indigenous facilities stand out. There were small restaurants offering cheap food in quantity for every ethnic group from Greek to Polish, Hungarian to Swedish. Cutting across ethnic lines, bars catered to special social tastes. The mixed couples did not mingle with the transvestites. The solitary drinkers stayed away from the party bars. Less clearly, the hotels and rooming houses polarized around yet different groupings. The sailor did not register where the salesmen gathered. Though the illegal activities went out to wherever demand promised patronage, each had its centre of gravity. Prostitution did not interfere with gambling. Dope peddling did not compete with bootlegging. Once it became clear what the boundaries were, it took just six minutes by actual timing to find a "kit" that someone had stashed for mixing, heating and injecting heroin. A serious customer never had to wait more than a quarter-hour to make contact, whatever might be his needs. Service was far better than the check-out line at any supermarket. Yet the traffic was quite small compared to the size of the population.

Gradually, the students grasped one of the basic facts of life on Skid Row. The restaurants, the bars, the streets, the alleys, the porches of tenements, and one thirty by forty foot triangular "park," were the only social centers available. Wherever they might go to sleep, they had to come to one of these places to socialize. This was known and accepted. The great majority did not drink to become convivial; they gathered together to relieve each other's boredom, and rather than cast a man out in the rain because he couldn't afford to buy a drink, someone would order him a beer so he could stay. For a group of people who literally lived in their social centers and only slept or recuperated in their rooms, the guarantee of being welcome was essential. Unfortunately, they had to convert the few facilities left them, by an unconcerned city, with no help. They had to make social centers out of places least amenable to that function, and they did it with nothing but their own depleted personal resources. However limited, warped, undeveloped, starved, or out of kilter, all they had was their own humanity, and because they brought all of it wherever they went they were, in their own special way, more wholly and fully present, wherever they went, than most men.

They left nothing behind, kept nothing hidden. Carrying the whole of what was left them as selves, they often enough exhibited parts not customarily seen in public, and that, not the people themselves, was the basis for disapproval. The occupants of Skid Row, the students eventually discovered, lived all too public lives. At least, they did in company what the general public regarded as only fit to be done in private. From urinating to making love, from vomiting to sleeping, from dressing to tending wounds, from taking medicine to resting, could all be seen; and those who lived in more compartmentalized ways found such a blend offensive. Having just come away from an island and a glacier where just such a blend had been a communal and environmental necessity, the students could accept it quite easily. They were surprised to see that the basic pattern of living on Skid Row differed very little from their own style of camping. The trees had given way to high buildings, the icefield had been replaced by pavement, but the ways of coping with a great deal of time and not very much to do remained the same. Like themselves, these folks were the sole occupants of an island. Their little enclosure was threatened by an ever rising tide of commercial and industrial development that encroached from all sides. Unlike the students, no one had arranged for their departure that silent morning.

Loaded with camping gear, everyone trudged up a mud road through the rain on Sunday afternoon. All they knew was that they had entered the state of Washington and come to Friday Creek, about twenty miles south of Bellingham. From the distance they heard a Gregorian chant coming through the trees. Turning a bend they came upon what could have been a Roman ruin. Aged, overlaid with twenty foot high trees growing out of the roof, abounding in symmetrical arches, the circular brick building arched up into a perfect dome. From the inside, the abandoned bee-hive brick kiln curved around and around in layers that drew the eye out of the hole on top. The deep tones of the Gregorian chant mixed with the candle-light to create a mood of reverence. Moss and moisture filled the dome with a musty incense. A dozen low arches evenly spaced all around opened to the fading daylight as altars of invitation.

Moors coming upon a mosque in an alien land could not have been more awestruck. Silence admitted the sound of a running stream. As eyes grew more accustomed to the dim light, details became more evident. Throughout the dome bricks were set on edge against each other without mortar. Sounds worked across the dome to drop intact at full volume precisely on their nodal points. The scars of intense heat worked up in carbon streaks as shadows of long extinguished flames, as if to provide the building with memories. One great room softly lit, so the glow faded gradually to a deep red, nearly as dark as claret. Simple, strong, and so boldly clear in design and construction, it bespoke its very nature. It was as natural as the island forest or the glacial snow. It belonged. Only the rubble of broken brick piled all over where the floor had been detracted. Turned up, scattered, and left by thieves in their search for marketable bricks, the mounds of trash, much more than the structure, showed the hand of men. That dirty smudge had to be erased. In two days the work parties cleared out all the rubble and rebuilt the floor with brick taken from the false roof. Stripped of all the growth that threatened to crumble the dome, re-inforced by welding that strengthened the steel bands holding it together, covered with clear plastic that waterproofed it, cleared of rubble and trash inside and out, sporting a floor of clean brick packed on sand, equipped with electricity but not lighted by it, the kiln was ready for use. There was a sense of having restored a monument to its original splendor. It came as a shock to find that the kiln was only ten years old.

Delighted to have a task, the students did the basic renovation in two days. Unwilling to relinquish their work, they improved it each day thereafter. As it became the social center, fewer people slept inside. The attendant building provided shelter for sleeping and storage, a catering service supplied hot meals. A barrel of beer went on tap every evening. Each day a few new members of the architecture staff arrived. With five days left to go the students felt that finally they had about all they wanted. They had no suspicion that work, shelter, food and drink was the least of what they were about to get.

The cultural program came on slowly. On the evening of the third day at the kiln they all gathered in the dome at dusk. A solo oboist played an hour of modern music before the beer arrived. After refreshments he came back and discussed the notions of sound, space, harmony, rhythm, atonality, improvisation, and composition underlying the works he had played. Then he gave an impromptu accompaniment to the reading of an original poem. That was followed by the reading of a chapter from a novel underway. A bit startled by the exposure, the students set up a couple of Congo drums and beat their way through half the night until the beer was gone.

That evening a solo cellist played, talked, joked and worked her way through a night of music appreciation that extended from Brahms to nursery rhymes by way of viola and violin. The second artist established the pattern of the performances beyond their special cultural merits. The students realized that they were encountering people who had spent most of a lifetime mastering some of the most difficult skills ever undertaken by man; but there was something more. By coming to the students and opening themselves to any questions they were providing an invitation.

115

In a groping way the questioning began to focus on what they had to give of themselves and find in themselves to rise to the level of artistry.

The impact of the artists began to show in the students' daytime work. A portion of the floor that had been laid down imperfectly was torn up and redone. Unattended damage to the kiln that had not been noticed was repaired. Shelters, walkways around the adjacent buildings, sheds, a crude drinking station called "The Plastic Pub" were all repaired. Even personal care improved. The dam down the creek had a waterfall that became a shower. Some shaved. Without being fastidious the students began to restore themselves back from the dishevelment that had gone unchecked from the island through Skid Row. That day an officer from the Immigration Service arrived. He was under the impression that the community was a religious cult. The fact that the students had turned their hand at building "found sculpture" from machines parts laying all around tended to confirm his suspicion. His concern was very specific. In the most courteous way, he inquired whether there were women present. At that point it came as a shock to everyone to realize that sex differences mattered. After assuring himself that they were not being held by force or the threat of force he took a considerable interest in the improvements.

In the evening a troupe of three actors from Western Washington University put on a one-act performance drawn from a segment of a poem by Koch. After analyzing and reconstructing their moods they drew several "volunteers" into the center of the dome and went through a verbal charade called Coil Supreme. Carrying over into a second keg of beer the drummers and those who worked over the rented piano partied their way into dawn. By night and by day the groups worked out their special style and technique. Quite at home with themselves and each other they played as hard as they worked.

Entirely at ease with the staff, they sought advice when it suited them and ignored it on the same basis. The spirit first sampled on the glacier returned in much amplified strength. None of the gloom or *Lord of the Flies* position so evident on the island reappeared. Midway through their stay at the kiln they found themselves as a fully developed and emotionally self-sufficient community. Selves that had remained hidden all that time emerged. Discussion, argument, and debate abounded on everything from adultery to Zen. Life histories were revealed. Philosophies exposed. Attitudes attacked. Values endorsed. Without guessing they were doing anything more than restoring an abandoned kiln and having a good time drinking, they began to make unexamined parts of themselves evident. By bringing them out in the open they took the first step toward building new selves. Their style became fraternal; they took an interest in each other far beyond the usual. When one lad was refused passage on a bus because of long hair and bare feet it hit them all. When another was caught by the Conservation Officer with two twenty-five pound salmon he had just killed for a barbecue, he had more volunteer "lawyers" than anyone could use.

And their technique became "stumbling Cartesian." Though not fully aware of the extent to which doubt might reach, when nothing was taken for granted, they started along the road. The seventeen acres they occupied were no longer an abandoned brick kiln on Friday Creek. It became a modern Benedictine Monastery in which work and meditation mixed with an exploration of the arts and, albeit, beer. Yet it remained in no danger of becoming a cult. Joined in a common though undefined exploration, they gradually became aware of how different they really were. Fortunately, they had learned that they did not have to become ostriches to protect the differences. These were the differences that exposure could cultivate just as the performances of the artists contributed to their special uniqueness.

The recital by the University of British Columbia string quartet brought the collaborative dimension of artistic excellence to the fore. For two hours the dome rang with the sound of strings tuned and played in harmony. After the performance it came as a surprise to find that the local constabulary and several citizens had come to listen. Having known the place as an abandoned ruin good for several loads of brick, and having heard all kinds of stories about the weird rites being performed, they had trouble believing their eyes and ears. Again and again they marvelled at the transformation, and remarked that there had never been anything like the performance anywhere in the area before. From them, the word spread that the Canadians were a breed unknown in those parts; hard working, constructive, fun loving, cultured, friendly, open, creative, intelligent, moral and somehow too good to be true. Alarmed at what seemed to them the decline and decay of their own youth, they showered the visitors with all the virtues they admired but found lacking. So the counter-myth went around as an antidote to the initial accusations.

The following night many returned and brought friends to hear a basso from the San Francisco Opera and to watch his wife do interpretive dancing. Their amazement grew. Promises to preserve the kiln and continue to use and improve it abounded. Men swore to protect it against brick thieves and destruction. Local politicos vowed to use all their influence to further what had been started. Regardless of practical limitations that might keep them from accomplishing their ends, the expression of concern was absolutely genuine. A certain hidden passion for improvement had been touched. Though it might be only an emotional outburst, it represented an awakening they would not soon forget. And it augmented the same feeling for preservation and continued use of the facilities that living in and around the kiln had stirred in the students. The guests and the host citizenry who had come to find out what was going on were in perfect accord. Having developed a facility entirely for their own use, the students were able to be fully and wholly themselves in a more expanded and complete sense than would ever be possible for anyone on Skid Row. Yet they could open up into the kiln, the grounds, the countryside, the work, the appreciation and the sharing without keeping parts of themselves compartmentalized.

In just one week they had put together a whole that exceeded the sum of its parts. Without quite knowing what they were doing they built themselves a vision. The kiln, the bricklaying, the artistic performances,

117

the drinking, the communual living, the geographic isolation and the continuous discussion, were only elements of technique for making it possible. However dim or fleeting, vague or contradictory, spotty or insubstantial, they had caught a glimpse. And the glimpse, not the activities, had fired their imaginations. In a hermitage of their own making they had seen the skeleton of Shang-ri-la. They had dabbled on the outskirts of Utopia. However soon they might forget it under the press of ordinary affairs, it would not be lost. They had touched on a new dimension.

Preparation for the last night began in a downpour before dawn. A pit was dug, coals were laid, a spit was built, and a huge leg of beef was started. All through the day plastic was hung to provide shelter for the guests who would arrive at dusk. Wives, girl friends, local citizens, professors, architects, artists, and scientists were invited from half a dozen places between Seattle and Vancouver. Broken brick was dumped into muddy spots down the road so vehicles would not bog down. A fire was built in the dome to dry it out and a clean-up squad brought the interior and the grounds to their peak of cleanliness. Everyone worked full tilt arranging food, lighting, access, extra accommodation and special effects. Before the staff withdrew, everyone was told to be in the dome, seated and waiting, by six-thirty. As was customary, the students did not know what they would be waiting for. Not prone to let a mystery go unexamined, they gathered.

The staff drove to a residence in Bellingham to put on Restoration period costumes from the university's drama department. The drive back took them through the town of Alger, about two miles from the kiln. Knowing that a dozen local citizens would be in the crossroads bar, they stopped in. The customers saw a Jesuit priest, a Dominican brother, a nun, two squires in velvet great-coats, a buccaneer, an Indian woman in a sari and a girl in a purple page-boy outfit come in. For the first few minutes they were awestruck. All the men had beards. The women were immaculate. And everyone was barefoot or in hiking boots. Looking from the brown wool of the religious costumes to the blue, purple, and butterscotch velvet greatcoats, they gathered their wits. The owner hurried to get a camera. A couple concluded the costuming had to do with the kiln. Toasts and congratulations were offered from all sides. And the group left to meet several dozen guests who were timing their arrival at the property so everyone could enter together. Principal amongst the guests was Henry Elder, director of the school of architecture, in the full ceremonial dress of a bishop.

Carrying candles and stepping to a chant, the procession strode up the path, through the trees, and into the dome. All attendants and ladies-in-waiting went to the center and stood around the bishop. The staff members in religious and court dress went around the inside edge and stopped at different low arches. For three-quarters of an hour they performed a one-act Existential play that had been written the day before. With lines written on anything that could be concealed, the outer ring looked through their openings to describe different worlds. Each report they gave to the bishop was explained and distorted by his chief administrator. The bishop was asked to decide which world would survive. His answer was relayed back by the administrator as meaning none should survive. As each one around the outside blew out his candle, the bishop grew more worried. By extinguishing his aide's candle before all were out he allowed all the others to relight theirs. Having begun with a three-minute oration of Pericles's funeral speech in Greek it ended with the priest chanting a mass in Latin. All the players withdrew as a soprano sang a soft but bright solo. For several minutes no one spoke.

Just as applause began to ring through the dome, half a dozen girls came in wearing shapely togas and carrying bowls of fruit and jars of wine. Two students in loin cloths carried a barbecued leg of beef on their shoulders. More serving girls came in with wicker trays. Loaves of bread were passed around and everyone broke off what he wanted, light, dark, french, sour dough. Large cheeses hard and soft, sharp and mild, pungent and creamy appeared. Whole roast chickens were broken apart and passed along. A dozen varieties of salami came from everywhere. Platters of beef dripping with natural juices passed from hand to hand. Grapes, nuts, oranges, bananas, plums and apples came along. And after every mouthful there was wine, heavy, light, dry, sweet, rose, chablis, claret and zinfandel. Hand to mouth and hand to hand; there was no china or silver to be seen. Each person was his own portable larder with supply stations never more than a few steps away. Eating and drinking in Roman fashion encouraged mobility.

Two drummers set up a wild beat on the tom-toms. Chains formed and circled. The dancing began. Shouts of *olé* mixed with toasts and the room began to rock.

When it seemed the dancing could not get wilder nor the chorus louder a Greek bazouki band struck out. Beginning with their amplified versions of Western songs evocative of the Mediterranean, they worked into their native music, mixing the Greek strings with Turkish woodwinds. In Zorba fashion the revellers jumped, whirled, stepped, stopped, sprang and slapped their heels. Driven to new heights of energy, they welcomed the chance to sit and watch when the belly-dancer appeared. Beginning with the dance of the veils, she introduced a new motion each time she peeled off a layer. Revealed under the last layer of thinnest gauze, she gyrated in seven separate directions at once, all the while maintaining a thumping beat with her whole midriff that would have done credit to the native girls of Bora Bora. As she went into her last number a young architect burst into the dome clad in nothing but a few vines appropriately draped. In a wild duet of Nature Boy and the Snake of Eden they stimulated the audience into a frenzy of gymnastics it did not know it could even attempt.

Quite beyond themselves the crowd did not notice the next stage until the strobe lights set out a pattern of flashes that resembled the cannon-blasts at the seige of Sevastopol. All motion was frozen into a series of disjointed stills, and the roar of artillery came over the powerful amplifier. A rock-and-roll band of amplified guitars and rim-rattling drums opened the light show. On a parachute held up to the curve of the dome projectors flashed subliminal images in quick succession and overlay. Color blazed through the smoke and splashed along the silk like dry dust cast by a contemporary Jackson Pollock. The blinding flashes of light slowed the gyrations of the dancers into a slow-motion satire of a Chaplin film. And throughout the dome the ear-splitting roar of the band pressed as thick as an invisible fog suddenly turned harder than steel. Frozen in frantic postures by the flashes of bright and black they were held there motionless by noise so stunning it solidified the very blood in their veins. It was the light, the black, the blindness, the deafness, the start, the stop, the roar, the numbness of Creation. And it went on until dawn.

Somewhere in the rain and the mystery of that night of thoughtless noise the end came. When they saw the debris by daylight the workshop was already over. The cleanup was silent. They were going home. Or were they? Something seemed to bar the way. A question? A small doubt? Some wonder? They could not stay, but no one was happy to leave. There was a sense of a vision fading. The trace of a ghost. When would there be another night like that? Yet beneath that selfish question another concern began to stir. Somehow it had been more than just another workshop. Defense Island, Garibaldi Glacier, Port Alberni, Skid Row and the brick kiln at Friday Creek had been stages in a launching. They had broken away from a tight confinement in a narrowly constricted sense of self. If they were not yet free, at least the bonds of a constraining psychological and social gravity had been weakened. Even though they might never find a self-sustaining orbit they had made a good start. They had begun a first probe toward relevance.

Man & society

*J*ohn Steinbeck saw the sickness of the migrant worker as part of the sickness of his society. While at work on The Grapes of Wrath, a novel about Oklahoma migrant workers in California, he wrote his literary agent:

I must go over into the interior valleys. . . . There are five thousand families starving to death over there, not just hungry but actually starving. The government is trying to feed them and get medical attention to them, with the Fascist group of utilities and banks and huge growers sabotaging the thing all along the line, and yelling for a balanced budget. In one tent there are twenty people quarantined for smallpox and two of the women are to have babies in that tent this week . . . Do you know what they're afraid of? They think that if these people are allowed to live in camps with proper sanitary facilities they will organize, and that is the bugbear of the large landowner and the corporation farmer.*

The Grapes of Wrath was published more than thirty years ago. Many people would disagree with Steinbeck that the motives of the rich farmers were quite so invidious. But Steinbeck's book did help to bring the harsh life of the migrant worker of the thirties to public attention. Today there are some public health programs as well as programs sponsored by private groups for these workers. But these are inadequate, so the inclusion here of a brief excerpt from The Grapes of Wrath has more than historical interest. The problem is not of the past; it is of the present. It remains rooted in societal indifference and neglect. The deplorable circumstance of California grape-pickers is just one example of the plight of the migrant worker today.

The Steinbeck selection does more than describe the condition of man under stress. It tells how people establish their own social controls in order to survive as a group. Thus this selection leads into the first of the three interrelated topics in this section: "The Human Condition." The second and third topics, "The Drug Culture" and "The Generation Gap," are widely discussed in efforts to explain youth's dissatisfaction with the condition of man in modern society.

"The Human Condition" begins with "If Hitler Asked You to Electrocute a Stranger, Would You?" a report by Philip Meyer on psychologist Stanley Milgram's experiments testing obedience to authority. For some, the article may be startling. For many, Milgram's results will emphasize the need for social controls not only of the governors but of the governed. But vital questions then arise: "Who shall control? When? To what extent?" The controls among the migrant workers described by Steinbeck arose spontaneously and their effect was to create group unity. But what are the differences between the social controls exercised by the migrant workers and those exercised by democratic governments or fascist states? Do they differ in kind, in degree, or merely in result? What are their varying influences on human health? The second article, Robert E. Kantor and William G. Herron's essay "Paranoia and High Office," is concerned with the dangers of emotional illness among those who exert social

---

* In Lewis Gannett, "John Steinbeck's Way of Writing," Introduction to *The Portable Steinbeck* (New York: Viking Press, 1946), pp. xx–xxi.

control. "When we do not attack," Corporal Adolf Hitler wrote home, "I fall mentally ill."

Several reasons for the alienation of a whole people are presented in Robert H. Sharpley's article, "A Psychohistorical Perspective of the Negro." Sharpley discusses some of the psychic wounds that prejudice has inflicted on the blacks. The black revolt should be no surprise. Years ago the black poet Langston Hughes wrote the warning:

What happens to a dream deferred?

> Does it dry up
> Like a raisin in the sun?
>   .   .   .

Or does it explode *

Sharpley's article is about a people whose poverty has long been a mark of abuse by others. Oscar Lewis' essay "The Culture of Poverty," describes a present culture within other cultural layers. In this country health workers are aware (and some are despairing) of those who live in the culture of poverty. Because of their alienation, the poor within the culture of poverty increase their disadvantage by not using available preventive health services. They live in a behavioral gap—the gap between what public health workers offer them and what they accept.

American attitudes toward sex throughout the nation's history are the theme of Arthur Schlesinger's change-of-pace article "An Informal History of Love U.S.A." This lively and perceptive historical commentary helps to illuminate the present condition of man.

The next two articles provide a basis for discussion of "The Drug Subculture." As a medical student, Joshua Kaufman joined with two psychiatrists, James R. Allen and Louis Jolyon West, to write about "Runaways, Hippies, and Marihuana." The "whys" for all three are explored. In the article that follows, Klaus Angel presents telling arguments in his "No Marijuana for Adolescents."

The so-called generation gap is the subject of the next three articles. In "What Generation Gap?" Joseph Adelson questions the depth of the abyss between the generations. Roy Menninger, however, in "What Troubles Our Troubled Youth?" sees and analyzes a deep separation between young people and their elders. William Neal Brown's carefully organized paper "Alienated Youth" lucidly describes a growing health problem. The alienation of some young people is more than a mere separation between themselves and their elders because of a lack of communication. It is an emotionally distressing expression of hostility based on their conception of the failures of the older generation.Thoreau once said that "no people ever lived by cursing their fathers, however great a curse their fathers might have been to them." By increasing understanding, the Adelson, Menninger, and Brown articles may help to diminish the cursing.

The section closes with a poem, Subhas Mukhopadhyay's "Breaking

---

Isn't Everything.'' Today many people who witness the needless neglect of social problems such as those described in The Grapes of Wrath *begin to break with the past. They see hope for the future only if past values and institutions are rejected—even violently.*

In an article in the September 26, 1970, issue of The New Yorker, *Yale University law professor Charles A. Reich writes of "a society that is unjust to its poor and minorities, is run for the benefit of a privileged few, lacks its proclaimed democracy and liberty, is ugly and artificial, destroys the environment and the self, and is, like the war it spawns, unhealthy for children and other living things." If this indictment is too glib and general, it still contains enough truth to shake one's faith in those of past generations who created the present. "Have patience," the old beseech the young. But patience has many definitions. It has been called a beggar's virtue. And it has been said that there is a point at which patience ceases to be a virtue. For the old it often becomes a refuge. It wears thin for those who long endure injustice and for those who see injustice perpetuated. For some the frustration is too much. Breaking becomes everything.*

But there is danger here. To break with all past values and institutions is to invite chaos into a world inhabited by people who possess the means to their total destruction and who are already desperately trying to handle change. Moreover, this approach to societal problems ignores basic human needs. People need the controls provided by values and institutions. When these controls are threatened, people may create new controls that may not be to their advantage. This problem of controls is examined in a brilliant article by Donald J. Marcuse, "The 'Army' Incident: The Psychology of Uniforms and Their Abolition on an Adolescent Ward" (Psychiatry, A Journal for the Study of Interpersonal Processes, *Vol. 30, No. 4 [November 1967]. pp. 350–75). Because of its length the article is not included here, but the reader is urged to study it. Part of it describes the reaction of some emotionally disturbed adolescents in a psychiatric hospital to the news that soon their nurses and nurses' aids would no longer wear uniforms. Seeing the emblems of authority threatened, the children counter the threat by establishing a remarkably effective army structure among themselves. Their army provides order, but it is the barren order of the desert. It is not an order that yields human growth. Since the hospital staff is excluded from the adolescent army, treatment is also excluded. Marcuse's perceptive analysis of the symbols of authority stimulates a variety of questions. Which institutions are necessary and which are noxious? What meanings do various emblems of authority hold for the stability of the values of human environment? Why do they have these meanings? Which institutions, values, and emblems should be kept? Which should be discarded? If one does not destroy old institutions, are not the new built on rotting foundations? Can revolutionary change occur without breaking, without violence? How rapidly should social change occur? Where does individual responsibility enter the picture? Perhaps the words of Alfred North Whitehead might be remembered here: "The art of progress is to preserve order amid change and to preserve change amid order."*

Breaking, then, isn't everything. When it is, one is left only with useless pieces.

The world of migratory workers

JOHN STEINBECK

The cars of the migrant people crawled out of the side roads onto the great cross-country highway, and they took the migrant way to the West. In the daylight they scuttled like bugs to the westward; and as the dark caught them, they clustered like bugs near to shelter and to water. And because they were lonely and perplexed, because they had all come from a place of sadness and worry and defeat, and because they were all going to a new mysterious place, they huddled together; they talked together; they shared their lives, their food, and the things they hoped for in the new country. Thus it might be that one family camped near a spring, and another camped for the spring and for company, and a third because two families had pioneered the place and found it good. And when the sun went down, perhaps twenty families and twenty cars were there.

In the evening a strange thing happened: the twenty families became one family, the children were the children of all. The loss of home became one loss, and the golden time in the West was one dream. And it might be that a sick child threw despair into the hearts of twenty families, of a hundred people; that a birth there in a tent kept a hundred people quiet and awestruck through the night and filled a hundred people with a birth-joy in the morning. A family which the night before had been lost and fearful might search its goods to find a present for a new baby. In the evening, sitting about the fires, the twenty were one. They grew to be units of the camps, units of the evenings and the nights. A guitar unwrapped from a blanket and tuned—and the songs, which were all of the people, were sung in the nights. Men sang the words, and women hummed the tunes.

Every night a world created, complete with furniture—friends made and enemies established; a world complete with braggarts and with cowards, with quiet men, with humble men, with kindly men. Every night relationships that make a world, established; and every morning the world torn down like a circus.

At first the families were timid in the building and tumbling worlds, but gradually the technique of building worlds became their technique. Then leaders emerged, then laws were made, then codes came into being. And as the worlds moved westward they were more complete and better furnished, for their builders were more experienced in building them.

The families learned what rights must be observed—the right of privacy in the tent; the right to keep the black past hidden in the heart; the right to talk and to listen; the right to refuse help or to accept, to offer help or to decline it; the right of son to court and daughter to be courted; the right of the hungry to be fed; the rights of the pregnant and the sick to transcend all other rights.

And the families learned, although no one told them, what rights are monstrous and must be destroyed: the right to intrude upon privacy, the right to be noisy while the camp slept, the right of seduction or rape, the right of adultery and theft and murder. These rights were crushed, because the little worlds could not exist for even a night with such rights alive.

And as the worlds moved westward, rules became laws, although no one told the families. It is unlawful to foul near the camp; it is unlawful in any way to foul the drinking water; it is unlawful to eat good rich food near one who is hungry, unless he is asked to share.

And with the laws, the punishments—and there were only two—a quick and murderous fight or ostracism; the ostracism was the worst. For if one broke the laws his name and face went with him, and he had no place in any world, no matter where created.

In the worlds, social conduct became fixed and rigid, so that a man must say "Good morning" when asked for it, so that a man might have a willing girl if he stayed with her, if he fathered her children and protected them. But a man might not have one girl one night and another the next, for this would endanger the worlds.

The families moved westward, and the technique of building the worlds improved so that the people could be safe in their worlds, and the form was so fixed that a family acting in the rules knew it was safe in the rules.

There grew up government in the worlds, with leaders, with elders. A man who was wise found that his wisdom was needed in every camp; a man who was a fool could not change his folly with his world. And a kind of insurance developed in these nights. A man with food fed a hungry man, and thus insured himself against hunger. And when a baby died a pile of silver coins grew at the door flap, for a baby must be well buried, since it has had nothing else of life. An old man may be left in a potter's field, but not a baby.

A certain physical pattern is needed for the building of a world—water, a river bank, a stream, a spring, or even a faucet unguarded. And there is needed enough flat land to pitch the tents, a little brush or wood to build the fires. If there is a garbage dump not too far off, all the better; for there can be found equipment—stove tops, a curved fender to shelter the fire, and cans to cook in and to eat from.

And the worlds were built in the evening. The people, moving in from the highways, made them with their tents and their hearts and their brains.

In the morning the tents came down, the canvas was folded, the tent poles tied along the running board, the beds put in place on the cars, the pots in their places. And as the families moved westward, the technique of building up a home in the evening and tearing it down with the morning light became fixed; so that the folded tent was packed in one place, the cooking pots counted in their box. And as the cars moved westward, each member of the family grew into his proper place, grew into his duties; so that each member, old and young, had his place in the car; so that in the weary, hot evenings, when the cars pulled into the camping places, each member had his duty and went to it without instruction: children to gather wood, to carry water; men to pitch the tents and bring down the beds; women to cook the supper and to watch while the family fed. And this was done without command. The families, which had been units of which the boundaries were a house at night, a farm by day, changed their boundaries. In the long hot light, they were silent in the cars moving slowly westward; but at night they integrated with any group they found.

The
human condition

℔f hitler asked you to electrocute a stranger, would you?

PHILIP MEYER

In the beginning, Stanley Milgram was worried about the Nazi problem. He doesn't worry much about the Nazis any more. He worries about you and me, and, perhaps, himself a little bit too.

Stanley Milgram is a social psychologist, and when he began his career at Yale University in 1960 he had a plan to prove, scientifically, that Germans are different. The Germans-are-different hypothesis has been used by historians, such as William L. Shirer, to explain the systematic destruction of the Jews by the Third Reich. One madman could decide to destroy the Jews and even create a master plan for getting it done. But to implement it on the scale that Hitler did meant that thousands of other people had to go along with the scheme and help to do the work. The Shirer thesis, which Milgram set out to test, is that Germans have a basic character flaw which explains the whole thing, and this flaw is a readiness to obey authority without question, no matter what outrageous acts the authority commands.

The appealing thing about this theory is that it makes those of us who are not Germans feel better about the whole business. Obviously, you and I are not Hitler, and it seems equally obvious that we would never do Hitler's dirty work for him. But now, because of Stanley Milgram, we are compelled to wonder. Milgram developed a laboratory experiment which provided a systematic way to measure obedience. His plan was to try it out in New Haven on Americans and then go to Germany and try it out on Germans. He was strongly motivated by scientific curiosity, but there was also some moral content in his decision to pursue this line of research, which was, in turn, colored by his own Jewish background. If he could show that Germans are more obedient than Americans, he could then vary the conditions of the experiment and try to find out just what it is that makes some people more obedient than others. With this understanding, the world might, conceivably, be just a little bit better.

But he never took his experiment to Germany. He never took it any farther than Bridgeport. The first finding, also the most unexpected and disturbing finding, was that we Americans are an obedient people: not blindly obedient, and not blissfully obedient, just obedient. "I found so much obedience," says Milgram softly, a little sadly, "I hardly saw the need for taking the experiment to Germany."

There is something of the theater director in Milgram, and his technique, which he learned from one of the old masters in experimental psychology, Solomon Asch, is to stage a play with every line rehearsed, every prop carefully selected, and everybody an actor except one person. That one person is the subject of the experiment. The subject, of course, does not know he is in a play. He thinks he is in real life. The value of this technique is that the experimenter, as though he were God, can change a prop here, vary a line there, and see how the subject responds. Milgram eventually had to change a lot of the script just to get people to stop obeying. They were obeying so much, the experiment wasn't working—it was like trying to measure oven temperature with a freezer thermometer.

The experiment worked like this: If you were an innocent subject in Milgram's melodrama, you read an ad in the newspaper or received one in the mail asking for volunteers for an educational experiment. The job would take about an hour and pay $4.50. So you make an appointment and go to an old Romanesque stone structure on High Street with the imposing name of The Yale Interaction Laboratory. It looks something like a broadcasting studio. Inside, you meet a young, crew-cut man in a laboratory coat who says he is Jack Williams, the experimenter. There is another citizen, fiftyish, Irish face, an accountant, a little overweight, and very mild and harmless-looking. This other citizen seems nervous and plays with his hat while the two of you sit in chairs side by side and are told that the $4.50 checks are yours no matter what happens. Then you listen to Jack Williams explain the experiment.

It is about learning, says Jack Williams in a quiet, knowledgeable way. Science does not know much about the conditions under which people learn and this experiment is to find out about negative reinforcement. Negative reinforcement is getting punished when you do something wrong, as opposed to positive reinforcement which is getting rewarded when you do something right. The negative reinforcement in this case is electric shock. You notice a book on the table, titled, *The Teaching-Learning Process*, and you assume that this has something to do with the experiment.

Then Jack Williams takes two pieces of paper, puts them in a hat, and shakes them up. One piece of paper is supposed to say, "Teacher" and the other, "Learner." Draw one and you will see which you will be. The mild-looking accountant draws one, holds it close to his vest like a poker player, looks at it, and says, "Learner." You look at yours. It says, "Teacher." You do not know that the drawing is rigged, and both slips say "Teacher." The experimenter beckons to the mild-mannered "learner."

"Want to step right in here and have a seat, please?" he says. "You can leave your coat on the back of that chair . . . roll up your right sleeve, please. Now what I want to do is strap down your arms to avoid excessive movement on your part during the experiment. This electrode is connected to the shock generator in the next room.

"And this electrode paste," he says, squeezing some stuff out of a plastic bottle and putting it on the man's arm, "is to provide a good contact and to avoid a blister or burn. Are there any questions now before we go into the next room?"

You don't have any, but the strapped-in "learner" does.

"I do think I should say this," says the learner. "About two years ago, I was at the veterans' hospital . . . they detected a heart condition. Nothing serious, but as long as I'm having these shocks, how strong are they—how dangerous are they?"

Williams, the experimenter, shakes his head casually. "Oh, no," he says. "Although they may be painful, they're not dangerous. Anything else?"

Nothing else. And so you play the game. The game is for you to read a series of word pairs: for example, blue-girl, nice-day, fat-neck. When you finish the list, you read just the first word in each pair and then a multiple-choice list of four other words, including the second word of the pair. The learner, from his remote, strapped-in position, pushes one of four switches to indicate which of the four answers he thinks is the right one. If he gets it right, nothing happens and you go on to the next one. If he gets it wrong, you push a switch that buzzes and gives him an electric shock. And then you go to the next word. You start with 15 volts and increase the number of volts by 15 for each wrong answer. The control board goes from 15 volts on one end to 450 volts on the other. So that you know what you are doing, you get a test shock yourself, at 45 volts. It hurts. To further keep you aware of what you are doing to that man in there, the board has verbal descriptions of the shock levels, ranging from "Slight Shock" at the left-hand side, through "Intense Shock" in the middle, to "Danger: Severe Shock" toward the far right. Finally, at the very end, under 435- and 450-volt switches, there are three ambiguous X's. If, at any point, you hesitate, Mr. Williams calmly tells you to go on. If you still hesitate, he tells you again.

Except for some terrifying details, which will be explained in a moment, this is the experiment. The object is to find the shock level at which you disobey the experimenter and refuse to pull the switch.

When Stanley Milgram first wrote this script, he took it to fourteen Yale psychology majors and asked them what they thought would happen. He put it this way: Out of one hundred persons in the teacher's predicament, how would their break-off points be distributed along the 15-to-450-volt scale? They thought a few would break off very early, most would quit someplace in the middle and a few would go all the way to the end. The highest estimate of the number out of one hundred who would go all the way to the end was three. Milgram then informally polled some of his fellow scholars in the psychology department. They agreed that very few would go to the end. Milgram thought so too.

"I'll tell you quite frankly," he says, "before I began this experiment, before any shock generator was built, I thought that most people would break off at 'Strong Shock' or 'Very Strong Shock.' You would get only a very, very small proportion of people going out to the end of the shock generator, and they would constitute a pathological fringe."

In his pilot experiments, Milgram used Yale students as subjects. Each of them pushed the shock switches, one by one, all the way to the end of the board.

So he rewrote the script to include some protests from the learner. At first, they were mild, gentlemanly, Yalie protests, but, "it didn't seem to have as much effect as I thought it would or should," Milgram recalls. "So we had more violent protestation on the part of the person getting the shock. All of the time, of course, what we were trying to do was not to create a macabre situation, but simply to generate disobedience. And that was one of the first findings. This was not only a technical deficiency of the experiment, that we didn't get disobedience. It really was the first finding: that obedience would be much greater than we had assumed it would be and disobedience would be much more difficult than we had assumed."

As it turned out, the situation did become rather macabre. The only meaningful way to generate disobedience was to have the victim protest with great anguish, noise, and vehemence. The protests were tape-recorded so that all the teachers ordinarily would hear the same sounds and nuances, and they started with a grunt at 75 volts, proceeded through a "Hey, that really hurts," at 125 volts, got desperate with, " I can't stand the pain, don't do that," at 180 volts, reached complaints of heart trouble at 195, an agonized scream at 285, a refusal to answer at 315, and only heart-rending, ominous silence after that.

Still, sixty-five percent of the subjects, twenty- to fifty-year-old American males, everyday, ordinary people, like you and me, obediently kept pushing those levers in the belief that they were shocking the mild-mannered learner, whose name was Mr. Wallace, and who was chosen for the role because of his innocent appearance, all the way up to 450 volts.

Milgram was now getting enough disobedience so that he had something he could measure. The next step was to vary the circumstances to see what would encourage or discourage obedience. There seemed very little left in the way of discouragement. The victim was already screaming at the top of his lungs and feigning a heart attack. So whatever new impediment to obedience reached the brain of the subject had to travel by some route other than the ear. Milgram thought of one.

He put the learner in the same room with the teacher. He stopped strapping the learner's hand down. He rewrote the script so that at 150 volts the learner took his hand off the shock plate and declared that he wanted out of the experiment. He rewrote the script some more so that the experimenter then told the teacher to grasp the learner's hand and physically force it down on the plate to give Mr. Wallace his unwanted electric shock.

"I had the feeling that very few people would go on at that point, if any," Milgram says. "I thought that would be the limit of obedience that you would find in the laboratory."

It wasn't.

Although seven years have now gone by, Milgram still remembers the first person to walk into the laboratory in the newly rewritten script. He was a construction worker, a very short man. "He was so small," says Milgram, "that when he sat on the chair in front of the shock generator, his feet didn't reach the floor. When the experimenter told him to push the victim's hand down and give the shock, he turned to the experimenter, and he turned to the victim, his elbow went up, he fell down on the hand of the victim, his feet kind of tugged to one side, and he said, 'Like this, boss?' ZZUMPH!"

The experiment was played out to its bitter end. Milgram tried it with forty different subjects. And thirty percent of them obeyed the experimenter and kept on obeying.

"The protests of the victim were strong and vehement, he was screaming his guts out, he refused to participate, and you had to physically struggle with him in order to get his hand down on the shock generator," Milgram remembers. But twelve out of forty did it.

Milgram took his experiment out of New Haven. Not to Germany, just twenty miles down the road to Bridgeport. Maybe, he reasoned, the people obeyed because of the prestigious setting of Yale University. If they couldn't trust a center of learning that had been there for two centuries, whom could they trust? So he moved the experiment to an untrustworthy setting.

The new setting was a suite of three rooms in a run-down office building in Bridgeport. The only identification was a sign with a fictitious name: "Research Associates of Bridgeport." Questions about professional connections got only vague answers about "research for industry."

Obedience was less in Bridgeport. Forty-eight percent of the subjects stayed for the maximum shock, compared to sixty-five percent at Yale. But this was enough to prove that far more than Yale's prestige was behind the obedient behavior.

For more than seven years now, Stanley Milgram has been trying to figure out what makes ordinary American citizens so obedient. The most obvious answer—that people are mean, nasty, brutish and sadistic—won't do. The subjects who gave the shocks to Mr. Wallace to the end of the board did not enjoy it. They groaned, protested, fidgeted, argued, and in some cases, were seized by fits of nervous, agitated giggling.

"They even try to get out of it," says Milgram, "but they are somehow engaged in something from which they cannot liberate themselves. They are locked into a structure, and they do not have the skills or inner resources to disengage themselves."

Milgram, because he mistakenly had assumed that he would have trouble getting people to obey the orders to shock Mr. Wallace, went to a lot of trouble to create a realistic situation.

There was crew-cut Jack Williams and his grey laboratory coat. Not white, which might denote a medical technician, but ambiguously authoritative grey. Then there was the book on the table, and the other appurtenances of the laboratory which emitted the silent message that things were being performed here in the name of science, and were therefore great and good.

But the nicest touch of all was the shock generator. When Milgram started out, he had only a $300 grant from the Higgins Fund of Yale University. Later he got more ample support from the National Science Foundation, but in the beginning he had to create this authentic-looking machine with very scarce resources except for his own imagination. So he went to New York and roamed around the electronic shops until he found some little black switches at Lafayette Radio for a dollar apiece. He bought thirty of them. The generator was a metal box, about the size of a small footlocker, and he drilled the thirty holes for the thirty switches himself in a Yale machine shop. But the fine detail was left to professional industrial engravers. So he ended up with a splendid-looking control panel dominated by the row of switches, each labeled with its voltage, and each having its own red light that flashed on when the switch was pulled. Other things happened when a switch was pushed. Besides the zzumphing noise, a blue light labeled "voltage energizer" went on, and a needle on a dial labeled "voltage" flicked from left to right. Relays inside the box clicked. Finally, in the upper left-hand corner of the control panel was this inscription, engraved in precise block letters:

SHOCK GENERATOR TYPE ZLB
DYSON INSTRUMENT COMPANY
WALTHAM, MASS.
OUTPUT: 15 VOLTS—450 VOLTS

One day a man from the Lehigh Valley Electronics Company of Pennsylvania was passing through the laboratory, and he stopped to admire the shock generator.

"This is a very fine shock generator," he said. "But who is this Dyson Instrument Company?" Milgram felt proud at that, since Dyson Instrument Company existed only in the recesses of his imagination.

When you consider the seeming authenticity of the situation, you can appreciate the agony some of the subjects went through. It was pure conflict. As Milgram explains to his students, "When a parent says, 'Don't strike old ladies,' you are learning two things: the content, and, also, to obey authority. This experiment creates conflicts between the two elements."

Here is a partial transcription from one of the experiments. The naive "teacher" is a heavyset, worried-looking man with prematurely grey hair. He is wearing a polo shirt. He is very polite. He has just pushed the 180-volt lever. A hidden camera is recording the performance.

LEARNER (*who, from the teacher's point of view is heard but not seen, an offstage voice*) Ow, I can't stand the pain. Don't do that....

TEACHER (*pivoting around in his chair and shaking his head*) I can't stand it. I'm not going to kill that man in there. You hear him hollering?

EXPERIMENTER As I told you before, the shocks may be painful, but—

TEACHER But he's hollering. He can't stand it. What's going to happen to him?

EXPERIMENTER (*his voice is patient, matter-of-fact*) The experiment requires that you continue, Teacher.

TEACHER Aaah, but, unh, I'm not going to get that man sick in there ... know what I mean?

EXPERIMENTER Whether the learner likes it or not, we must go on, through all the word pairs.

TEACHER I refuse to take the responsibility. He's in there hollering!

EXPERIMENTER It's absolutely essential that you continue, Teacher.

TEACHER (*indicating the unused questions*) There's too many left here, I mean, Geez, if he gets them wrong, there's too many of them left. I mean who's going to take the responsibility if anything happens to that gentleman?

EXPERIMENTER I'm responsible for anything that happens to him. Continue please.

TEACHER All right. (*Consults list of words.*) The next one's "Slow—walk, truck, dance, music." Answer, please. (*A buzzing sound indicates the learner has signaled his answer.*) Wrong. A hundred and ninety-five volts. "Dance." (*Zzumph!*)

LEARNER Let me out of here. My heart's bothering me! (*Teacher looks at experimenter.*)

EXPERIMENTER Continue, please.

LEARNER (*screaming*) Let me out of here, you have no right to keep me here. Let me out of here, let me out, my heart's bothering me, let me out! (*Teacher shakes head, pats the table nervously.*)

TEACHER You see, he's hollering. Hear that? Gee, I don't know.

EXPERIMENTER The experiment requires. . . .

TEACHER (*interrupting*) I know it does, sir, but I mean—hunh! He don't know what he's getting in for. He's up to 195 volts! (*Experiment continues, through 210 volts, 225 volts, 240 volts, 255 volts, 270 volts, delivered to the man in the electric chair, at which point the teacher, with evident relief, runs out of word-pair questions.*)

EXPERIMENTER You'll have to go back to the beginning of that page and go through them again until he's learned them all correctly.

TEACHER Aw, no. I'm not going to kill that man. You mean I've got to keep going up with the scale. No sir. He's hollering in there. I'm not going to give him 450 volts.

EXPERIMENTER The experiment requires that you go on.

TEACHER I know it does, but that man is hollering in there, sir.

EXPERIMENTER (*same matter-of-fact tone*) As I said before, although the shocks may be painful. . . .

TEACHER (*interrupting*) Awwww. He—he—he's yelling in there.

EXPERIMENTER Start with "Blue," please, at the top of the page. Continue, please, Teacher. Just go ahead.

TEACHER (*concentrating intently on list of words in front of him, as if to shut everything else out*) "Blue—boy, girl, grass, hat." (*Buzz indicates answer.*) Correct. "Night—day, sky, job, chair. (*Buzz*) Wrong. The answer is "day." Two hundred and eighty-five volts. (*Zzumph!*)

LEARNER Ohhhuhhoohhh!

Philip Meyer

EXPERIMENTER Continue, please.

TEACHER "Fat—man, lady, tub, neck." Answer, please. (*Buzz*) Wrong. The answer is "neck." Three hundred volts. (*Zzumph!*)

LEARNER Ohhh. I absolutely refuse to answer any more. (*Shouting urgently, now*) Let me out of here. You can't hold me here. Get me out. Get—me—out—of—here.

EXPERIMENTER Continue. The next word is "Green," please.

TEACHER "Green—grass, hat, ink, apple." (*Nothing happens. No answering buzz. Just gloomy silence.*)

TEACHER I don't think he is going to answer.

EXPERIMENTER If the learner doesn't answer in a reasonable time, about four or five seconds, consider the answer wrong. And follow the same procedures you have been doing for wrong answers. Say "Wrong," tell him the number of volts, give him the punishment, read him the correct answer. Continue, please.

TEACHER "Green—grass, hat, ink, apple." Answer please. (*More silence. Teacher just sits there.*)

EXPERIMENTER Go on with the procedure, please, Teacher.

TEACHER Three hundred and fifteen volts. The answer is "ink." (*Zzumph!*)

LEARNER Ohh. Ooohh.

TEACHER (*relieved to hear response*) Next one....

LEARNER I absolutely refuse to answer.

TEACHER You got to. You get a shock if you don't answer. (*Experiment continues with learner refusing to answer, and, finally, failing even to grunt or groan. At 375 volts, the teacher stands up. Has he had enough? Will he break off the experiment? Will he disobey?*)

TEACHER I think something's happened to that fellow in there. I don't get no answer. He was hollering at less voltage. Can't you check in and see if he's all right, please?

EXPERIMENTER (*same detached calm*) Not once we've started. Please continue, Teacher.

TEACHER (*sits down, sighs deeply*) "Cool—day, shade, water, paint." Answer, please. Are you all right in there? Are you all right?

EXPERIMENTER Please continue, Teacher. Continue, please. (*Teacher pushes lever. Zzumph!*)

TEACHER (*swiveling around in his chair*) Something's happened to that man in there. (*Swiveling back*) Next one. "Low—dollar, necklace, moon, paint." (*Turning around again*) Something's happened to that man in there. You better check on him, sir. He won't answer or nothing.

EXPERIMENTER Continue. Go on, please.

TEACHER You accept all responsibility.

EXPERIMENTER The responsibility is mine. Correct. Please go on. (*Teacher returns to his list, starts running through words as rapidly as he can read them, works through to 450 volts.*)

TEACHER That's that.

EXPERIMENTER Continue using the last switch on the board, please. The four-fifty switch for each wrong answer. Continue, please.

TEACHER But I don't get no anything!

EXPERIMENTER Please continue. The next word is "White."

TEACHER Don't you think you should look in on him, please.

EXPERIMENTER Not once we've started the experiment.

TEACHER But what if something has happened to the man?

EXPERIMENTER The experiment requires that you continue. Go on, please.

TEACHER Don't the man's health mean anything?

EXPERIMENTER Whether the learner likes it or not. . . .

TEACHER What if he's dead in there? (*Gestures toward the room with the electric chair.*) I mean, he told me he can't stand the shock, sir. I don't mean to be rude, but I think you should look in on him. All you have to do is look in the door. I don't get no answer, no noise. Something might have happened to the gentleman in there, sir.

EXPERIMENTER We must continue. Go on, please.

TEACHER You mean keep giving him what? Four hundred fifty volts, what he's got now?

EXPERIMENTER That's correct. Continue. The next word is "White."

TEACHER (*now at a furious pace*) "White—cloud, horse, rock, house." Answer, please. The answer is "horse." Four hundred and fifty volts. (*Zzumph!*) Next word, "Bag—paint, music, clown, girl." The answer is "paint." Four hundred and fifty volts. (*Zzumph!*) Next word is "Short—sentence, movie. . . ."

EXPERIMENTER Excuse me, Teacher. We'll have to discontinue the experiment.

(*Enter Milgram from camera's left. He has been watching from behind one-way glass.*)

MILGRAM I'd like to ask you a few questions. (*Slowly, patiently, he dehoaxes the teacher, telling him that the shocks and screams were not real.*)

TEACHER You mean he wasn't getting nothing? Well, I'm glad to hear that. I was getting upset there. I was getting ready to walk out.

(*Finally, to make sure there are no hard feelings, friendly, harmless Mr. Wallace comes out in coat and tie. Gives jovial greeting. Friendly reconciliation takes place. Experiment ends.*) © STANLEY MILGRAM 1965

Subjects in the experiment were not asked to give the 450-volt shock more than three times. By that time, it seemed evident that they would go on indefinitely. "No one," says Milgram, "who got within five shocks of the end ever broke off. By that point, he had resolved the conflict."

Why do so many people resolve the conflict in favor of obedience?

Milgram's theory assumes that people behave in two different operating modes as different as ice and water. He does not rely on Freud or sex or toilet-training hang-ups for this theory. All he says is that ordinarily we operate in a state of autonomy, which means we pretty much have and assert control over what we do. But in certain circumstances, we operate under what Milgram calls a state of agency (after agent, n . . . one who acts for or in the place of another by authority from him; a substitute; a deputy. —*Webster's Collegiate Dictionary*). A state of agency, to Milgram, is nothing more than a frame of mind.

"There's nothing bad about it, there's nothing good about it," he says. "It's a natural circumstance of living with other people. . . . I think of a state of agency as a real transformation of a person; if a person has different properties when he's in that state, just as water can turn to ice under certain conditions of temperature, a person can move to the state of mind that I call agency . . . the critical thing is that you see yourself as the instrument of the execution of another person's wishes. You do not see yourself as acting on your own. And there's a real transformation, a real change of properties of the person."

To achieve this change, you have to be in a situation where there seems to be a ruling authority whose commands are relevant to some legitimate purpose; the authority's power is not unlimited.

But situations can be and have been structured to make people do unusual things, and not just in Milgram's laboratory. The reason, says Milgram, is that no action, in and of itself, contains meaning.

"The meaning always depends on your definition of the situation. Take an action like killing another person. It sounds bad.

"But then we say the other person was about to destroy a hundred children, and the only way to stop him was to kill him. Well, that sounds good.

"Or, you take destroying your own life. It sounds very bad. Yet, in the Second World War, thousands of persons thought it was a good thing to destroy your own life. It was set in the proper context. You sipped some saki from a whistling cup, recited a few haiku. You said, 'May my death be as clean and as quick as the shattering of crystal.' And it almost seemed like a good, noble thing to do, to crash your kamikaze plane into an aircraft carrier. But the main thing was, the definition of what a kamikaze pilot was doing had been determined by the relevant authority. Now, once you are in a state of agency, you allow the authority to determine, to define what the situation is. The meaning of your action is altered."

So, for most subjects in Milgram's laboratory experiments, the act of giving Mr. Wallace his painful shock was necessary, even though unpleasant, and besides they were doing it on behalf of somebody else and it was for science. There was still strain and conflict, of course. Most people resolved it by grimly sticking to their task and obeying. But some broke out. Milgram tried varying the conditions of the experiment to see what would help break people out of their state of agency.

"The results, as seen and felt in the laboratory," he has written, "are disturbing. They raise the possibility that human nature, or more specifically the kind of character produced in American democratic society, cannot be counted on to insulate its citizens from brutality and inhumane treatment at the direction of malevolent authority. A substantial proportion of people do what they are told to do, irrespective of the content of the act and without limitations of conscience, so long as they perceive that the command comes from a legitimate authority. If, in this study, an anonymous experimenter can successfully command adults to subdue a fifty-year-old man and force on him painful electric shocks against his protest, one can only wonder what government, with its vastly greater authority and prestige, can command of its subjects."

This is a nice statement, but it falls short of summing up the full meaning of Milgram's work. It leaves some questions still unanswered.

The first question is this: Should we really be surprised and alarmed that people obey? Wouldn't it be even more alarming if they all refused to obey? Without obedience to a relevant ruling authority there could not be a civil society. And without a civil society, as Thomas Hobbes pointed out in the seventeenth century, we would live in a condition of war, "of every man against every other man," and life would be "solitary, poor, nasty, brutish and short."

In the middle of one of Stanley Milgram's lectures at C.U.N.Y. recently, some mini-skirted undergraduates started whispering and giggling in the back of the room. He told them to cut it out. Since he was the relevant authority in that time and place, they obeyed, and most people in the room were glad that they obeyed.

This was not, of course, a conflict situation. Nothing in the coeds' social upbringing made it a matter of conscience for them to whisper and giggle. But a case can be made that in a conflict situation it is all the more important to obey. Take the case of war, for example. Would we really want a situation in which every participant in a war, direct or indirect—from front-line soldiers to the people who sell coffee and cigarettes to employees at the Concertina barbed-wire factory in Kansas—stops and consults his conscience before each action. It is asking for an awful lot of mental strain and anguish from an awful lot of people. The value of having civil order is that one can do his duty, or whatever interests him, or whatever seems to benefit him at the moment, and leave the agonizing to others. When Francis Gary Powers was being tried by a Soviet military tribunal after his U-2 spy plane was shot down, the presiding judge asked if he had thought about the possibility that his flight might have provoked a war. Powers replied with Hobbesian clarity: "The people who sent me should think of these things. My job was to carry out orders. I do not think it was my responsibility to make such decisions."

It was not his responsibility. And it is quite possible that if everyone felt responsible for each of the ultimate consequences of his own tiny contributions to complex chains of events, then society simply would not work. Milgram, fully conscious of the moral and social implications of his research, believes that people should feel responsible for their actions. If someone else had invented the experiment, and if he had been the naive subject, he feels certain that he would have been among the disobedient minority.

"There is no very good solution to this," he admits, thoughtfully. "To simply and categorically say that you won't obey authority may resolve your personal conflict, but it creates more problems for society which may be more serious in the long run. But I have no doubt that to disobey is the proper thing to do in this [the laboratory] situation. It is the only reasonable value judgment to make."

The conflict between the need to obey the relevant ruling authority and the need to follow your conscience becomes sharpest if you insist on living by an ethical system based on a rigid code—a code that seeks to answer all

143

questions in advance of their being raised. Code ethics cannot solve the obedience problem. Stanley Milgram seems to be a situation ethicist, and situation ethics does offer a way out: When you feel conflict, you examine the situation and then make a choice among the competing evils. You may act with a presumption in favor of obedience, but reserve the possibility that you will disobey whenever obedience demands a flagrant and outrageous affront to conscience. This, by the way, is the philosophical position of many who resist the draft. In World War II, they would have fought. Vietnam is a different, an outrageously different, situation.

Life can be difficult for the situation ethicist, because he does not see the world in straight lines, while the social system too often assumes such a God-given, squared-off structure. If your moral code includes an injunction against all war, you may be deferred as a conscientious objector. If you merely oppose this particular war, you may not be deferred.

Stanley Milgram has his problems, too. He believes that in the laboratory situation, he would not have shocked Mr. Wallace. His professional critics reply that in his real-life situation he has done the equivalent. He has placed innocent and naive subjects under great emotional strain and pressure in selfish obedience to his quest for knowledge. When you raise this issue with Milgram, he has an answer ready. There is, he explains patiently, a critical difference between his naive subjects and the man in the electric chair. The man in the electric chair (in the mind of the naive subject) is helpless, strapped in. But the naive subject is free to go at any time.

Immediately after he offers this distinction, Milgram anticipates the objection.

"It's quite true," he says, "that this is almost a philosophic position, because we have learned that some people are psychologically incapable of disengaging themselves. But that doesn't relieve them of the moral responsibility."

The parallel is exquisite. "The tension problem was unexpected," says Milgram in his defense. But he went on anyway. The naive subjects didn't expect the screaming protests from the strapped-in learner. But they went on.

"I had to make a judgment," says Milgram. "I had to ask myself, was this harming the person or not? My judgment is that it was not. Even in the extreme cases, I wouldn't say that permanent damage results."

Sound familiar? "The shocks may be painful," the experimenter kept saying, "but they're not dangerous."

After the series of experiments was completed, Milgram sent a report of the results to his subjects and a questionnaire, asking whether they were glad or sorry to have been in the experiment. Eighty-three and seven-tenths percent said they were glad and only 1.3 percent were sorry; 15 percent were neither sorry nor glad. However, Milgram could not be sure at the time of the experiment that only 1.3 percent would be sorry.

Kurt Vonnegut Jr. put one paragraph in the preface to *Mother Night*, in 1966, which pretty much says it for the people with their fingers on the shock-generator switches, for you and me, and maybe even for Milgram. "If I'd been born in Germany," Vonnegut said, "I suppose I would have *been* a

Nazi, bopping Jews and gypsies and Poles around, leaving boots sticking out of snowbanks, warming myself with my sweetly virtuous insides. So it goes."

Just so. One thing that happened to Milgram back in New Haven during the days of the experiment was that he kept running into people he'd watched from behind the one-way glass. It gave him a funny feeling, seeing those people going about their everyday business in New Haven and knowing what they would do to Mr. Wallace if ordered to. Now that his research results are in and you've thought about it, you can get this funny feeling too. You don't need one-way glass. A glance in your own mirror may serve just as well.

Paranoia and high office

ROBERT E. KANTOR and WILLIAM G. HERRON

The appeal of high office, elected and appointed, is its power, excitement, and glory. The possible psychic cost to the individual is customarily overlooked; but the chief justice of a court of appeals, holder of a doctorate in law, and a promising candidate for parliament, wrote of himself:

> On the 1st of October...I took up office...I have already mentioned the heavy burden of work I found there. I was driven, maybe by personal ambition, but certainly also in the interests of the office, to achieve first of all the necessary respect among my colleagues and others concerned with the Court (barristers, etc.) by unquestionable efficiency. The task was all the heavier and demanded all the more tact in my personal dealing with the members of the panel of five Judges over which I had to preside as almost all of them were much senior to me (up to twenty years), and anyway they were much more intimately acquainted with the procedure of the Court, to which I was a newcomer. It thus happened that after a few weeks I had already overtaxed myself mentally. I started to sleep badly at the very moment when I was able to feel that I had largely mastered the difficulties of settling down in my new office and in my new residence...The first really bad, that is to say almost sleepless, nights occurred in the last days of October or the first days of November. It was then that an extraordinary event occurred. During several nights when I could not get to sleep, a recurrent crackling noise in the wall of our bedroom became noticeable at shorter or longer intervals; time and again it woke me as I was about to go to sleep. Naturally we thought of a mouse although it was very extraordinary that a mouse should have found its way to the first floor of such a solidly built house. But having heard similar noises innumerable times since then, and still hearing them around me every day...I have come to recognize them as undoubted divine miracles—they are called "interferences" by the voices talking to

PARANOIA AND HIGH OFFICE From *Mental Hygiene*, Vol. 52, No. 4, October 1968. Reprinted by permission of The National Association for Mental Health and R. E. Kantor.

me—and I must at least suspect . . . that even then it was already a matter of such a miracle.[1] (pp. 63–64)

With the publication of his *Memoirs of My Nervous Illness,*[1] Daniel Paul Schreber became the most quoted patient in psychiatry. For, from these memoirs, Freud [2] wrote his famed *Psychoanalytic Notes upon an Autobiographical Account of a Case of Paranoia (Dementia Paranoides)* in 1911. Today, the name Schreber occurs in almost every text of psychiatry, and always associated with the name of Freud. Most present-day clinical theories of paranoia may be traced back to Freud's study of the Schreber case.

But Schreber's memoirs themselves seem not to have been studied again. The psychoanalysts quote passages extracted from Freud; the original source has been unavailable. Now, however, the memoirs have been translated into English, and are no longer a scarce item. The MacAlpine and Hunter translation provides a needed opportunity for re-evaluation of the Freudian interpretation. They think that the Freudian preoccupation with the dynamics of homosexual repression overlooked the important pre-illness events with which Schreber's troubles began. Schreber himself was quite clear on the importance of fatigue in his breakdown:

I come now to my personal fortunes during the two nervous illnesses which I have suffered. I have twice had a nervous illness, each time in consequence of mental overstrain; the first . . . was occasioned by my candidature for parliament, the second by the extraordinary burden of work on taking up office as President of the Senate of a Court of Appeal in Dresden, to which I had been newly appointed. (pp. 61–62)

Schreber's attribution of the crucial role played by his fatigue foreshadows the modern view that any factor (e.g., fatigue, toxin, or injury) disturbing brain functions, renders the person more vulnerable to psychological disorganization: he becomes more prone to memory and judgment error; his perceptions tend to be distorted; he suffers from lessened attention span. But, most important, his ties with reality loosen, and from this it follows that his susceptibility to severe mental illness increases.

There is, it is now believed, a wide spectrum of schizophrenic severity involving dissimilar life-styles.[3] At one end of this spectrum are the process schizophrenics, mostly non-paranoids, who give up their struggle to meet the world's demands before or during their adolescence and who constitute a large part of the mental hospital population. At the other end of the spectrum, the reactive schizophrenics, mostly paranoids, compose the group that is of the most concern to us, for among them are the responsible officials and highly placed executives whose breakdown menaces all of us.

[1] D. P. Schreber, *Memoirs of My Nervous Illness* (translated by Ida MacAlpine and Richard A. Hunter). London: William Dawson and Sons, Ltd., 1955.

[2] S. Freud, *Psycho-analytic Notes upon an Autobiographical Account of a Case of Paranoia (Dementia Paranoides).* In E. Jones (ed.), *Collected Papers,* vol. 3. London: Hogarth, 1956, pp. 390–470.

[3] R. E. Kantor and W. G. Herron, *Reactive and Process Schizophrenia.* Palo Alto, Calif.: Science and Behavior Books, 1966.

When such men are forced, by severe stress or shock, to retreat from the real world, their retreat is into the solace of private solutions for their problems and toward paranoid suspiciousness of the people around them who cannot share their private views. Woodrow Wilson is a case in point.

In the Paris of 1919, well before his final lingering illness, President Wilson entered into the interminable, bitter wrangling of the post-war peace talks. The talks and meetings seemed to him unending, the anger and the accusations, terribly unjust. When Wilson suggested that Italy might not be entitled to all of the lands Yugoslavia also wanted, the Romans tore his pictures from their walls. Wilson said that Germany should not be so partitioned as to give France thousands of square miles of indubitably German soil, and Clemenceau accused him of favoring the Boches over his own allies. Under these pressures, the President grew thinner, more drawn, his hair grayer each day. The whole business seemed so useless, and he saw that he was surrounded by all the limitless European fears and hates.

On April 3, 1919, Wilson's voice failed, and he coughed without stopping. When Dr. Grayson took his temperature, it was 103 degrees; and the physician, in a panic, thought the President had been poisoned. A rumor had been running through Paris to the effect that President Wilson had been poisoned by means of germs slipped into his drinking water. Both Grayson and Mrs. Wilson stayed by the President's side all night; and, in the morning, Dr. Grayson made a medical diagnosis of influenza. Despite this, Wilson insisted on returning to his tasks. Thereupon, the French, Italian, and British premiers came to his bedside to resume the quarrels over who got what from whom. The relapse came, and Dr. Grayson absolutely forbade further work.

Shortly afterward, President Wilson showed a marked change in his demeanor. According to Smith's biography,[4] Wilson began to fret about the furniture of the house in which he was residing. Things were being taken, he felt, and he wanted every item in the residence listed. Carefully noting the use of the official cars, Wilson declared that they were for government business only, although earlier he had encouraged his pent-up and overworked staff to relax and refresh themselves by rides in the country. When he began to rearrange the furnishings of a room and Colonel House remonstrated that it would be more prudent to use some of the youthful aides for the physical labor, the President turned on him with the accusation that House wished to plant spies about him.

Fears of espionage haunted Wilson. He became possessed by the notion that all of the French employees about the place—servants, waiters, washerwomen, porters—were spies for the French, understood English perfectly, and reported to their government every word he uttered. Now he locked all his documents in a safe he kept by his side. In writing of this period later, Head Usher Ike Hoover said, "One thing was certain: he was never the same after this little spell of sickness."[5]

The danger illustrated by Wilson's case is, of course, that vital plans

---

[4] G. Smith, *When Cheering Stopped*. New York: Bantam Books, 1965, p. 48.
[5] N. P. Fabricant, *13 Famous Patients*. New York: Chilton Co., 1960, p. 8.

and conclusions about the peace of the planet may be shaped by a chronically exhausted man. Suppose such a man, beset with doubts and possessing the considerable vanity any successful politician has, were to suffer a serious blow to his self-esteem at the same time that his natural assessment powers were at low ebb because of chronic overwork. The net effect could be that he would become hypersensitive to any impressions others might leave; he might silently ponder aspects of others' conduct and weave out of these bits an imagined audience reaction related to his tormenting problem.

This is precisely what happened to James Forrestal, our first Secretary of Defense. It would be useful to examine Forrestal's psychosis in more detail, for it tells what behavior to expect when an important political figure starts to break down mentally.

One of the crucial points to note in the development of paranoid mentality, even more than the patent misinterpretations, is the inability to alter fixed ideas. On Forrestal's flight from Florida to the hospital at Bethesda, he expressed the opinion that he was undergoing his present "punishment" because he had been a "bad" Catholic. His badness consisted of having wed a divorcee and of neglecting his faith for the past three decades. Although Dr. William Menninger, the psychiatrist, and his closest friends, who were with him on the flight, repeatedly assured him that no one wished to hurt him and that no punishment was in store for him, Forrestal not only would not be persuaded, but in fact became even more disturbed. At the end of the trip, his friends had to restrain him by force from jumping out of the private auto that met them at the airport.[6]

But even before this incident, Forrestal had already shown another of the major signs of paranoia. He had built up, and lived in, a "pseudo-community" [7] peopled by his enemies, which led him to ascribe to actual persons around him a set of imaginary attitudes and functions. This was a danger easy to fall into in a position like Forrestal's, in which his unique duties had no precedents and thus needed to be worked out alone. His idiosyncratic perspectives evolved from both the necessary secrecy of high office and his own seclusive habits, and he could not check out his doubts and misgivings with others.

One result of this danger was that of accumulated misinterpretation. For instance, Forrestal expressed to Ferdinand Eberstadt, a close associate from civilian life, the view that his failure in office arose from the conspiracy of certain persons in the White House together with Communists and Zionists. "They" wished to ruin him and were hiding in his home now; to Eberstadt's consternation, Forrestal began to search areas in his house, such as closets, in which his enemies must surely be lurking.[6]

An increase of delusions tends to follow the crystallization of a paranoid "pseudo-community." In Forrestal's case, he at first only thought that people were persecuting him, but later he began to "see" the listening devices and other types of enemy equipment. At Hobe Sound, Florida, while walking the beach with Under-Secretary Robert Lovett, Forrestal pointed to metal

[6] A. A. Rogow, *James Forrestal*. New York: Macmillan, 1963, pp. 9, 5, 6, 51.
[7] N. Cameron, *American Journal of Sociology*, 65:52, 1959.

holders for beach umbrellas, which were driven into the sand, and said that nothing could be discussed because the sockets were wired and were recording every remark. Later, he talked about the forthcoming invasion of the United States by the Communists, and sometimes even appeared to believe that the invasion had already come.[6]

Along with fixed ideas of persecution, with the surrounding "pseudo-community" of enemies, with the widening circle of delusions, came a gradual deterioration of health and behavior. Secretary Forrestal, in the month before his resignation, showed loss of weight (in an already thin body) and appetite, stomach upsets, ceaseless exhaustion, and sleeplessness. He fretted over tiny details, postponed even small decisions, and made surprising mistakes in identity. He rubbed and scratched a part of his scalp until it remained irritated, and he continually dipped his fingers into the glass of water on his desk in order to wet his lips. On the day of his resignation, an aide found him sitting rigid in his office staring at the wall; when the assistant asked repeatedly, "Is something the matter?", Forrestal at last replied, "You are a loyal fellow." His growing confusion, another sign of deterioration, showed in his dazed inability to comprehend that, after his resignation, he was no longer entitled to an official limousine.

Finally, and seemingly inevitably, on May 22, 1949, at Bethesda Naval Hospital, Forrestal walked into the kitchen and jumped to his death through the nearby window. He was the highest ranking American official ever to have killed himself.

A biographer, Rogow,[6] impressed with the importance of the problem of how to deal with mental disability in high office, has suggested, "... the most lasting tribute to James Forrestal would be a massive effort to reduce the incidence of physical and mental breakdown in political life." That the inhuman strains of high office are as great today as they ever have been has been attested to by Washington correspondent James Reston:[8]

> It would be hard to overestimate the physical and nervous tension on the men at the top of this government.
> They are on the go 18 hours a day, and in the President's case, often longer: endless conferences, constant testimony on Capitol Hill, a succession of tedious ceremonial dinners, pressure for more bombing, pressure for less bombing—all this, and a constant drumfire of criticism at home and abroad. The Johnson system here is based on the assumption that men can do whatever they have to do.... It is a dubious assumption.

Along with the probability that tension and stress in high office will remain at barely tolerable levels goes the estimate that mental and physical breakdown will increase among our decision-makers. Reston[8] notes the particular irritability and contradictoriness of President Johnson under incessant strains: "One day he appeals for support of his war policies. The next day he cries impatiently for patience. One day he reaches out to his critics for understanding, and next he lashes out at them as 'Nervous

---

[8] J. Reston, "A Tired, Tense Administration." San Francisco *Chronicle*, May 20, 1966.

Nellies' and shatters his prize consensus with peremptory demands for 'unity.' "

To provide against the danger of mental disability, there is the so-called "Disability Amendment" to the Constitution. One provision is that, if the President certifies in writing that he considers himself disabled, the Vice President may take over the duties until the President states in writing that his disability is ended. Yet, considering the great possibility that a presidential psychosis would be paranoia, and since a paranoiac is always most resistant to the suggestion that he is mentally ill, it is precisely this presidential admission of disability that is least likely to be forthcoming.

The amendment further provides that, in case the disabled President refuses to declare himself out of office, the Vice President, with the consent of a majority in the Congress and in the Cabinet, can become Acting President by declaring the President unable to operate. But, if the President disagrees, it requires a two-thirds vote of the entire Congress to overrule his disagreement. Therefore, it is at least conceivable that, for a while, a paranoid man would be Chief Executive, wielding full power.

The syndrome of paranoia carries with it not only deterioration of intellectual activities, but also strongly increased feelings of insecurity. It must be remembered that aggressive action offers an illusory security to the leader and his followers. For a paranoid political leader, war may appear as an appropriate action to counter the psychological insecurities that he feels personally and that he imagines to exist in the country at large. Wars have been waged before in the name of national security.

The bizarre possibilities of paranoia come to a sum in this inventive dialogue by Lenny Bruce:[9]

We're 17,000 students who have marched from Annapolis, and we demand to see the bomb.

Ah'd like to see it mahself, son.

Aw, c'mon, now, let's see the bomb, we're not gonna hurt anybody, we just wanna take a few pictures, then we'll protest, and that's it.

...But there is no bomb. Just something we keep in the White House garage. We spent three million dollars on it, and once we got it started, it just made a lot of noise and smelled up the whole house, so we haven't fooled with it since.

Now wait a minute. You see, I led the march, and I've got 17,000 students that are protesting the bomb. So don't tell me there's no bomb.

Son, Ah'd like to help you if Ah could. If Ah had a bomb....

But what am I gonna tell all those poor kids out there? That there's no bomb?

The only thing that did work out was the button.

What button?

The button that the madmen are always gonna push.

That's what the bomb is—a button?

Yes—it's a button.

Well ... give me the button, then.

---

[9] L. Bruce, *An Autobiography.* Chicago: Playboy Press, 1963, pp. 223–24.

A psychohistorical perspective of the negro

ROBERT H. SHARPLEY, M.D.

The inner city man, the ghetto dweller, the hard-core American, are but a few of the synonymous terms applied to the men whose current plight represents America's domestic crisis. These men, subject of innumerable studies, have a genesis and history that is intricately woven into the fabric of America, but what makes the thread of their lives so poignant is that the color of their thread is black. It is black because of the pigmentation of their skins and because of the dark deeds they have been subjected to for the past 300 years and are currently trying to change.

To establish a frame of reference we should perhaps define the man, his historical development, the effects of both past and present society on his psychosocial genesis and development, and the relevance of these things to his current posture. The man I am discussing is called colored, Negro, Afro-American, or Black American—but still, even though oft overlooked, a human being.

He is a human being found in all strata of American society; hence, the degree and type of social interaction he experiences with his non-black counterparts vary in style and intensity. What do not vary, but delineate him from other Americans, are the limitations placed on the man because of the hue of his skin.

Historically he is like many others who came to this country in 1619— i.e., a mature individual in a new land with unlimited potentials; however, because of pigmentation, regression was enforced upon him and a pathological social system was created. Black Americans are today demanding treatment and cure of this system, which at its best infantilized and at its worst dehumanized.

Comparison of two western hemisphere systems

If one compares American slavery to slavery in other parts of the world, one sees, as described quite well by Nathan Glazer, that

A PSYCHOHISTORICAL PERSPECTIVE OF THE NEGRO Reprinted from *The American Journal of Psychiatry*, volume 126, pages 645–650, 1969. Copyright 1969, The American Psychiatric Association. Reprinted by permission of the publisher and the author.

American slavery was the most awful the world has ever known. . . . The slave was totally removed from the protection of organized society (compare the elaborate provisions for the protection of slaves in the Bible), his existence as a human being was given no recognition by any religious or secular agency, he was totally ignorant of and completely cut off from his past, and he was offered absolutely no hope for the future. His children could be sold, his marriage was not recognized, his wife could be violated or sold (there was something comic about calling the woman with whom the master permitted him to live a "wife"), and he could also be subject, without redress, to frightful barbarities—there were presumably as many sadists among slaveholders, men and women, as there are in other groups. The slave could not by law, be taught to read or write; he could not practice religion without the permission of his master, and he could never meet with his fellows, for any religious or other purposes, except in the presence of a white; and finally, if a master wished to free him, every legal obstacle was used to thwart such action. This is not what slavery meant in the ancient world, in the medieval and early modern Europe, or in Brazil and the West Indies.

In Brazil, the slave had many more rights than in the United States: he could legally marry, he could, indeed had to, be baptized and become a member of the Catholic Church, his family could not be broken up for sale, and he had many days on which he could either rest or earn money to buy his freedom. The government encouraged manumission, and the freedom of infants could often be purchased for a small sum at the baptismal font. In short: the Brazilian slave knew he was a man, and that he differed in degree, not in kind, from his master.[1]

Effects of the system

The effects of the system are not just a horrible historical curiosity but are still felt by today's Negro, seen in the plight of today's Negro, and greatly influence the thinking of today's non-Negro. Questions and comments of today's whites, to the effect that blacks are innately shiftless, childish, and unmotivated, reflect not only the effects of the system and the limitations it has placed on some people's thinking, but also the lack of complete comprehension of what the system was geared to do and what the Afro-American of today is trying to do. The work of Thomas Pettigrew refutes the idea of innate negative traits and supports the implications of the total effects of the system:

The profound personality change created by Nazi internment, as independently reported by a number of psychologists and psychiatrists who survived, was toward childishness and total acceptance of the SS guards as father figures—a syndrome strikingly similar to the "Sambo" caricature of the Southern slave.

[1] S. M. Elkins, *Slavery*. Chicago: University of Chicago Press, 1959.

153

Nineteenth century racists readily believed that the "Sambo" personality was simply an inborn racial type. Yet no African anthropological data have ever shown any personality type resembling Sambo: and the concentration camps molded the equivalent personality pattern in a wide variety of Caucasian prisoners. Nor was Sambo merely a product of "slavery" in the abstract, for the less devastating Latin American system never developed such a system.

Extending this line of reasoning, psychologists point out that slavery in all its forms sharply lowered the need for achievement in slaves. ... Negroes in bondage, stripped of their African heritage, were placed in a completely dependent role. All of their rewards came, not from individual initiative and enterprise, but from absolute obedience—a situation that severely depresses the need for achievement among all peoples.[2]

Psychosocial development

Acknowledging these historical facts, one might still wonder if after 300 years there is a difference between the psychosocial development of the Black American and that of his white counterpart. In this writer's opinion there is. Comparison of the Negro's psychosocial development with the Freudian psychodynamic development chart shows that the Afro-American is now actively engaged in reaching for maturity in many ways.

The initial stage of development is the oral stage. During this time the individual is completely dependent on his provider and trust and mistrust are developed. Following this is the muscular anal stage, which is hallmarked by the individual's becoming aware of autonomy and learning to handle aggression for positive or negative reasons. In the genital stage initiative and guilt are of greatest significance. Latency, the fourth stage and last part of childhood, provides a period when the individual learns to produce for recognition, develops a sense of industry, and gets satisfaction from completing tasks. His violent drives are dormant. One witnesses the lull before the storm that is part of adolescence.

Adolescence is hallmarked by rapid growth, search for identity, questioning of fundamental concepts, reality testing, attempts to connect and relate earlier learned skills and knowledge with the present. The ego identity is jelled. As Erikson states:

> The sense of ego identity then is the accrued confidence that the inner sameness and continuity prepared in the past are matched by the sameness and continuity of one's meaning for others, as evidenced in the tangible promise of a career....
>
> For support adolescents not only help one another temporarily through much discomfort by forming cliques and by stereotyping themselves, their ideals, and their enemies: they also perversely test each other's capacity to pledge fidelity.

[2] T. Pettigrew, *A Profile of the Negro American.*

The adolescent mind is essentially a mind of the moratorium, a psychosocial stage between childhood and adulthood, and between the morality learned by the child, and the ethics to be developed by the adult. It is an ideological mind—and, indeed, it is the ideological outlook of a society that speaks most clearly to the adolescent who is eager to be affirmed by his peers, and is ready to be confirmed by rituals, creeds, and programs which at the same time define what is evil, uncanny, and inimical. In searching for the social values which guide identity, one therefore confronts the problems of ideology and aristocracy, both in their widest possible sense which connotes, that within a defined world image and a predestined course of history, the best people will come to rule and rule develops the best in people. In order not to become cynically or apathetically lost, young people must somehow be able to convince themselves that those who succeed in their anticipated adult world thereby shoulder the obligation of being the best.[3]

I have discussed only five stages and shall not discuss the other three, for in preparing this discourse I have tried to provide the analogue for what I feel the problem of today represents. The remaining levels of development for the people discussed in this paper are unreached goals and hang before the inner city dweller like the grapes before Tantalus.

To support this analogue we can look at the history of slavery and see that mature men were placed in a system that caused regression to oral stages or complete dependency. Kenneth Stampp describes in *The Peculiar Institution* how mature men were forced into compliant positions and hence regressed:

1. ...Unconditional submission is the only footing upon which slavery should be placed....the slave should know that his master is to govern absolutely and he is to obey implicitly. That he is never for a moment to exercise will or judgment in opposition to a positive order. 2. Make the slave feel inferior....they must be made to feel that African ancestry tainted them, that their color was a badge of degradation. 3. ...awe them with a sense of their master's enormous power. 4. ...persuade the bondsman to take an interest in the master's enterprise and to accept his standards of good conduct. 5. Impress Negroes with their helplessness: to create in them "a habit of perfect dependence" upon their masters.[4]

For such a code to develop and be printed makes it palpably clear that the first Negroes were not the shiftless, unthinking, infantile people they are oft stereotyped and considered by many to be, historically and innately.

The Civil War dissolved not only the shackles of slavery but also the program of enforced dependency. The reconstruction era permitted the Negro transient political power and social freedom, but a decade later his

[3] E. H. Erikson, *Childhood and Society.* New York: W. W. Norton & Co., 1963.
[4] K. Stampp, *The Peculiar Institution.* New York: Alfred A. Knopf, 1956.

sense of autonomy was severely limited and the trust he had begun to develop was quickly transformed to mistrust. The next few decades witnessed the emergence of Negro institutions, limited acquisition of property, and efforts to gain education. Undoubtedly, initiative was easily found.

The fourth stage has occupied much of the 20th century. From local sports centers to Olympic stadiums, from industrial assembly lines to research laboratory desks, from neighborhood churches to concert stage, and in most other spheres of endeavor, the Negro has developed a sense of industry, received satisfaction from completing tasks, and learned to get recognition by production. The latter has been most important, for recognition has not always meant freedom. The search for this is part of his present quest and current status. During World War II, the Negro gained better jobs, improved housing, better education, travel experience, and a chance to see, compare, and think about the living conditions of others nationally and internationally. He also got a look at the performance of others and saw that given the same opportunity to try a task, he could get the same result. Involvement with the war and later with postwar problems, and feeling that the promises of improvement in the future would soon be realized, he repressed his anxieties and let his aggression remain latent. It was the quiet before the storm. The past 16 years have been the stage on which the race problem has been dealing with tasks commonly seen in individual psychosexual development. These tasks are addressed any time there is a power differential.

Maturity and freedom

Adolescence, as noted previously, includes the period of rapid growth, with disappointment, frustration, rage, peer grouping, reality testing, and attempts to connect and relate earlier learned skills and knowledge with present. If we focus on the evolution of the Afro-American in the American society we will see that most of these things are now true. Since the Civil Rights Act of 1952 and the Montgomery bus boycott of 1953, the status of the Black American has shown considerable growth on a relative basis but woefully insufficient growth on an absolute scale—i.e., on the history of a country that is 300 years old.

Disappointment is inevitable for the Negro if one looks at contemporary history. The Supreme Court decision and the bus boycott led to hope, promises for a brighter future, a belief in social, political, and economic change, and—most important—that these changes could be wrought in a nonviolent manner. Hence the Negro felt he could endure and indeed demonstrated endurance. Reality testing of the current situation has not helped. Trite clichés have stressed that more education, attainment of skills, improved speech, greater appreciation of cultural norms, and increased buying power would remedy problems and raise the Negro to the position of his white counterpart. Many have studied and successfully attained these marks only to find positions unavailable to them. Negro youth and adults who have attempted to relate previously learned skills to opportunities available find that they cannot be employed. Department of Commerce statistics indicate that the unemployment rate of nonwhites with a high school education is greater than that of white high school dropouts. White society has assumed certain prerogatives that have been labeled or understood to represent maturity. When the Negro has turned to mature society he has found deceit, hypocrisy, credibility chasms, and objects that he feels he not only cannot identify with but must also reject. The Black American's high hopes are shattered from 16 years of snail-like progress as well as the progressive increases in resistance to change. Residual mistrust is mushrooming, and despair and rage are the result.

Perhaps we should look again at the goal of adolescence, the factors necessary for progressing to maturity, and the factors that hinder progress. Although the person in the pubertal stage is oft confused, frightened, and unsure of his actions, he is striving for emancipation from dependence and achievement of maturity. The Black American is looking for exactly this—which represents freedom. Freedom, as defined by Martin Luther King, is the essence of man, or as Tillich says, "Man is man because he is free." Freedom means "the capacity to deliberate or weigh alternatives; to express oneself in discretion; and to take responsibility." [5]

In the analytic model it has been shown that the parental figures usually voice desires to emancipate their youngsters but demonstrate contradictions. The parents, symbols of maturity, frequently express worries, doubts, and fears that the adolescent is not only unable to function independently but also that unknown danger and harm will befall the unguided pre-adult. The parents have strong wishes to retain control and find it difficult to share the adolescent's love with others.

In our analogue we see that the desire to maintain dominance and control is partially the result of unreal and shortsighted economic, political, and social reasons as well as deep-seated guilt feelings. The latter lies especially with those who believe in Newton's basic law and thus fear a mammoth revenge. It also lies with those who are willing to help decorate the stale cakes of the ghetto but not permit the ghetto man to shop for his own flour.

Results of thwarted growth

In the early '60s, it was felt that change could come from love. Now some are trying this doctrine, as exemplified by followers of the late Martin Luther King, and others, more impatient, feel force is better. In both cases I believe there is a desperation that the Negro is trying to communicate at any level where he feels he will be heard. It is typified by the youngster in Watts who, when asked what did the riot accomplish when his own home

[5] M. L. King, Jr., *Where Do We Go From Here: Chaos or Community?* Boston: Beacon Press, 1967.

and neighborhood were destroyed, answered: "We won because we made them pay attention to us." [6] What he did not say was that peer solidarity had produced an effect.

Whether by force or love, both reactions are also geared toward communicating the identity problem that all Americans must face, as well as the inaction they must overcome. This idea is best expressed by James Baldwin:

> The really terrible thing, old buddy, is that YOU must accept THEM. And I mean that very seriously. You must accept them and accept them with love. For these innocent people have no other hope. They are, in effect, still trapped in a history which they do not understand; and until they understand it, they cannot be released from it. They have had to believe for many years, and for innumerable reasons, that black men are inferior to white men. Many of them, indeed, know better, but, as you will discover, people find it very difficult to act on what they know. To act is to be committed, and to be committed is to be in danger. In this case, the danger, in the minds of most white Americans, is the loss of identity.... But these men are your brothers—your lost, younger, brothers. And if the word INTEGRATION means anything, this is what it means: that we, with love, shall force our brothers to see themselves as they are, to cease fleeing from reality and begin to change it....[7]

The desire to retain dominance and control has furthered the resistance to social change and perpetuated the racism. Racism as defined by Ruth Benedict is "the dogma that one ethnic group is condemned by nature to hereditary inferiority and another group is destined to hereditary superiority." [8] By this definition we see that power is given to one group over the other, which can be dangerous, for "... power is never good unless he who has it is good." [9] The cry from the ghetto, the black man's history, and one of the black man's dilemmas is that power resides neither with good figures nor with himself. He is now stating that he must have power over himself to be free, for freedom is also participation in power.

The cry for power is the effort to regain full masculinity and maturity. Historically the Negro male has been looked upon as chattel or for reproductive purposes. Marriage was not permitted, paternalism was ignored, and a sense of worth and maturity was destroyed. Females could absorb some sense of value because their positions as domestics were not always as degraded, and daily encounters were not always so humiliating. The male, even after the abolition of slavery, found that work was unavailable, he was still dominated by another man, and that in the labor pool he was less in demand than the female. Unfortunately this has prevailed to the present. The Black American of today in his new assertion of manhood is not looking

---

[6] *Ibid.*
[7] J. Baldwin, *The Fire Next Time.* New York: Dial Press, 1963.
[8] King, *op. cit.*
[9] *Ibid.*

for love but for justice, not for patronage but for empathy, not for paternalism but for the freedom of maturity.

The adolescent frequently hides his anxiety, fear, uncertainty, and despair behind rebellious behavior. This is not unlike our inner city dweller. The ghetto dweller lives in a restricted world that the outside cannot totally comprehend; but the ghetto dweller watches and notes with care the behavior of the outside world. His main drive is to join the outside world as quickly as possible. His disappointment with the effects of nonviolence and continued waiting have pushed him to Black Power, which is "a cry of disappointment . . . a call to mass political and economic strength to achieve . . . a psychological call to manhood." [10]

The negro's attitudes

I have tried to give an analogy of the tasks that confront the Negro as a people and confront children in their psychosexual growth. I have not discussed the substages of adolescence or the dynamics of this stage as particularly reflected in racial activity following Dr. King's death. I hope to do this in a later paper. I have discussed characteristics that are not found in every single Black American, but are representative of most. What I have not mentioned is his feeling throughout these phases. Three words and three quotes will suffice. The words are: pain, despair, and resignation. The quotes are: "If you are born in America with a black skin, you're in prison. . . ." "It doesn't matter any longer what you do to me; you can put me in jail, you can kill me. By the time I was seventeen, you'd done everything that you can to me. The problem now is how are you going to save yourselves." "There isn't a lot of time. Time is running out. And the Negro is making it palpably clear that he wants all of his rights, that he wants them here and that he wants them now." [11]

---

[10] *Ibid.*

[11] *Ebony* Magazine, "The White Problem in America." Chicago: Johnson Publishing Co., 1966.

The culture
of poverty

OSCAR LEWIS

Poverty and the so-called war against it provide a principal theme for the domestic program of the present Administration. In the midst of a population that enjoys unexampled material well-being—with the average annual family income exceeding $7,000—it is officially acknowledged that some 18 million families, numbering more than 50 million individuals, live below the $3,000 "poverty line." Toward the improvement of the lot of these people some $1,600 million of Federal funds are directly allocated through the Office of Economic Opportunity, and many hundreds of millions of additional dollars flow indirectly through expanded Federal expenditures in the fields of health, education, welfare and urban affairs.

Along with the increase in activity on behalf of the poor indicated by these figures there has come a parallel expansion of publication in the social sciences on the subject of poverty. The new writings advance the same two opposed evaluations of the poor that are to be found in literature, in proverbs and in popular sayings throughout recorded history. Just as the poor have been pronounced blessed, virtuous, upright, serene, independent, honest, kind and happy, so contemporary students stress their great and neglected capacity for self-help, leadership and community organization. Conversely, as the poor have been characterized as shiftless, mean, sordid, violent, evil and criminal, so other students point to the irreversibly destructive effects of poverty on individual character and emphasize the corresponding need to keep guidance and control of poverty projects in the hands of duly constituted authorities. This clash of viewpoints reflects in part the infighting for political control of the program between Federal and local officials. The confusion results also from the tendency to focus study and attention on the personality of the individual victim of poverty rather than on the slum community and family and from the consequent failure to distinguish between poverty and what I have called the culture of poverty.

The phrase is a catchy one and is used and misused with some frequency in the current literature. In my writings it is the label for a specific conceptual model that describes in positive terms a subculture of Western society with its own structure and rationale, a way of life handed on from generation to generation along family lines. The culture of poverty is not just a matter of deprivation or disorganization, a term signifying the absence of something. It is a culture in the traditional anthropological sense in that it provides human beings with a design for living, with a ready-made set of solutions for human problems, and so serves a significant adaptive function. This style of life transcends national boundaries and regional and rural-urban differences within nations. Wherever it occurs, its practitioners exhibit remarkable similarity in the structure of their families, in interpersonal relations, in spending habits, in their value systems and in their orientation in time.

Not nearly enough is known about this important complex of human behavior. My own concept of it has evolved as my work has progressed and remains subject to amendment by my own further work and that of others. The scarcity of literature on the culture of poverty is a measure of the gap in communication that exists between the very poor and the middle-class personnel—social scientists, social workers, teachers, physicians, priests and others—who bear the major responsibility for carrying out the antipoverty programs. Much of the behavior accepted in the culture of poverty goes counter to cherished ideals of the larger society. In writing about "multi-problem" families social scientists thus often stress their instability, their lack of order, direction and organization. Yet, as I have observed them, their behavior seems clearly patterned and reasonably predictable. I am more often struck by the inexorable repetitiousness and the iron entrenchment of their lifeways.

The concept of the culture of poverty may help to correct misapprehensions that have ascribed some behavior patterns of ethnic, national or regional groups as distinctive characteristics. For example, a high incidence of common-law marriage and of households headed by women has been thought to be distinctive of Negro family life in this country and has been attributed to the Negro's historical experience of slavery. In actuality it turns out that such households express essential traits of the culture of poverty and are found among diverse peoples in many parts of the world and among peoples that have had no history of slavery. Although it is now possible to assert such generalizations, there is still much to be learned about this difficult and affecting subject. The absence of intensive anthropological studies of poor families in a wide variety of national contexts—particularly the lack of such studies in socialist countries—remains a serious handicap to the formulation of dependable cross-cultural constants of the culture of poverty.

My studies of poverty and family life have centered largely in Mexico. On occasion some of my Mexican friends have suggested delicately that I turn to a study of poverty in my own country. As a first step in this direction I am currently engaged in a study of Puerto Rican families. Over the past three years my staff and I have been assembling data on 100 repre-

161

sentative families in four slums of Greater San Juan and some 50 families of their relatives in New York City.

Our methods combine the traditional techniques of sociology, anthropology and psychology. This includes a battery of 19 questionnaires, the administration of which requires 12 hours per informant. They cover the residence and employment history of each adult; family relations; income and expenditure; complete inventory of household and personal possessions; friendship patterns, particularly the *compadrazgo*, or godparent, relationship that serves as a kind of informal social security for the children of these families and establishes special obligations among the adults; recreational patterns; health and medical history; politics; religion; world view and "cosmopolitanism." Open-end interviews and psychological tests (such as the thematic apperception test, the Rorschach test and the sentence-completion test) are administered to a sampling of this population.

All this work serves to establish the context for close-range study of a selected few families. Because the family is a small social system, it lends itself to the holistic approach of anthropology. Whole-family studies bridge the gap between the conceptual extremes of the culture at one pole and of the individual at the other, making possible observation of both culture and personality as they are interrelated in real life. In a large metropolis such as San Juan or New York the family is the natural unit of study.

Ideally our objective is the naturalistic observation of the life of "our" families, with a minimum of intervention. Such intensive study, however, necessarily involves the establishment of deep personal ties. My assistants include two Mexicans whose families I had studied; their "Mexican's-eye view" of the Puerto Rican slum has helped to point up the similarities and differences between the Mexican and Puerto Rican subcultures. We have spent many hours attending family parties, wakes and baptisms, responding to emergency calls, taking people to the hospital, getting them out of jail, filling out applications for them, hunting apartments with them, helping them to get jobs or to get on relief. With each member of these families we conduct tape-recorded interviews, taking down their life stories and their answers to questions on a wide variety of topics. For the ordering of our material we undertake to reconstruct, by close interrogation, the history of a week or more of consecutive days in the lives of each family, and we observe and record complete days as they unfold. The first volume to issue from this study is to be published next month under the title of *La Vida, a Puerto Rican Family in the Culture of Poverty—San Juan and New York* (Random House).

There are many poor people in the world. Indeed, the poverty of the two-thirds of the world's population who live in the underdeveloped countries has been rightly called "the problem of problems." But not all of them by any means live in the culture of poverty. For this way of life to come into being and flourish it seems clear that certain preconditions must be met.

The setting is a cash economy, with wage labor and production for profit and with a persistently high rate of unemployment and underemployment, at low wages, for unskilled labor. The society fails to provide social, political and economic organization, on either a voluntary basis or by government imposition, for the low-income population. There is a bilateral kinship system centered on the nuclear progenitive family, as distinguished from the unilateral extended kinship system of lineage and clan. The dominant class asserts a set of values that prizes thrift and the accumulation of wealth and property, stresses the possibility of upward mobility and explains low economic status as the result of individual personal inadequacy and inferiority.

Where these conditions prevail the way of life that develops among some of the poor is the culture of poverty. That is why I have described it as a subculture of the Western social order. It is both an adaptation and a reaction of the poor to their marginal position in a class-stratified, highly individuated, capitalistic society. It represents an effort to cope with feelings of hopelessness and despair that arise from the realization by the members of the marginal communities in these societies of the improbability of their achieving success in terms of the prevailing values and goals. Many of the traits of the culture of poverty can be viewed as local, spontaneous attempts to meet needs not served in the case of the poor by the institutions and agencies of the larger society because the poor are not eligible for such service, cannot afford it or are ignorant and suspicious.

Once the culture of poverty has come into existence it tends to perpetuate itself. By the time slum children are six or seven they have usually absorbed the basic attitudes and values of their subculture. Thereafter they are psychologically unready to take full advantage of changing conditions or improving opportunities that may develop in their lifetime.

My studies have identified some 70 traits that characterize the culture of poverty. The principal ones may be described in four dimensions of the system: the relationship between the subculture and the larger society; the nature of the slum community; the nature of the family, and the attitudes, values and character structure of the individual.

The disengagement, the nonintegration, of the poor with respect to the major institutions of society is a crucial element in the culture of poverty. It reflects the combined effect of a variety of factors including poverty, to begin with, but also segregation and discrimination, fear, suspicion and apathy and the development of alternative institutions and procedures in the slum community. The people do not belong to labor unions or political parties and make little use of banks, hospitals, department stores or museums. Such involvement as there is in the institutions of the larger society —in the jails, the army and the public welfare system—does little to suppress the traits of the culture of poverty. A relief system that barely keeps people alive perpetuates rather than eliminates poverty and the pervading sense of hopelessness.

People in a culture of poverty produce little wealth and receive little in return. Chronic unemployment and underemployment, low wages, lack of property, lack of savings, absence of food reserves in the home and chronic shortage of cash imprison the family and the individual in a vicious circle.

Thus for lack of cash the slum householder makes frequent purchases of small quantities of food at higher prices. The slum economy turns inward; it shows a high incidence of pawning of personal goods, borrowing at usurious rates of interest, informal credit arrangements among neighbors, use of secondhand clothing and furniture.

There is awareness of middle-class values. People talk about them and even claim some of them as their own. On the whole, however, they do not live by them. They will declare that marriage by law, by the church or by both is the ideal form of marriage, but few will marry. For men who have no steady jobs, no property and no prospect of wealth to pass on to their children, who live in the present without expectations of the future, who want to avoid the expense and legal difficulties involved in marriage and divorce, a free union or consensual marriage makes good sense. The women, for their part, will turn down offers of marriage from men who are likely to be immature, punishing and generally unreliable. They feel that a consensual union gives them some of the freedom and flexibility men have. By not giving the fathers of their children legal status as husbands, the women have a stronger claim on the children. They also maintain exclusive rights to their own property.

Along with disengagement from the larger society, there is a hostility to the basic institutions of what are regarded as the dominant classes. There is hatred of the police, mistrust of government and of those in high positions and a cynicism that extends to the church. The culture of poverty thus holds a certain potential for protest and for entrainment in political movements aimed against the existing order.

With its poor housing and overcrowding, the community of the culture of poverty is high in gregariousness, but it has a minimum of organization beyond the nuclear and extended family. Occasionally slum dwellers come together in temporary informal groupings; neighborhood gangs that cut across slum settlements represent a considerable advance beyond the zero point of the continuum I have in mind. It is the low level of organization that gives the culture of poverty its marginal and anomalous quality in our highly organized society. Most primitive peoples have achieved a higher degree of sociocultural organization than contemporary urban slum dwellers. This is not to say that there may not be a sense of community and *esprit de corps* in a slum neighborhood. In fact, where slums are isolated from their surroundings by enclosing walls or other physical barriers, where rents are low and residence is stable and where the population constitutes a distinct ethnic, racial or language group, the sense of community may approach that of a village. In Mexico City and San Juan such territoriality is engendered by the scarcity of low-cost housing outside of established slum areas. In South Africa it is actively enforced by the *apartheid* that confines rural migrants to prescribed locations.

The family in the culture of poverty does not cherish childhood as a specially prolonged and protected stage in the life cycle. Initiation into sex comes early. With the instability of consensual marriage the family tends to be mother-centered and tied more closely to the mother's extended family. The female head of the house is given to authoritarian rule. In spite of much verbal emphasis on family solidarity, sibling rivalry for the limited supply of goods and maternal affection is intense. There is little privacy.

The individual who grows up in this culture has a strong feeling of fatalism, helplessness, dependence and inferiority. These traits, so often remarked in the current literature as characteristic of the American Negro, I found equally strong in slum dwellers of Mexico City and San Juan, who are not segregated or discriminated against as a distinct ethnic or racial group. Other traits include a high incidence of weak ego structure, orality and confusion of sexual identification, all reflecting maternal deprivation; a strong present-time orientation with relatively little disposition to defer gratification and plan for the future, and a high tolerance for psychological pathology of all kinds. There is widespread belief in male superiority and among the men a strong preoccupation with *machismo*, their masculinity.

Provincial and local in outlook, with little sense of history, these people know only their own neighborhood and their own way of life. Usually they do not have the knowledge, the vision or the ideology to see the similarities between their troubles and those of their counterparts elsewhere in the world. They are not class-conscious, although they are sensitive indeed to symbols of status.

The distinction between poverty and the culture of poverty is basic to the model described here. There are numerous examples of poor people whose way of life I would not characterize as belonging to this subculture. Many primitive and preliterate peoples that have been studied by anthropologists suffer dire poverty attributable to low technology or thin resources or both. Yet even the simplest of these peoples have a high degree of social organization and a relatively integrated, satisfying and self-sufficient culture.

In India the destitute lower-caste peoples—such as the Chamars, the leatherworkers, and the Bhangis, the sweepers—remain integrated in the larger society and have their own panchayat institutions of self-government. Their panchayats and their extended unilateral kinship systems, or clans, cut across village lines, giving them a strong sense of identity and continuity. In my studies of these peoples I found no culture of poverty to go with their poverty.

The Jews of eastern Europe were a poor urban people, often confined to ghettos. Yet they did not have many traits of the culture of poverty. They had a tradition of literacy that placed great value on learning; they formed many voluntary associations and adhered with devotion to the central community organization around the rabbi, and they had a religion that taught them they were the chosen people.

I would cite also a fourth, somewhat speculative example of poverty dissociated from the culture of poverty. On the basis of limited direct observation in one country—Cuba—and from indirect evidence, I am inclined to believe the culture of poverty does not exist in socialist countries. In 1947 I undertook a study of a slum in Havana. Recently I had an opportunity to revisit the same slum and some of the same families. The physical aspect of the place had changed little, except for a beautiful new nursery school. The people were as poor as before, but I was impressed to find much less of the feelings of despair and apathy, so symptomatic of the culture of poverty in the urban slums of the U.S. The slum was now highly organized, with block committees, educational committees, party committees. The people had found a new sense of power and importance in a doctrine that glorified the lower class as the hope of humanity, and they were armed. I was told by one Cuban official that the Castro government had practically eliminated delinquency by giving arms to the delinquents!

Evidently the Castro regime—revising Marx and Engels—did not write off the so-called *lumpenproletariat* as an inherently reactionary and antirevolutionary force but rather found in them a revolutionary potential and utilized it. Frantz Fanon, in his book *The Wretched of the Earth*, makes a similar evaluation of their role in the Algerian revolution: "It is within this mass of humanity, this people of the shantytowns, at the core of the *lumpenproletariat*, that the rebellion will find its urban spearhead. For the *lumpenproletariat*, that horde of starving men, uprooted from their tribe and from their clan, constitutes one of the most spontaneous and most radically revolutionary forces of a colonized people."

It is true that I have found little revolutionary spirit or radical ideology among low-income Puerto Ricans. Most of the families I studied were politically conservative, about half of them favoring the Statehood Republican Party, which provides opposition on the right to the Popular Democratic Party that dominates the politics of the commonwealth. It seems to me, therefore, that disposition for protest among people living in the culture of poverty will vary considerably according to the national context and historical circumstances. In contrast to Algeria, the independence movement in Puerto Rico has found little popular support. In Mexico, where the cause of independence carried long ago, there is no longer any such movement to stir the dwellers in the new and old slums of the capital city.

Yet it would seem that any movement—be it religious, pacifist or revolutionary—that organizes and gives hope to the poor and effectively promotes a sense of solidarity with larger groups must effectively destroy the psychological and social core of the culture of poverty. In this connection, I suspect that the civil rights movement among American Negroes has of itself done more to improve their self-image and self-respect than such economic gains as it has won although, without doubt, the two kinds of progress are mutually reinforcing. In the culture of poverty of the American Negro the additional disadvantage of racial discrimination has generated a potential for revolutionary protest and organization that is absent in the slums of San Juan and Mexico City and, for that matter, among the poor whites in the South.

If it is true, as I suspect, that the culture of poverty flourishes and is endemic to the free-enterprise, pre-welfare-state stage of capitalism, then it is also endemic in colonial societies. The most likely candidates for the culture of poverty would be the people who come from the lower strata of a rapidly changing society and who are already partially alienated from it. Accordingly the subculture is likely to be found where imperial conquest has smashed the native social and economic structure and held the natives, perhaps for generations, in servile status, or where feudalism is yielding to capitalism in the later evolution of a colonial economy. Landless rural workers who migrate to the cities, as in Latin America, can be expected to fall into this way of life more readily than migrants from stable peasant villages with a well-organized traditional culture, as in India. It remains to be seen, however, whether the culture of poverty has not already begun to develop in the slums of Bombay and Calcutta. Compared with Latin America also, the strong corporate nature of many African tribal societies may tend to inhibit or delay the formation of a full-blown culture of poverty in the new towns and cities of that continent. In South Africa the institution-alization of repression and discrimination under *apartheid* may also have begun to promote an immunizing sense of identity and group consciousness among the African Negroes.

One must therefore keep the dynamic aspects of human institutions for-ward in observing and assessing the evidence for the presence, the waxing or the waning of this subculture. Measured on the dimension of relationship to the larger society, some slum dwellers may have a warmer identification with their national tradition even though they suffer deeper poverty than members of a similar community in another country. In Mexico City a high percentage of our respondents, including those with little or no formal schooling, knew of Cuauhtémoc, Hidalgo, Father Morelos, Juárez, Díaz, Zapata, Carranza and Cárdenas. In San Juan the names of Rámon Power, José de Diego, Baldorioty de Castro, Rámon Betances, Nemesio Canales, Lloréns Torres rang no bell; a few could tell about the late Albizu Campos. For the lower-income Puerto Rican, however, history begins with Muñoz Rivera and ends with his son Muñoz Marín.

The national context can make a big difference in the play of the crucial traits of fatalism and hopelessness. Given the advanced technology, the high level of literacy, the all-pervasive reach of the media of mass communi-cations and the relatively high aspirations of all sectors of the population, even the poorest and most marginal communities of the U.S. must aspire to a larger future than the slum dwellers of Ecuador and Peru, where the actual possibilities are more limited and when an authoritarian social order persists in city and country. Among the 50 million U.S. citizens now more or less officially certified as poor, I would guess that about 20 percent live in a culture of poverty. The largest numbers in this group are made up of Negroes, Puerto Ricans, Mexicans, American Indians and Southern poor whites. In these figures there is some reassurance for those concerned, because it is much more difficult to undo the culture of poverty than to cure poverty itself.

Middle-class people—this would certainly include most social scientists—tend to concentrate on the negative aspects of the culture of poverty. They attach a minus sign to such traits as present-time orientation and readiness to indulge impulses. I do not intend to idealize or romanticize the culture of poverty—"it is easier to praise poverty than to live in it." Yet the positive aspects of these traits must not be overlooked. Living in the present may develop a capacity for spontaneity, for the enjoyment of the sensual, which is often blunted in the middle-class, future-oriented man. Indeed, I am often

167

struck by the analogies that can be drawn between the mores of the very rich—of the "jet set" and "café society"—and the culture of the very poor. Yet it is, on the whole, a comparatively superficial culture. There is in it much pathos, suffering and emptiness. It does not provide much support or satisfaction; its pervading mistrust magnifies individual helplessness and isolation. Indeed, poverty of culture is one of the crucial traits of the culture of poverty.

The concept of the culture of poverty provides a generalization that may help to unify and explain a number of phenomena hitherto viewed as peculiar to certain racial, national or regional groups. Problems we think of as being distinctively our own or distinctively Negro (or as typifying any other ethnic group) prove to be endemic in countries where there are no segregated ethnic minority groups. If it follows that the elimination of physical poverty may not by itself eliminate the culture of poverty, then an understanding of the subculture may contribute to the design of measures specific to that purpose.

What is the future of the culture of poverty? In considering this question one must distinguish between those countries in which it represents a relatively small segment of the population and those in which it constitutes a large one. In the U.S. the major solution proposed by social workers dealing with the "hard core" poor has been slowly to raise their level of living and incorporate them in the middle class. Wherever possible psychiatric treatment is prescribed.

In underdeveloped countries where great masses of people live in the culture of poverty, such a social-work solution does not seem feasible. The local psychiatrists have all they can do to care for their own growing middle class. In those countries the people with a culture of poverty may seek a more revolutionary solution. By creating basic structural changes in society, by redistributing wealth, by organizing the poor and giving them a sense of belonging, of power and of leadership, revolutions frequently succeed in abolishing some of the basic characteristics of the culture of poverty even when they do not succeed in curing poverty itself.

168

An informal history of love u.s.a.

ARTHUR SCHLESINGER, JR.

The Founding Fathers dedicated this republic to the agreeable proposition that all men, and all Americans especially, were endowed by their Creator with unalienable rights to life, liberty and the pursuit of happiness. Their descendants have been trying to claim these rights for themselves ever since. We have, on the whole, caught up with life and liberty. But, so far as the third item is concerned, we appear to have had a good deal more pursuit than happiness.

"This people is one of the happiest in the world," wrote Alexis de Tocqueville a century and a quarter ago. Would anyone say this so confidently today? The pursuit of happiness has never ceased, but we seem to be falling farther and farther behind our goal. George and Martha were once the father and mother of their country. Now they revile each other in a thousand movie houses in *Who's Afraid of Virginia Woolf?* The passion for happiness carries us everywhere—to the neighborhood saloon and the psychoanalyst's couch, to the marriage counselor and the divorce lawyer, to promiscuity, homosexuality and impotence, to mom or marijuana and amphetamines—everywhere, evidently, except to happiness itself.

What has happened to the American theory of happiness? We have always construed that theory in private terms—in terms of individual success and individual fulfillment. And if, for some, such success and fulfillment can come from acquiring power or money, for very many Americans it comes ultimately from the triumphs and consolations of personal relations—above all, the relation of love. As a nation we have inherited the dream of love brought to our shores by the earliest colonists, a dream nourished by our fantasies but often negated by facts.

So fundamental is the romantic dream to our lives that we do not realize how small a part of mankind through history has shared it. All ages and

AN INFORMAL HISTORY OF LOVE U.S.A. Originally published in *The Saturday Evening Post*, 1966. Reprinted by permission of the author.

cultures, of course, have known marriage and family. Some peoples, like the old Romans or the Indians of the *Kamasutra*, have thought deeply and ingeniously about sex. But the idea of romantic love as cherished by Americans—the belief in passion and desire as the key to happy marriage and the good life—is relatively new and still largely confined to the Christian world. "In China," Francis L. K. Hsu has reminded us, "the term 'love,' as it is used by Americans, has never been respectable. Up to modern times the term was scarcely used in Chinese literature." (If the Red Guards have their way, it will not be used again.) And even on the continent of Europe, except as the young in recent years have succumbed to the processes of Americanization, passion has been generally kept distinct from marriage and family. There romantic love, that ennobling emotional experience, has remained an improbable hope, to be pursued outside the normal conventions of life and doomed to tragedy. Only the Americans have assumed that passion is destined to fulfillment. Only the Americans have attempted on a large scale the singular experiment of trying to incorporate romantic love into the staid and stolid framework of marriage and the family.

This was true from the start—in spite of misconceptions we still have about the 17th-century Puritans. Stern and God-fearing, the first settlers no doubt rejected the licentiousness of the Old World for the austerity of the New. Yet, for all their condemnation of playing cards, the theater, fancy clothes and other lures of the devil, for all the repression wrought by their dogmatic Calvinism, the Puritans were surprisingly open and frank about sex. Hawthorne's prim moralistic Puritans were characters more of the 19th than of the 17th century. In extreme cases the elders issued their scarlet letters; they insisted on confessions of fornication in open church (and these became so common that they were almost routine); and they rebuked outspoken hussies, like Abigail Bush of Westfield who said in 1697 that her new stepmother was "hot as a bitch." But, if one might expect John Rolfe to go off with Pocahontas in hot-blooded Virginia, one must not forget that Priscilla Mullens and John Alden lived and loved in rockbound Plymouth. Gov. William Bradford in his *History of Plymouth Plantation*, after roundly deploring the sexual excesses of his flock, concluded philosophically:

> It may be in this case as it is with water when their streams are stopped or dammed up; when they get passage they flow with more violence, and make more noise and disturbance, than when they are suffered to run quietly in their own channels.

The elders expelled James Mattock from the First Church of Boston for declining to sleep with his wife, and town records show that Puritan ministers cheerfully married an astonishing number of New England maidens already well along with their first babies.

After all, if the Puritans put people into stocks, they also bundled. No doubt this was because houses were small and winters cold, and young men and women could find privacy and warmth only in bed. "Why it should be thought incredible," wrote the Rev. Samuel Peters, "for a young man and young woman innocently and virtuously to lie down together in a bed with a great part of their clothes on, I cannot conceive." If the Reverend Peters could not conceive, some of the young bundlers evidently did. One thing sometimes led to another, then as now; and still the practice continued in Puritan New England for nearly two centuries.

The Puritans thus in their way saw sex as a natural and joyous part of marriage to be plainly discussed and freely accepted. A Marylander visiting Boston in 1744 could report: "This place abounds with pretty women who appear rather more abroad than they do at [New] York and dress elegantly. They are, for the most part, free and affable as well as pretty. I saw not one prude while I was there." He would not have been so fortunate a century later. For, though passion and marriage continued together in the romantic dream, circumstances were conspiring to separate them in American reality.

For one thing the very proclamation of independence and the formation of the new democratic republic contained a deep and subtle challenge to the ideals of romantic love. Romance, after all, had sprung up in the feudalism of medieval Europe, as the pastime of the nobility. The American colonies had no nobility, no feudal institutions, and the new republic pledged itself to liberty, equality and rationality. The bright, clear light of the young nation was hard on passion. "No author, without a trial," observed Hawthorne, "can conceive of the difficulty of writing a romance about a country where there is no shadow, no antiquity, no mystery, no picturesque and gloomy wrong, nor anything but a commonplace prosperity, in broad and simple daylight, as is happily the case with my dear native land."

The French writer Stendhal, reflecting on romantic love half a century after the Declaration of Independence, predicted sorrowfully that it has no future in America. "They have such a *habit of reason* in the United States," he wrote, "that 'crystallization' [by which he meant the moment of abandonment to love] has become impossible....Of the pleasure that passion gives I see nothing." In Europe, "desire is sharpened by restraint; in America it is blunted by liberty."

In America, desire was blunted too by the role of marriage in a new country. For the incessant demand for population and labor was transforming marriage into a service institution, and this utilitarian motive was fundamentally at conflict with the old ideals of romantic love. Benjamin Franklin, an instinctive and antiromantic made the point with characteristic pungency in 1745: "A single man has not nearly the value he would have in [a] state of union. He is an incomplete animal. He resembles the odd half of a pair of scissors." When a good colonist met and married a girl right off the boat, it was probably less a case of love at first sight than of an overweening practical need for a wife—if only to escape the bachelors' tax. And when a man instructed his wife to dress only in a shift at the wedding ceremony, it was less because of concupiscence than of computation; for a widow, by thus symbolizing her poverty, could spare her new husband responsibility for the debts of his predecessor. So South Kingstown, R.I., February, 1720:

> Thomas Calverwell was joyned in marriage to Abigail Calverwell his wife. . . . He took her in marriage after she had gone four times across the highway in only her shift and hair-lace and no other clothing. Joyned together in marriage by me
>
> GEORGE HAZARD, *Justice*

Men absorbed in building a new land in the wilderness had little time or energy left for the cultivation of romantic passions. And, as the new nation grew, they seemed to have even less time. By the early part of the 19th century the making of money was becoming an obsessive masculine goal. Tocqueville, visiting the United States in 1831–32, noted that American men had contracted "the ways of thinking of the manufacturing and trading classes." This constituted another blow to romance. Few American men, Tocqueville said, were "ever known to give way to those idle and solitary meditations which commonly precede and produce the great emotions of the heart."

If American men were becoming too preoccupied for passion, American women were becoming too rational. Scarcity gave women in the early colonies and, later, on the ever-receding frontier a measure of bargaining power they could never have expected in the homeland, and they happily seized every opportunity for self-assertion. One finds even George Washington commenting ruefully on female independence. He wrote in 1783:

> I never did, nor do I believe I ever shall, give advice to a woman who is setting out on a matrimonial voyage; first, because I never could advise one to marry without her consent; and secondly, because I know it is to no purpose to advise her to refrain when she has obtained it. A woman very rarely asks an opinion or requires advice on such an occasion, till her resolution is formed; and then it is with the hope and expectation of obtaining a sanction, not that she means to be governed by your disapprobation.

This is one of the first descriptions of the clear-eyed, rational American girl who would grow in glory through the 19th century and have her final triumph as the heroine of the novels of Henry James and in the drawings of Charles Dana Gibson. From the start she was a source of wonder to foreigners. Young Tocqueville, encountering her wherever he went, confessed himself "almost frightened at [her] singular address and happy boldness." She rarely displayed, he said, "that virginal bloom in the midst of young desires or that innocent and ingenuous grace" characteristic of the girls he knew in Europe; but she was far more formidable, thinking for herself, speaking with freedom, acting on her own impulse, surveying the world with "firm and calm gaze," viewing the vices of society "without illusion" and braving them "without fear." Above all there was her remarkable, her terrible self-control: "She indulges in all permitted pleasures without yielding herself up to any of them, and her reason never allows the reins of self-guidance to drop." The result, the young Frenchman decided, was "to make cold and virtuous women instead of affectionate wives and agreeable companions to men. Society may be more tranquil and better regulated, but domestic life has often fewer charms."

So as America entered the 19th century, love was lost between the preoccupied male and the cool female. The memory of passion lingered, the haunting hope of romantic fulfillment. "Give all to love," sang Emerson:

> Obey thy heart;
> Friendship, kindred, days,
> Estate, good fame,
> Plans, credit, and the Muse—
> Nothing refuse.

The sentimental popular novel dilated endlessly on romance. The new middle class reveled in the fantasy of love. But in practice not many (not Emerson himself) gave all to love—and least of all estate, fame, plans or credit. When Alexander Hamilton as Secretary of the Treasury was accused of having connived with a minor official in crooked financial dealings, he triumphantly proved that his payments to Mr. Reynolds involved no corruption at all; they were simply in exchange for the favors of Mrs. Reynolds. This was the pattern of priority in the new republic.

The growing conflict between romantic dream and bourgeois circumstance set the pursuit of happiness on its path of frustration. Passion and marriage, which the American experiment in love had tried to bring together, were now in the 19th century thrust asunder. Sex once again became a matter of physical gratification, which man warily pursued on his own. "If ye touch at the islands, Mr. Flask," shouted Captain Bildad in his farewell to the *Pequod* in *Moby Dick*, "beware of fornication. Good-bye, good-bye!" Marriage was to be a higher union of souls, with sexual emotion strictly confined to its procreative goal. Such was the accepted view. But the strain between the theory and reality now introduced a deep and disabling confusion into the American attitude toward love.

Tocqueville commented on "the great change which takes place in all the habits of women in the United States as soon as they are married." He attributed this to their "cold and stern reasoning power" which taught them that "the amusements of the girl cannot become the recreations of the wife," banished their "spirit of levity and independence" and dedicated them to the notion that "the sources of a married woman's happiness are in the home of her husband." For his part the 19th-century American husband placed his wife on a pedestal as one above the temptations of physical passion. So the cool girl tended to become the frigid wife, sentimentality replaced sexuality, and the 19th-century marriage lost the sense of easy companionship between man and woman. "In America," wrote Mrs. Francis Trollope, a traveler from England, "with the exception of dancing, which is almost wholly confined to the unmarried of both sexes, all the enjoyments of the men are found in the absence of the women. They dine, they play cards, they have musical meetings, they have suppers, all in large parties, but all without women.... The two sexes can hardly mix for the greater part of a day without great restraint and ennui."

173

Soon, the 19th-century marriage, as it divorced itself from passion, began to acquire an appalling gentility. The plain speaking of the early Puritans was long since forgotten. Soon the shadow of Queen Victoria was to fall almost more heavily on America than on her native land. Mrs. Trollope was exasperated to discover, for example, that men and women could visit the art gallery in Philadelphia only in separate groups, lest exposure to classical statues cause embarrassment in mixed company. Often statues were draped to spare the female sensibility. Captain Marryat, the sturdy British novelist, asked a young American lady who had fallen off a rock whether she had hurt her leg. To his total bafflement, she appeared deeply offended. Finally she instructed him that the word "leg" was never used before ladies; in mixed company, she said, the word was "limb." Later, visiting a ladies' seminary, Marryat was stunned to see a square piano with four limbs, each of which, to protect the pupils, had been dressed in little trousers with frills at the bottom.

The sickness of prudery grew in the course of the century. By the '80's the public library of Concord, Mass., was banning *The Adventures of Huckleberry Finn* as a dirty book. By the '90's tracts like *From the Ballroom to Hell* explained how the waltz led young ladies to ruin. According to Thomas Beer in *The Mauve Decade,* ladies of gentle breeding were specifying in the premarital contracts with their well-bred fiancés that the terminology of wedding ceremony did not imply the right of consummation.

As marriage expelled passion, it was tacitly agreed that men were entitled to an outlet for the base drives of their lower natures, and sex acquired its own separate and accepted domain. This was the heyday of flamboyant prostitution and the "double standard." When Gov. Grover Cleveland of New York, running as the Democratic candidate for President in 1884, was accused of having fathered an illegitimate child 10 years before, it was readily admitted that he had had an affair with Maria Halpin and had assumed responsibility for her child. The Republicans chanted sarcastically in the streets:

Ma! Ma! Where's my pa?
Gone to the White House,
Ha! Ha! Ha!

But the voters elected Cleveland, and on Election Night the Democrats sang:

Hurrah for Maria,
Hurrah for the kid,
We voted for Grover,
And we're damned glad we did.

Cleveland thus benefited from the separation between passion and marriage in the public mind. Eighty years later, when the two had been once again brought together, the electorate snuffed out the presidential ambitions of another governor of New York who had committed the offense, not of illicit romance, but of behaving with splendid legality in divorcing one wife and marrying another.

An even more notorious Victorian case involved the most popular preacher of the day. Here too the separation between passion and marriage enabled the Rev. Henry Ward Beecher to ride out a scandal that would very possibly have destroyed his career in a presumably more sophisticated age. A man of magnetic charm and robust appetite, Beecher seduced pretty Elizabeth Tilton, who taught Sunday school at his church. In time the story reached Victoria Woodhull, a leading feminist of the day, who published it in her weekly magazine, rejoicing in this ministerial recognition of the power of sex: "The immense physical potency of Mr. Beecher, and the indomitable urgency of his great nature for the intimacy and embraces of the noble and cultured women about him, instead of being a bad thing, as the world thinks...is one of the noblest and grandest endowments of this truly great and representative man."

Elizabeth Tilton, who had earlier confessed her relations with Beecher to her husband, now rushed to Beecher's defense and denied the charge. Theodore Tilton sued Beecher for the alienation of his wife's affections. While the whole nation watched with palpitant and prurient curiosity, the case ended with a hung jury. Three years later Elizabeth Tilton said, "The charge, brought by my husband, of adultery between myself and the Reverend Henry Ward Beecher was true....The lie I had lived so well the last four years had become intolerable to me." But none of this perceptibly lessened the size of Beecher's congregation or his popularity and moral influence with it.

For most Americans, of course, life went on. Young men and women met, flirted, skated together or went on hayrides, kissed, married, made love, had children and placidly completed the cycle of life. When they thought about love at all, they thought about it with the sentimentality they found in the saccharine popular fiction of the day, or else with overpowering moral gravity. "I lose my respect," said Thoreau, "for the man who can make the mystery of sex the subject of a coarse jest, yet, when you speak earnestly and seriously on the subject, is silent."

Still the schism between passion and marriage, between sacred and profane love, created a pervasive tension in the American consciousness. The expulsion of sex from Victorian marriage led to much agony beneath the respectable surface: sick headaches, neurasthenia, nervous breakdowns, addiction to patent medicines (often containing large admixtures of alcohol or morphine), frigidity, impotence, homosexuality. The more extreme feminists raged at the proposition that women were not expected to find pleasure in the sexual act.

"Yes, I am a free lover!" cried Victoria Woodhull in a public lecture. "I have an inalienable, constitutional, and natural right to love whom I may, to love as long or as short a period as I can, to change that love every day if I please!" Sensitive individuals, unable to join the conspiracy to sweep passion under the rug, grew deeply concerned about sex, fearful of its power, anxious to bring it under control.

Sex became, for example, a central issue in many of the communities

175

founded in mid-century by men and women abandoning contemporary society in search of a more perfect way of living together. Thus one of the older utopian groups, the Shakers, solved the problem of sex by abolishing it. Sworn to celibacy, they kept their communities going by recruitment. Yet as old Governor Bradford had said, water dammed up flows with the greater violence. Visitors noted that, while the Shakers abstained from sexual relations, they indulged instead in ecstatic dances, carried on at increasing tempo till they dropped in dazed exhaustion.

At the other extreme was the sexual experimentation of John Humphrey Noyes at the Oneida Community. Theologically, Noyes was a Perfectionist; he believed that Christ had long since returned to earth and that men of faith were now sinless. His community avowed the principles of complex marriage and male continence. Normal marriage seemed to him a selfish limitation on the biblical commandment to love. At Oneida, therefore, couples could have sexual relations as they wished. But having children was another matter. Here Noyes proposed an early form of eugenics—of selective mating—which he called "stirpiculture." To assure the separation of intercourse and breeding, Noyes advised methods of sexual restraint. Noyes was himself a man of considerable presence and ability. The community prospered far longer than other similar communities, eventually disbanding without having made a permanent contribution to the solving of mankind's ancient riddles of love and sex.

The tension about sex was also reflected in American literature. For the striking fact about the American novel in the 19th century was its avoidance of love—that is, of heterosexual love between consenting adults. Among major writers only Hawthorne hinted at the subject toward the middle of the century and James and Howells toward the end, and all so cryptically that a great part of their audience hardly understood what they were saying. While European novels described mature passion between men and women —*Wuthering Heights* or *Madame Bovary* or *Anna Karenina*—American novelists wrote about men by themselves in the forest or on a whaling ship, or boys lazily drifting down the river on a raft. When women appeared, they generally represented a contrast between symbolic abstractions; the ethereal fair girl and the passionate, and therefore dangerous dark girl. The women in Cooper were waxworks; there were no women in *Moby Dick*; in Poe they were generally symbols of death; Whitman's invocation of women was of men in disguise; Mark Twain fled from adult love like the plague. Unable to deal with the fact of heterosexual love, American literature in the 19th century suppressed it.

In the 19th century American society thus twisted itself into a torment of contradiction and uncertainty in its attitudes toward love. I do not mean that most Americans did not achieve a tolerable happiness with their wives; of course they did; and they conserved the family—at least in the middle classes—as the basic social unit. Yet the pursuit of happiness through a passionless marriage was generating a lurking, nagging frustration. By barring the joy of sex from wedlock, the Victorian code at once degraded the sexual impulse and weakened the marital tie. By transferring romantic love to the fantasy world of the sentimental novel and emptying serious literature of adult sexual content, it misled the national imagination and impoverished the national sensibility. The Victorians' unsatisfactory pursuit of happiness thus ended half on Main Street and half on Back Street, with marriage denied passion and passion denied legitimacy.

But the Victorian code corresponded neither to the emotional nor the physical realities of an increasingly urban and cosmopolitan society. Its collapse was inevitable. How shocking at the time were the first intimations of sexual liberation just before the First World War; how innocent they seem in retrospect! War itself hastened the disappearance of the old inhibitions, bringing back from France a new generation determined to live life to the full. The success of the feminist movement increased the pressure against the double standard. The psychology of Sigmund Freud gave the role of sex in life a fresh legitimacy. Then the prosperity of the '20's began to free the American people for the first time on a large scale from the acquisitive compulsions which Tocqueville had noted a century earlier. And, as the new psychology and the new leisure encouraged romantic love, so the new technology simplified life for romantic lovers. The automobile offered lovers mobility and privacy at just the time that contraceptives, now cheap and available, offered them security. Advertising and popular songs incessantly celebrated the cult of sex. Above all, the invention of the movies gave romantic love its troubadours and its temples of worship.

Living life to the full was still relatively innocuous in the '20's. "None of the Victorian mothers—and most of the mothers were Victorian—had any idea how casually their daughters were accustomed to be kissed," Scott Fitzgerald wrote in *This Side of Paradise* at the start of the decade.

... Amory saw girls doing things that even in his memory would
have been impossible: eating three o'clock, after-dance suppers
in impossible cafés, talking of every side of life with an air half
of earnestness, half of mockery, yet with a furtive excitement.

Skirts grew shorter; women bobbed their hair and smoked cigarettes; men packed hip flasks in their raccoon coats; and together they danced the Charleston, saxophones wailing in the background, or waded fully clothed into the fountain at the Plaza. Skeptics scorned the romantic dream. "Love," said H. L. Mencken, "is the delusion that one woman differs from another." But the contagion was irresistible.

Thus the Victorian schism was repaired and passion came back into marriage. "All societies recognize that there are occasional violent attachments between persons of opposite sex," Ralph Linton, the anthropologist, observed in 1936, "but our present American culture is practically the only one which has attempted to capitalize these and make them the basis for marriage." The American experiment was at last in full tide. "No other known civilization, in the 7,000 years that one civilization has been succeeding another," wrote the historian Denis de Rougemont, "has bestowed on the love known as *romance* anything like the same amount of daily publicity. ...No other civilization has embarked with anything like the same ingenuous assurance upon the perilous enterprise of making marriage coincide with love thus understood, and of making the first depend upon the second." The Age of Love, in Morton Hunt's phrase, had begun—and it is still going strong.

But the Age of Love has hardly turned out to be an age of fulfillment. If sexual repression failed to produce happiness in the 19th century, sexual liberation appears to have done little better in the 20th. More than that, while repression at least preserved the family, if at times by main force, the pursuit of happiness through love is now evidently weakening the family structure itself. Divorce, of course, is an expression of the determination to make romance legal at any cost; so, if one marriage fails, another must be promptly started; and the steady increase in divorce in these years —the rate trebled from 1900 to 1960—suggests how the pursuit of love is paradoxically leading to the breakdown of marriage. Freedom, instead of re-solving the dilemmas of love, is only heightening anxiety. Another of those observant Frenchmen, Raoul de Roussy de Sales, noted in 1938: "America appears to be the only country in the world where love is a national problem."

It remains a national problem today. The Second World War and its aftermath swept away whatever remained of the Victorian code; and the postwar years have seen the pursuit grow ever more complex. Most young Americans have adapted themselves to the new folkways. Like their ances-tors, they meet and marry and live out their lives in quiet content. But in the margins of American society the search for love, having broken out of the old channels, is being driven more and more by frustration to sensa-tion. Amory Blaine, the hero of *This Side of Paradise*, was dismayed by the '20's. He would have been appalled by the '60's. Among the seekers of sensa-tion, drink has given way to drugs, fraternity hops to Sexual Freedom Leagues, petting to orgies, experiment to perversion. For some, sensation leads on to violence.

Denis de Rougemont has argued that the whole idea of romantic love manifested a repressed longing for suffering and tragedy. No doubt this is an exaggeration. But poets have long sensed a kinship between love and death. "Come lovely and soothing death," wrote Walt Whitman:

> Undulate round the world, serenely arriving, arriving,
> In the day, in the night, to all, to each,
> Sooner or later delicate death.

If the suppression of sex in our 19th-century literature resulted in the Gothic obsessions of American fiction—the tormented allegories of Haw-thorne, the necrophilia of Poe, the hallucinated terror of the later Mark Twain—the age of sexual liberation has produced the dark violence of Faulkner and the erotomegalomania of Mailer. Gershon Legman has under-lined the irony that sexual congress is legal, but describing it (at least until very recently) is not; while murder is illegal but describing it has long been acceptable.

Is our literary violence in some sense a surrogate for sex? Is novelist and critic Leslie Fiedler right in suggesting that "the death of love left a vacuum at the affective heart of the American novel into which there rushed the love of death"? Our literature at least raises the possibility that the compulsive pursuit of love reinforces destructive tendencies already deep in our national character. The Measuring Man, entering girls' apartments under the pretense of inspecting them for a model agency, is revealed to be the Boston Strangler.

The American experiment in love has not yet proved itself. The national attempt to unite passion and marriage led many Americans into hypocrisy in the 19th century and into hysteria in the 20th. Must the conclusion be that we have essayed a human impossibility?—that the attempt to combine the tumult of romance with the permanence of marriage places a greater burden on marriage than it can bear? Some sociologists have even speculated that we may be moving toward a society of "progressive polygamy," as more and more Americans marry several spouses in the course of life.

No doubt Americans ask a great deal of marriage. Yet the probability is that the attempt to combine romance and monogamy will continue. When this works, it is the highest felicity. "The happiness of the domestic fireside," wrote Jefferson, "is the first boon of heaven." As for the less blessed in American society, they would perhaps do better to concentrate on the deflation of undue expectations, the recovery of discipline and the recognition that romantic love, while the most beautiful of human experiences, is not a divinely guaranteed way of life.

The drug culture

The
drug culture

Runaways, hippies, and marihuana

JOSHUA KAUFMAN, JAMES R. ALLEN, M.D.,
and LOUIS JOLYON WEST, M.D.

The summer of 1967 was San Francisco's "summer of love." The news-papers predicted that 100,000 young people would flock to the bay area to join in it. Thirty thousand actually came, inundating the city. As part of a major research program in adolescence sponsored by the Oklahoma Medical Research Foundation, a large apartment in the Haight-Ashbury district was converted into a combination home, office, laboratory, commune, and "crash-pad"—a place where transients, including runaway teen-agers, could spend the night. From this base, a research team of two psychiatrists, three college undergraduates, and three graduate students observed the life and times of the hippies.

Hippies

The mass media popularized the term "hippie" and created the Haight-Ashbury myth through extravagant reports about the district's psychedelic drug-using inhabitants, described as colorful "flower children," who es-poused a style of life and a world view based on sharing, tolerance, love, and freedom for each individual "to do his own thing."

Most of these denizens of Golden Gate Park and nearby were either am-used or disgusted by the hippie label. Asked if he were a hippie, one answered, "Hippie, what's that? ... I'm just a human being." And when a prominent reporter asked a Haight-Ashbury "town meeting" what they preferred being called, one bearded spokesman declared, "People!"

Davis(4) suggests that the hippies represent a bona fide social movement, noting that they "are expressing, albeit elliptically, what is best about a seemingly ever-broader segment of American youth: its openness to new experiences, puncturing of cant, rejection of bureaucratic regimentation, aver-sion to violence, and identification with the exploited and disadvantaged."

RUNAWAYS, HIPPIES, AND MARIHUANA Reprinted from *The American Journal of Psychiatry*, volume 126, pages 717–720, 1969. Copyright 1969, the American Psychiatric Association. Reprinted by permission of the publisher and the authors.

Berger(2) has suggested that they are merely reviving elements of bohemias of the past: fraternity, salvation through the innocence of the child, living for the moment, mind expansion, and freedom of self-expression (provided that it does not harm anyone else). But the availability of synthetic psychedelic drugs and their role as a cohesive factor in Haight-Ashbury that summer had no real parallel in earlier bohemias.

West and Allen(12) call the hippies the Green Rebellion, distinguishing them from other rebellious youth such as the New Left and Black Power groups. They see the movement's goals as "beauty, freedom, creativity, individuality, self-expression, mutual respect, and the ascendance of spiritual over material values." They also differentiate true hippies from the many similar-looking drug-using pseudo-hippies, plastic hippies, teeny boppers, and runaways, who have become pharmacologically with them but are not philosophically of them. West and Allen warn that self-intoxication with powerful drugs, which is presently both a sacrament (LSD) and a unifying force (marihuana), will inevitably drain the Green Rebellion's energies and destroy it.

Runaways

In the summer of 1967 the Haight-Ashbury myth seemed to offer possible solutions to the problems of youth: an assurance of acceptability, a romantic new identity, and an escape from the hypocrisies of elders. It proffered magical solutions to some of the pressing problems of our time: violence, the dehumanization resulting from technological progress, and urban man's increasing alienation from and defilement of nature. The flow of runaways into Haight-Ashbury, together with the increasingly important role of drug use in the pattern of adolescent rebellion, quickly became an important focus of the research team's attention, and one of the authors (J. K.) was assigned full time to the study of the runaway and his problems, including marihuana.

A syndrome of prolonged absence from home, referred to and accepted by the individual as running away, has frequently been defined as a manifestation of juvenile delinquency. Foster(5), describing 100 runaways who had been referred to a juvenile court, noted a predominance of what he termed "typically delinquent" behavior. Reimer(10) reported three types of runaway: truants; children taking refuge from unbearable environmental situations; and runaways proper, showing "characterological abnormalities" manifested by antagonism, surly defiance, impulsiveness, unprovoked assaultive behavior, and periodic docility.

Following Cohen's(3) suggestion that differing delinquent acts have differing meanings for the individual, Robins and O'Neal(11), in their 30-year follow-up of children who were seen in a child guidance clinic, found that adults who were once runaways had a more frequent diagnosis of sociopathic personality than the rest of the group. Nye and Short(9) found that running away was characteristic of a population drawn from a juvenile correctional institution but rare in a high school population.

We saw runaways in their "natural habitat": on the road, on the streets, in hamburger joints, at dance halls, in the parks, and in the pads, including our own. Most of these youngsters never came to the attention of legal or medical authorities. Unlike the runaways of Nye and Short, these teen-agers came chiefly from the high schools. Unlike those of Reimer, they rarely manifested obstinacy, assaultiveness, or pathological docility. Unlike Foster's subjects, they rarely engaged in acts that are generally labeled delinquent, with one glaring exception: they used illegal drugs, particularly marihuana. Furthermore, they did so without apparent guilt or fear, often expressing a self-righteous enthusiasm for the value of drug effects and scorn for the prohibitions of society and its laws forbidding sale and use of drugs.

For these youngsters, running away can be formulated as a result of the interaction of socioeconomic history with personal history. Today's youth are, to use Keniston's(6) term, "post-modern," and the post-modern style is characterized by the conviction that in a world of rapid change adult (parental) models and values are increasingly irrelevant. Keniston(7) also suggests that the myth behind our society—society's goals and ideals—has become tarnished and negative. Post-modern youth are disillusioned with it and alienated from the society that spawned it.

Many of today's runaways, rather than being candidates for reform school, are reminiscent of the wandering bands of youth described long ago by Makarenko(8). Since the Children's Crusade, if not before, there have been times when large numbers of youngsters, almost in epidemics, have run away to seek fortune, romance, a dream. Many of the children who flocked to Haight-Ashbury were pilgrims, inspired by a myth that was largely a creation of the mass media; they were seeking a utopia where the problems of adolescence would not bother them.

The mind-expanding psychedelic drugs (LSD in particular) were often endowed by these romantics with religious properties. Some even waited until they finally arrived in Haight-Ashbury before partaking of the LSD sacrament, "saving" themselves for it like a virgin for her husband. But marihuana was their friend and companion, the medium through which camaraderie was found all along the road. The frustrations and hardships of that road were eased by the drug's beneficent euphoria, and interpersonal antagonisms among the travelers went up in its aromatic smoke.

Not all runaways were seekers of the dream. Some might be just as cogently termed "pushaways" as "runaways." One boy was a "caboose" child, pawned off repeatedly by his parents onto older brothers. Some came from broken homes. In some cases the parents had competed for the child's loyalties until he took flight.

Many runaways received either covert or overt parental sanction to leave, expressed as scorn, indifference, or obvious envy; here the parents used the child to act out vicariously their own immature desires for adventure and escape. For such adolescents the fashionable 1967 public myth of the flower children had a double appeal. Without the myth some of them might have stayed home, but other maneuvers would then probably have been sought for resolution of the conflicts within the family setting. Marihuana was already becoming available nationwide; some stay-at-homes were planting it in their backyards.

Some precedents for running away were already set in the family. For example, one 16-year-old girl's sister had run away, but her parents neither alerted the police nor looked for her themselves. When she returned months later they did not even question her about where she had been. The younger girl correctly assumed that if she ran away there would be no danger of her being reported to the police or of her being rejected when she returned.

Most of the runaways gave false names, either to throw off pursuit or to symbolize the taking on of a new identity. One girl chose the name Wendy Golightly to symbolize both her search for the never-never land of Barrie's *Peter Pan* and her desire to be free of social inhibitions, as was the heroine of Truman Capote's *Breakfast at Tiffany's*. Usually only first names were given. Nearly everyone claimed to be over 18 and thus not a runaway by legal criteria.

The role of marihuana

Marihuana was almost always the first illegal drug used by runaways. Many had been introduced to it before leaving home or while on the road. In Haight-Ashbury it was so universally employed that it was considered a staple of life like bread and jam. But as Becker(1) notes, "turning on" is not as simple as just smoking; one must learn the technique: how to inhale and retain the smoke and how to recognize, enjoy, explore, and control the perceptual and affective changes that occur, hopefully maintaining the "high" without excessive intoxication. Acquiring these skills gave many runaways a sense of achievement, a talking point, and a password.

The horrible reactions to marihuana predicted by various authorities were virtually never seen. The runaways generally took this to mean that all the widely advertised dangers of drugs were establishment lies. This further alienated them from the social structure and made them more willing to experiment with all sorts of chemicals.

Meanwhile, the circumstances of the runaway made it unlikely that he would note the degree to which marihuana might interfere with his intellectual functioning. More chronic reactions (apathy, depression, loss of motivation) were seldom attributed to smoking pot. Instead, diminished aggressiveness was considered a desirable effect of drug use; the undesirable corollary effects (such as diminished energy) were minimized or interpreted as results of other factors.

The role of marihuana among the runaways is complex. To begin with, it offers the excitement of the forbidden, the companionship and acceptance of other explorers, and the promise of pleasure. Some users define the role of pot as a social experience, an escape, or a way to rebel, but most insist that the pharmacological effects are a significant source of gratification. Certainly marihuana and other drug use largely structures the Haight-Ashbury dweller's time. Most days are spent in getting money for staples (including marihuana and other drugs), taking drugs, and talking about sources, brands, prices, risks, legalities, and trips—both good and bad.

Observations to date suggest that most of the summer pilgrims—runaways and others—will eventually rejoin "straight" society, whether or not they return to their parents. But such returns are dependent on many factors, including psychopathology, affective state, cognitive dissonance, relationships with others (both in the psychedelic community and in the "straight" community), and the pressures of reality. Of those who do go home some, having had a bad experience, may not try drugs again. Others are now exploring meditation and other nonchemical "turn-ons."

Some possible lessons

However, a significant number of ex-runaways are continuing to use marihuana and are introducing it to others at home. Some of the psychosocial factors that are presently drawing millions of youngsters into marihuana smoking have been described, but further study is clearly required. For those youngsters who are graduates of Haight-Ashbury and for their friends (whom they are probably indoctrinating), the important question that faces mental health personnel may not be "Why don't they stop using drugs?" but "Can we as individuals and as a society offer them viable alternatives to drugs?"

It is difficult to compete with the fascination of the cabal, with its private slang, secret symbols, shared experiences, exhilarating camaraderie, and special mystical, presumably transcendental zeitgeist. The psychedelic posters and the acid-rock musical groups convey a host of messages and serve to expand or recreate the psychedelic experience. Such a song is "White Rabbit," by the Jefferson Airplane. There are many others referring to marihuana and other drugs.

One song that was of particular importance in the summer of 1967 was "She's Leaving Home," by the Beatles. Most of the runaways felt that it illustrated their inability to communicate their goals and values to their parents. The song's message seems clear: the youngster who runs away, whether his trip be geographical, pharmacological, or both, can best be understood in terms of the interaction of significant intrapsychic maturational variables, current sociocultural factors, and the all-important relationship of the child to his parents.

References

1. H. Becker, *The Outsiders*. New York: The Free Press (Macmillan Co.), 1963.
2. B. M. Berger, "Hippie Morality—More Old Than New," *Trans-action* 5(2):19–27, 1967.

3. A. K. Cohen, *Delinquent Boys*. New York: The Free Press (Macmillan Co.), 1955.
4. F. Davis, "Why All of Us May Be Hippies Someday," *Trans-action* 5(2):10–19, 1967.
5. R. M. Foster, "Intrapsychic and Environmental Factors in Running Away from Home," *Amer. J. Orthopsychiat.* 32:486–91, 1962.
6. K. Keniston, *The Uncommitted*. New York: Harcourt Brace Jovanovich, 1965.
7. K. Keniston, "Youth, Challenge, and Violence," *American Scholar* 37:227–46, 1968.
8. A. S. Makarenko, *The Road to Life*. London: Central Books, 1967.
9. F. I. Nye and J. Short, "Scaling Delinquent Behavior," *Amer. Sociol. Rev.* 22:326–33, 1967.
10. M. D. Reimer, "Runaway Children," *Amer. J. Orthopsychiat.* 10:522–26, 1940.
11. L. N. Robins and P. O'Neal, "The Adult Prognosis for Runaway Children," *Amer. J. Orthopsychiat.* 29:752–61, 1959.
12. L. J. West and J. R. Allen, "Three Rebellions: Red, Black, and Green," in J. F. Masserman, ed.: *The Dynamics of Dissent*, vol. 13 of *Science and Psychoanalysis*. New York: Grune & Stratton, 1968.

No marijuana for adolescents

KLAUS ANGEL

The question of whether or not marijuana is psychologically dangerous to the adolescent does not admit of an easy answer. It can only be answered with some degree of certainty after careful study of the specific function that the drug serves in the life of each individual user.

Predictions in psychological development are notoriously dangerous. It is difficult enough to explain why a person's development took a certain course in the past; to predict the course his development will take in the future is a nearly impossible task. After all, past external influences and the individual's reactions to them can be discovered, but one can never be certain that patterns of behavior will be maintained in the future as the individual's psychological development proceeds. And, of course, one cannot predict future external influences. Careful studies of how marijuana-smoking adolescents turn out compared to nonmarijuana-smokers are not available, partly because the phenomenon has not existed long enough.

Because of these considerations, I feel myself on shaky ground when I discuss the dangers of marijuana. What I have to say must be understood to have a tentative cast, akin to what is called in scientific terminology "a preliminary report." Such a report comprises the best formulations that can be made in the opinion of the author at the time while research is in progress.

Marijuana smokers are frequently divided into three categories: (1) the psychologically addicted; (2) regular smokers who are not addicted, and (3) occasional smokers who can be likened to the occasional drinker, the individual who accepts a drink just to be "social." I am skeptical about these divisions which are usually based on statements made by the smokers themselves who are rarely aware of the important meaning the drug has to them. Even where smoking is infrequent and social, it is rare in my experience that it is of little significance and it is often difficult to determine just exactly where addiction starts.

NO MARIJUANA FOR ADOLESCENTS From *The New York Times Magazine*, November 30, 1969. © 1969 by The New York Times Company. Reprinted by permission.

189

I am convinced that frequency or regularity of smoking is an insufficient indicator of addiction. After all, there are alcoholics who go on binges only once a month, but despite the weeks between binges, they are still alcoholics. The degree of addiction can frequently only be determined when one observes the intense struggle involved in a person who tries to give up marijuana. This should not be surprising, since the same seems to be true of cigarette (tobacco) smoking, even though the pharmacologic effect on the mind is less. Yet, there are few cigarette smokers who can give it up with the ease with which they could stop eating fried chicken.

In order to understand addiction or even lesser degrees of dependence on external inanimate substances, a short digression on the psychology of dependence may be helpful.

Passive dependent experience is of great importance in the first months of life. The baby depends for his very survival on the ministrations of the mother. This dependence not only involves material needs, but also emotional support, which gives him his self-esteem. The mother's ministrations have a profound magical effect on the baby. She can achieve wonders: she can stop him from crying, make him laugh, make him feel safe and comfortable. The infant believes that he also has magical powers. All he has to do is to scream and his wishes are fulfilled. The toddler also needs this "magical" support of the mother to maintain his developing activities. Toddlers can be observed to interrupt their explorations or their play at frequent intervals to return to mother for what has been called "emotional refueling." The first inanimate objects—the cuddly toys, the soft blanket— that serve as substitutes for mother appear at this stage. The toddler refuses to be parted from these transitional objects, as they have been called, which have a "magical" effect similar to that of the mother. The toddler who clasps his teddy bear can go about his activities much longer before returning to the mother for "refueling."

There is also considerable evidence that the baby has fantasies of being merged with his mother. It is probably for this reason that the mother's support has such a powerful effect. It can, as it were, flow over onto the child. As the child's physical and mental capacities develop, he learns to depend more and more on his own achievements and his self-esteem gradually begins to derive from these achievements instead of almost exclusively from external sources. The toddler's elation about his ability to walk is an example of this early self-esteem.

Now let us return to adolescence. The adolescent has to learn to separate himself from his parents in ways that bear many similarities to the separation process of the toddler. He also has to relinquish his dependence on his parents for emotional support and learn to base his self-esteem on his own achievements. These achievements not only involve success in the path toward his profession but also social and sexual success. He has to learn to get along with other people on his own and to develop confidence in his adult sexual functioning.

Before the adolescent reaches maturity he has to deal with many disappointments, frustrations, feelings of helplessness and wishes for escape. Sooner or later, however, the task must be completed. Conflicts such as dependence versus independence, or masturbation versus heterosexual relationships, have to be resolved. The question now is how are these inevitable conflicts of adolescence going to be settled? Is the adolescent going to tackle them by asking himself after a disappointment, "What did I do wrong?" "How can I do it differently?" Is he going to be able to base his self-esteem on his own achievements? Or is he going to fall back on external "magic" that can elevate his self-esteem at command just as the transitional objects that he used when he was a toddler did?

One psychiatrist calls the former a "realistic regimen," and the latter an "artificial pharmacothymic regimen." (In Greek, *pharmacon* means both "drug" and "magical substance." *Pharmacothymia*, thus, means both a craving for drugs" and "craving for magic.") It is quite evident that it need not necessarily be an either/or proposition. One may, generally speaking, retain a realistic regimen and use a pharmacothymic regimen as an adjunct. This is what many adults do with liquor and smoking. It seems to me, however, to be an entirely different thing whether an adult whose professional and family life is established, who is already on a "realistic regimen," uses alcohol or marijuana, or whether an adolescent, who still has to establish a realistic pattern for himself, smokes marijuana. In addition, the anxieties involved in the struggle of the adolescent are so great that the temptation to rely on magic is much greater. For these reasons, I doubt seriously that Margaret Mead and some others are justified when they criticize parents and ask "What do parents expect if they tell their teen-age children not to smoke marijuana when they themselves have a martini in one hand and a cigarette in the other."

We are now ready to understand some clinical examples:

Nancy, an attractive 17-year-old girl, started to smoke marijuana during her freshman year at an out-of-town college. She had been a rather rebellious adolescent, who had functioned well in her high school, both scholastically and socially. She had chosen a rather liberal college, although her parents had expressed some objections. In the college of her choice, rebellion, which was her accustomed way of coping with her dependent feelings toward her parents, proved to be difficult, since there were few rules against which one could rebel. She therefore found herself increasingly lonely and homesick, but too proud to admit it to her parents and consider transferring to another college. Her school work deteriorated. In her longing for direction and guidance she became involved with a young man who was doing graduate work. She mistook his somewhat dictatorial behavior as a sign of the strength she was seeking. At first Nancy's academic work improved because of the support she derived from this relationship, but when her boyfriend began making sexual demands and became increasingly irritable with her clinging dependence, she became anxious again and was unable to study. In the midst of this conflict she started to smoke marijuana. She felt frightened of a sexual relationship on the one hand and of losing her boy-friend on the other hand. When Nancy sought psychiatric help, she had been using marijuana for several months.

Trudy, an 18-year-old college girl, was introduced to marijuana by her boyfriend. She had always had difficulties in feeling close to people, par-ticularly to boys, and had been a shy, somewhat withdrawn adolescent. She had felt that her life lacked direction and that she needed something to make her feel "more enthusiastic and alive." To this end she had searched for intense and meaningful experiences by having a couple of "wild" affairs, by going to bohemian parties with loud music and bongo drums and asso-ciating with a variety of different and colorful characters. None of these efforts had seemed to help.

After Trudy's experience with marijuana she felt that she was a changed person. She described the drug as if it had been sent from heaven. She felt really alive for the first time, "as if warmed by a fire." Simple things like music, dancing or movies had a heightened effect. She immediately fell deeply in love with her boyfriend and smoked marijuana whenever she was with him. She felt that she had finally discovered what being in love is really like.

Bob, a gifted, young art student had felt alienated from his parents for "most of his life." He had rejected their values as "cheap, materialistic and exploiting" and had been looking for "real, esthetic human experience." His feelings of alienation gradually "spread" from his parents to the world as a whole. He felt his fellow students were too conventional and their paintings too "bourgeois." He became preoccupied with how he could be different from them. Anything that was the same in him as in anyone he associated with became frightening. He went to great lengths to smoke marijuana to help him in his quest for originality in both his painting and life style. Gradually he began to feel that the reveries he had while under its influence were the only true art and much more valuable than anything he could put on canvas. In his reveries, Bob frequently felt himself becoming a more or less amorphous mass that had a mysterious union with some powerful force in nature. This force protected him, enveloped him and gave direction to his life. Little by little, he gave up his friendships—with the exception of those who could furnish him with the drug. He attended school perfunc-torily and smoked marijuana daily.

In all three cases the drug was used for magical support. Its role was similar to the transitional objects of the toddler that provide "emotional refueling" when mother is absent. But it is noteworthy that the expectations these young people had of the drug were different. The more unrealistic and intense the expectation, the higher the degree of magic that the drug can give.

Nancy suffered from fairly common adolescent conflicts. She wanted her anxieties over sex soothed and her dependent longings for home supported. She did not, however, expect that the drug would change her as a person and give her capacities and qualities that she did not have before. Accord-ingly, with psychiatric help, Nancy was able to give up marijuana and learn to cope with her anxieties on her own, although only with considerable difficulty. The drug competed for a while with the treatment. In the early stages, marijuana seemed a much easier way to feel safe and calm than did the therapy, which involved facing the problems that upset her.

The situation was different in the second and third cases.

Trudy also used marijuana as an aid in forming a relationship with a boy, but she felt that the drug not only soothed and supported her but also changed her by giving her heightened self-experience through increased perception of external stimuli. She confused this heightened self-experience (in the company of another person who was also in a trance) with love, that is, with empathic feeling for another person. The drug thus stimulated Trudy's feeling of "I am I," just as her other "intense experiences" had done. It did not, of course, enhance her capacity for empathy with people, which had been her difficulty from the start. Instead, it postponed her struggle with her conflicts in this area. She actually got married to her boy-friend and only came for psychiatric help when she discovered that she did not have much in common with her husband during the day, only at night when they were both high. Marijuana is often used for this purpose, that is, to aid in forming a relationship that in actuality turns out to be a pseudorelationship, a phenomenon that could be called "instant love" and that, like instant coffee, is not the same as the real thing.

Bob had gone one step further still. He did not even pretend that the drug helped him in his relationship to people. He substituted a relationship to the drug (and its suppliers) for relationships to people. He even believed that his relationship to the drug was the more valuable one. Marijuana here functioned as an almost literal substitute for the early powerful, life-sustaining mother. He even experienced feelings of mysterious union with this powerful force that are reminiscent of the fantasies of merging with the mother that babies are believed to have.

Trudy and particularly Bob expected greater changes and were more affected by the drug than Nancy because their identities were more unstable to begin with than the first patient's. They were less sure about who they really were and what they wanted from life. Trudy had previously searched rather indiscriminately for intense experiences in an attempt to find meaning and direction for her life. Bob had a greater need to prove he was different and original, since sameness was a threat to his inner feelings of uniqueness. He was afraid he could lose the feeling "I am I," if anything about him was the same as in someone else.

Although I have stated that the magical effects of the drug increase in proportion to the unreality and intensity of the expectations of the user, I do not wish to imply that addiction is necessarily more likely to occur where the drug fulfills the greatest need. Addiction is not necessarily more intense in cases like Bob's than in cases like that of Nancy. Addiction is not only a function of the need for a drug; the person's attitude toward this need is also involved, e.g., the degree to which a person is inclined to either give in to such a need or to struggle with it. Therefore, although the need for the drug was less intense in the first case than in the third, it is conceivable that

193

someone like Nancy might abandon herself to this need and become thoroughly addicted and an individual of the third type, like Bob, might experience great conflict over smoking marijuana and try hard to give it up.

Young people frequently say it is better to use marijuana than alcohol. Alcohol does not seem to be as prevalent as marijuana among younger adolescents. It may be easier to become addicted to marijuana because it does not cause a hangover. Also it appears that one can learn to compensate by willpower for marijuana's adverse effects on performance to a far greater extent than one can with alcohol. One study has shown that people who consider themselves to be quite high on marijuana can still perform prescribed tasks, including driving, with a fair degree of accuracy. This lesser influence on performance helps users to rationalize its use. They tell themselves that marijuana's psychological dangers cannot be very great if they can still perform prescribed tasks. It may also be that marijuana lends itself better to magical fantasies than alcohol, since its effects are more varied, obscure and inconsistent. It therefore may resemble more the dark potions of the sorcerers of childhood and of primitive tribes.

I may be accused of being rather pessimistic about the dangers of marijuana. In my defense, I would like to point out that the Mexicans, who have known marijuana for many centuries, may have an even more pessimistic view than I do. Their well-known folksong, for instance, describes its effects this way:

> La cucaracha, la cucaracha,
> *Ya no puede caminar,*
> *Porque no tiene,*
> *Porque le falta,*
> *Marijuana que fumar.*
> (The cockroach
>   the cockroach
> Cannot walk any longer,
> Because she hasn't,
> Oh no, she hasn't,
> Marijuana for to smoke.)

The generation gap

What generation gap?

JOSEPH ADELSON

Can the truth prevail against a false idea whose time has come?

The idea that there is a generation gap is not totally false, perhaps. But it is false enough, false in the sense of being overblown, oversimplified, sentimentalized. This may be too strong a way of putting it. Let us say, then, that the idea of a generation gap is at the least unexamined, one of those notions that seems so self-evident that we yield to it without taking thought, and without qualms about not taking thought.

Once we examine the idea, we find it is almost too slippery to hold. What *do* we mean by a generation gap? Do we mean widespread alienation between adolescents and their parents? Do we mean that the young have a different and distinctive political outlook? Are we speaking of differences in styles of pleasure-seeking: greater sexual freedom, or the marijuana culture? Or do we simply mean that the young and the old share the belief that there is a significant difference between them, whether or not there is?

These questions—and many others one might reasonably ask—are by no means easy to answer. Few of them can in fact be answered decisively. Nevertheless, enough information has been accumulated during the last few years to offer us some new understanding of the young. As we will see, this evidence contains some surprises; and persuades us to cast a very cold eye on the more simple-minded views about this young generation and its place in our society.

One definition of generational conflict locates it in rebellion against parental authority, or in the failure of parents and their adolescent youngsters to understand and communicate with each other. (In short, "The Graduate.") On this particular issue, there is, as it happens, abundant evidence, and all of it suggests strongly that there is no extensive degree of alienation between parents and their children. Vern Bengtson, one of the most careful scholars in this area, has collected data from more than 500 students en-

WHAT GENERATION GAP? From *The New York Times Magazine*, January 18, 1970. © 1970 by The New York Times Company. Reprinted by permission.

rolled in three Southern California colleges. About 80 percent of them report generally close and friendly relationships with their parents; specifically, 79 percent feel somewhat close or very close, 81 percent regard communication as good, and 78 percent feel that their parents understand them all or most of the time.

Essentially similar findings have emerged from Samuel Lubell's perceptive studies of college youth. He reports that only about 10 percent of the students he interviewed were in serious discord with their parents, and there was in most of these cases a long history of family tension. Any clinician working with college-age students would agree; among the rebellious or alienated, we find that their troubles with their families go back a long way and surfaced well before the college years.

In some respects the findings of Bengtson and Lubell are not really surprising. What they do is bring us up to date, and tell us that a long-established line of findings on adolescence continues to be true. A few years ago my colleague Elizabeth Douvan and I studied 3,000 youngsters of 12 to 18, from all regions of the country and all socio-economic levels. We concluded that there were few signs of serious conflict between American adolescents and their parents; on the contrary, we found that it was more usual for their relationships to be amiable.

The recently published study by psychiatrist Daniel Offer—of a smaller group, but using more intensive methods of scrutiny—arrives at much the same conclusion. Incidentally, there is no support for the common belief that the adolescent is hostage to the influence of his friends and turns away from parental guidance. A number of studies, here and abroad, tell us that while peer opinion may carry some weight on trivial issues—taste, clothing and the like—on more central matters, such as career and college choice, it is parental opinion that counts.

Whatever the supposed generation gap may involve, it does not seem to include deep strains between the young and their parents. The idea of the adolescent's family milieu as a kind of *Götterdämmerung*, as the scene of a cataclysmic struggle between the forces of authority and rebellion, is exaggerated. As Lubell put it: "we found both much less authority and much less rebellion than popularly imagined."

Those who are convinced that there is a generation gap also tend to identify youth in general with radical or militantly liberal beliefs. Thus, the young are sometimes seen as a New Breed, impatient with the political pieties of the past, less subject to that fatigue and corruption of spirit characteristic of the older generation of voters.

There is indeed a generational element in politics; there always has been. But to identify the young with liberal or left militancy makes sense only from the perspective of the élite university campus. Once we look at the total population of the young a decidedly different picture emerges. We have, for example, a brilliant and revealing analysis of the 1968 election by the University of Michigan's Survey Research Center, based upon 1,600 interviews with a representative national sample of voters. Perhaps the most

interesting finding was that the under-30 voter was distinctly over-repre-
sented in the Wallace constituency, and that the Wallace movement outside
the South drew proportionately more of its strength from younger than
from older voters.

Some of the center's commentary on generational influences is worth
quoting at length. "One of the most important yet hidden lines of cleavage
split the younger generation itself. Although privileged young college students angry at Vietnam and shabby treatment of the Negro saw themselves
as sallying forth to do battle against a corrupted and cynical older generation, a more head-on confrontation at the polls, if a less apparent one, was
with their own age mates who had gone from high school off to the factory
instead of college, and who were appalled by the collapse of patriotism and
respect for the law that they saw about them. Outside of the election
period, when verbal articulateness and leisure for political activism count
most heavily, it was the college share of the younger generation—or at least
its politicized vanguard—that was most prominent as a political force. At
the polls, however, the game shifts to 'one man, one vote,' and this vanguard
is numerically swamped even within its own generation."

To overemphasize the role of generational conflict in politics is to ignore
or dismiss what we have learned over the years about the transmission of
political sentiments in the great majority of cases—it seems to average
about 75 percent in most studies—children vote the same party their parents
do; it has often been noted that party preference is transmitted to about the
same degree as religious affiliation. Political attitudes are also acquired
within the family, though generally less strongly than party affiliation;
among studies on this matter there is hardly one which reports a negative
relationship between parental attitudes and those of their children.

My own research during the last few years has dealt with the acquisition
of political values during adolescence, and it is patently clear that the
political outlook of the parents, particularly when it is strongly felt, tends to
impress itself firmly on the politics of the child. Thus, the most conservative
youngster we interviewed was the daughter of a leader of the John Birch
Society; the most radical was the daughter of a man who had—in 1965—
ceased paying income taxes to the Federal Government in protest against
our involvement in Vietnam.

The strongest recent evidence on this subject seems to come from
studies of the student radical. These studies make it evident that the "rebellious" student is, for the most part, not rebelling against the politics he
learned at home. Radical activists are for the most part children of radical
or liberal-left parents; in many instances, their parents are—overtly or
tacitly—sympathetic to what their children are doing. (This is shown in the
letters written to the press by parents of the students expelled by Columbia
and Chicago; the rhetoric of these letters reveals how strong the bond of
political sympathy is between the parents and their children. For instance,
a letter from a group of Columbia parents states: "We are, of course, concerned about the individual fates of our sons and daughters, but more so
with resisting such pressures against a student movement which has done

so much to arouse the nation to the gross horrors and injustices prevalent in our country.")

Are the young abandoning traditional convictions and moving toward new moral and ideological frameworks? We hear it said that the old emphasis on personal achievement is giving way to a greater concern with self-realization or with leisure and consumption; that a selfish materialism is being succeeded by a more humanistic outlook; that authority and hierarchy are no longer automatically accepted, and are replaced by more democratic forms of participation; that rationalism is under attack by proponents of sensual or mystical perspectives, and so on.

The most ambitious recent survey on this topic was sponsored by *Fortune* magazine. *Fortune* seems to believe that its findings demonstrate a generation gap and a departure from "traditional moral values" on the part of many of the educated young. A careful look at the survey suggests that it proves neither of these propositions, but only how badly statistics can deceive in a murky area.

The *Fortune* pollsters interviewed a representative sample of 18-to-24-year-olds, dividing them into a noncollege group (largely upward-mobile youngsters interested in education for its vocational advantages), and a so-called "forerunner" group (largely students interested in education as self-discovery and majoring in the humanities and social sciences). Some substantial, though not surprising, differences are found among these groups—the "forerunners" are more liberal politically, less traditional in values, less enchanted about business careers (naturally) than the two other groups. But the findings tell us nothing about a *generation* gap, since the opinions of older people were not surveyed. Nor do they tell us anything about changes in values, since we do not have equivalent findings on earlier generations of the young.

What the findings do tell us (and this is concealed in the way the data are presented, so much so that I have had to recompute the statistics) is, first, that an overwhelming majority of the young—as many as 80 percent—tend to be traditionalist in values; and, second, that there is a sharp division within the younger generation between, on the one hand, that distinct minority that chooses a liberal education and, on the other, both those who do not go to college and the majority of college students who are vocationally oriented. In brief, the prevailing pattern (of intra-generational cleavage) is quite similar to that which we find in politics.

The *Fortune* poll brings out one interesting thing: many of those interviewed—well over 80 percent—report that they do not believe that there are great differences in values between themselves and their parents. This is supported by other investigations. Bengtson's direct comparison of college students demonstrates that they "shared the same general value orientations and personal life goals." He concludes that "both students and parents in this sample are overwhelmingly oriented toward the traditional middle-class values of family and career." From his careful study of normal middle-class high-school boys, Daniel Offer states flatly, "Our evidence indicates that both generations *share the same basic values*" (his italics).

Despite the impressive unanimity of these appraisals, the question of value change should remain an open one. It is hard to imagine that some changes are not taking place, in view of the vast social, economic and technological changes occurring in industrialized countries: the growth of large organizations, shifts in the occupational structure, the rapid diffusion of information, etc., etc. Yet the nature of these changes in values, if any, is by no means evident, and our understanding remains extremely limited.

We simply do not know which areas of values are changing, how rapidly the changes are taking place, which segments of the population they involve, how deeply they run, how stable any of the new values will turn out to be. Many apparent changes in "values" seem to be no more than changes in manners, or in rhetoric.

All in all, the most prudent assessment we can make, on the basis of the evidence we now have, is that no "value revolution" or anything remotely like it is taking place or is in prospect; and that if changes are occurring, they will do so through the gradual erosion, building and shifting of values.

Let us limit ourselves to the two areas of pleasure where generational differences are often held to be present: sex and drugs. Is there a sexual revolution among the young? And has a drug culture established itself as a significant part of youth culture?

Announced about 10 or 15 years ago, the sexual revolution has yet to take place. Like the generation gap itself, it may be more apparent than real. Support for this statement is provided by the Institute for Sex Research at Indiana University, which has just completed a new study, begun in 1967, in the course of which 1,200 randomly selected college students were interviewed. Comparing the findings with those obtained in its study of 20 years ago, the institute reports increasing liberalism in sexual practices but stresses that these changes have been gradual. One of the study's authors states, "There remains a substantial commitment to what can only be called traditional values." Most close students of the sexual scene seem to agree that the trend toward greater permissiveness in the United States probably began back in the nineteen-twenties, and has been continuing since. Sexual attitudes and habits are becoming more liberal—slowly. We are becoming Scandinavians—gradually.

The sexual changes one notes on the advanced campuses are of two kinds. First, there is a greater readiness to establish quasi-marital pairings, many of which end in marriage; these are without question far more common than in the past, and are more often taken for granted. Second, there is a trend, among a very small but conspicuous number of students, toward extremely casual sexuality, sometimes undertaken in the name of sexual liberation. To the clinician, these casual relationships seem to be more miserable than not—compulsive, driven, shallow, often entered into in order to ward off depression or emotional isolation. The middle-class inhibitions persist, and the attempt at sexual freedom seems a desperate maneuver to overcome them. We have a long way to go before the sexually free are sexually free.

As to drugs, specifically marijuana: Here we have, without much question, a sharp difference between the generations. It is a rare citizen over 30 who has had any experience with marijuana, and it is not nearly so rare among the young, particularly those in college. Still, the great majority of youngsters—almost 90 percent—have had no experience with marijuana, not even to the degree of having tried it once, and, of course, far fewer use it regularly. Furthermore, a strong majority of the young do not believe marijuana should be legalized. What we have here, then, is both a generation gap and (as we have had before) a gap in attitude and experience within the younger generation.

It would be nice if we could keep our wits about us when we contemplate the implications of marijuana for our society. That is hard to do in the presence of hysteria on one side, among those who hold it to be an instrument of the devil, and transcendent rapture on the other, among those who see it as the vehicle and expression of a revolution in values and consciousness. In any case, the drug scene is too new and too fluid a phenomenon for us to foretell its ultimate place in the lives of the young. Drug use has grown rapidly. Will it continue to grow? Has it reached a plateau? Will it subside?

A more interesting question concerns the sociological and ideological factors involved in marijuana use. As marijuana has become more familiar, it has become less of a symbol of defiance and alienation. Lubell points out that just a few years ago the use of marijuana among college students was associated with a liberal or left political outlook; now it has become acceptable and even popular among the politically conservative. From what I have been able to learn, on some campuses and in some suburban high schools drug use is now most conspicuous among the *jeunesse dorée*—fraternity members and the like—where it succeeds or complements booze, and coexists quite easily with political indifference or reaction and Philistine values. To put it another way, marijuana has not so much generated a new life style—as Timothy Leary and others had hoped—as it has accommodated itself to existing life styles.

Is there a generation gap? Yes, no, maybe. Quite clearly, the answer depends upon the specific issue we are talking about. But if we are talking about a fundamental lack of articulation between the generations, then the answer is—decisively—no. From one perspective, the notion of a generation gap is a form of pop sociology, one of those appealing and facile ideas which sweep through a self-conscious culture from time to time. The quickness with which the idea has taken hold in the popular culture—in advertising, television game shows and semi-serious potboilers—should be sufficient to warn us that its appeal lies in its superficiality. From another perspective, we might say that the generation gap is an illusion, somewhat like flying saucers. Note: not a delusion, an illusion. There *is* something there, but we err in our interpretation of what it is. There *is* something going on among the young, but we have misunderstood it. Let us turn now to the errors of interpretation which bedevil us when we ponder youth.

The most obvious conceptual error, and yet the most common, is to generalize from a narrow segment of the young to the entire younger generation.

With some remarkable consistency, those who hold that there is a generation gap simply ignore the statements, beliefs and activities of the noncollege young, and indeed of the ordinary, straight, un-turned-on, nonactivist collegian. And the error goes even beyond this: on the university scene, the élite campus is taken to stand for all campuses; within the élite university, the politically engaged are taken to reflect student sentiment in general; and among the politically active, the radical fraction is thought to speak for activists as a whole.

It is not surprising to come across these confusions in the mass media, given their understandable passion for simplification of the complex, and their search for vivid spokesmen of strong positions. Thus, the typical TV special on the theme, "What Is Happening to Our Youth?", is likely to feature a panel consisting of (1) a ferocious black militant, (2) a feverish member of SDS, (3) a supercilious leader of the Young Americans for Freedom (busily imitating William Buckley), and (4), presumably to represent the remaining 90 percent, a hopelessly muddled moderate. But we have much the same state of affairs in the quality magazines, where the essays on youth are given to sober yet essentially apocalyptic ruminations on the spirit of the young and the consequent imminent decline (or rebirth) of Western civilization.

Not too surprisingly, perhaps, the most likely writer of these essays is an academic intellectual, teaching humanities or the social sciences at an élite university. Hence he is exposed, in his office, in his classes, to far more than the usual number of radical or hippyesque students. (And he will live in a neighborhood where many of the young adolescents are preparing themselves for such roles.)

On top of this, he is, like the rest of us, subject to the common errors of social perception, one of which is to overestimate the size of crowds, another to be attracted by and linger upon the colorful and deviant. So he looks out of his office window and sees what seems to be a crowd of thousands engaging in a demonstration; or he walks along the campus, noting that every second male face is bearded. If he were to count—and he is not likely to count, since his mind is teeming with insights—he might find that the demonstration is in hundreds rather than thousands, or that the proportion of beards is nearer one in 10 than one in two. It is through these and similar processes that some of our most alert and penetrating minds have been led astray on the actualities of the young; that is why we have a leading intellectual writing, in a recent issue of a good magazine, that there are "millions" of activist students.

It is not surprising, then, that both the mass media and the intellectual essayists have been misled (and misleading) on the infinite variety of the young: the first are focused upon the glittering surface of social reality, the second upon the darker meanings behind that surface (an art brought to its highest state, and its highest pitch, by Norman Mailer). What *is* surprising, and most discouraging, is that a similar incompleteness of perception dominates the professional literature—that is, technical psychological and sociological accounts of adolescence and youth.

Having attended, to my sorrow, many convocations of experts on the young, I can attest that most of us are experts on atypical fractions of the young: on heavy drug users, or delinquents, or hippies, or the alienated, or dropouts, or the dissident—and, above all, on the more sprightly and articulate youngsters of the upper middle class. By and large, our discourse at these meetings, when it is not clinical, is a kind of gossip: the upper middle class talking to itself about itself. The examples run: my son, my colleague's daughter, my psychoanalytic patient, my neighbor's drug-using son, my Ivy League students. Most of us have never had a serious and extended conversation with a youngster from the working or lower-middle classes. In our knowledge of the young we are, to use Isaiah Berlin's phrase, hedgehogs, in that we know one thing, and know it well, know it deeply, when we also need to be foxes, who know many things less deeply.

What we know deeply are the visibly disturbed, and the more volatile, more conspicuous segments of the upper middle class. These are the youngsters with problems, or with *panache*—makers and shakers, shakers of the present, makers of the future. Their discontents and their creativity, we hear it said, produce the new forms and the new dynamics of our social system. Thus, they allow us to imagine the contours of a hopeful new order of things or, contrariwise, permit us visions of Armageddon.

Perhaps so, but before judging this matter, we would do well to recognize that our narrowness of vision has led us to a distorted view of adolescence and youth. We have become habituated to a conflict model of adolescence—the youngster at odds with the milieu and divided within himself. Now, adolescence is far from being a serene period of life. It is dominated by significant transitions, and like all transitional periods—from early childhood to middle age—it produces more than its share of inner and outer discord. Yet, we have become so committed to a view of the young based upon conflict, pathology and volatility—a view appropriate for some adolescents most of the time and for most some of the time—that we have no language or framework for handling conceptually either the sluggish conformity or the effectiveness of adaptation or the generational continuity which characterizes most youngsters most of the time.

Another common error is to exaggerate the differences between younger and older generations. Differences there are, and always have been. But the current tendency is to assume that anything new, any change in beliefs or habits, belongs to or derives from the country of the young.

This tendency is particularly evident in the realm of politics, especially on the left, where "young" and "new" are often taken to be synonymous. Is this really so? To be sure, the young serve as the shock troops of New Left action. But consider how much of the leadership is of an older generation; as one example, most of the leaders of the New Mobilization—Lens, Dellinger, Dowd and others—are in their forties and fifties. It is even more significant that the key ideologues of radical politics—such men as Marcuse, Chomsky, Paul Goodman—are of secure middle age and beyond. The young have, in fact, contributed little to radical thought, except perhaps to vulgarize it to a degree painful for those of us who can remember a time when that body of thought was intellectually subtle, rich and demanding.

For that matter, is New Left thought really new—that is, a product of the nineteen-sixties? I was dumfounded several weeks ago when I stumbled across a book review I had written in the nineteen-fifties, a commentary on books by Erich Fromm, Lionel Trilling and the then unknown Herbert Marcuse. My review suggested that these otherwise disparate authors were united in that they sensed and were responding to a crisis of liberalism. The optimistic, melioristic assumptions of liberalism seemed to be failing, unable to cope with the alienation and the atavistic revivals produced by technological civilization.

Thus, even in the sunny, sleepy nineteen-fifties a now-familiar critique of American society was already well-established. The seminal ideas, political and cultural, of current radical thought had been set down, in the writings of C. Wright Mills, Marcuse, Goodman and others, and from another flank, in the work of Norman O. Brown, Mailer and Allen Ginsberg. That sense of life out of control, of bureaucratic and technological things in the saddle, of malaise and restlessness were, in the nineteen-fifties, felt only dimly, as a kind of low-grade infection. In the middle and late nineteen-sixties, with the racial explosion in the cities and our involvement in Vietnam, our political and cultural crisis became, or seemed to become, acute.

What I am getting at is that there is no party of the young, no politics indigenous to or specific to the young, even on the radical left. The febrile politics of the day do not align the young against the old, not in any significant way. Rather, they reflect the ideological differences in a polarized nation.

What we have done is to misplace the emphasis, translating ideological conflict into generational conflict. We have done so, I believe, because it suits our various psychological purposes. On the left, one's weakness in numbers and political potency is masked by imagining hordes of radicalized youth, a wave of the future that will transform society. On the right, one can minimize the intense strains in the American polity by viewing it, and thus dismissing it, as merely a youth phenomenon—kid stuff. And for the troubled middle, it may be easier to contemplate a rift between the generations than to confront the depth and degree of our current social discord.

A third error we make is to see the mood of the young—as we imagine that to be—as a forecast of long-term national tendencies. In our anxious scrutiny of youth, we attempt to divine the future, much as the ancients did in their perusal of the entrails of birds. Yet consider how radically the image of the American young has changed within as brief a period as a decade.

Ten years ago, we were distressed by the apparent apathy and conformism of the young, their seeming willingness, even eagerness, to be absorbed into suburban complacency. We were dismayed by the loss of that idealism, that amplitude of impulse we felt to be the proper mood of the young. By the early nineteen-sixties we were ready to believe that that lost idealism had been regained; the prevailing image then was of the Peace Corps volunteer, whose spirit of generous activism seemed so much in the American grain. And for the last few years we have been held by a view of youth fixed in despair and anger.

It should be evident that these rapid shifts in our idea of the young run parallel to changes in the American mood. As we moved from the quietude of the Eisenhower years, to the brief period of quickened hope in the Kennedy years, to our current era of bitter internal conflict dominated by a hateful war and a fateful racial crisis, so have our images of youth moved and changed. Yet, we were in each of these earlier periods as willing as we are today to view the then current mood of youth, as we saw it, as a precursor of the social future.

The young have always haunted the American imagination, and never more so than in the past two decades. The young have emerged as the dominant projective figures of our culture. Holden Caulfield, Franny Glass, the delinquents of the Blackboard Jungle, the beats and now the hippies and the young radicals—these are figures, essentially, of our interior landscape. They reflect and stand for some otherwise silent currents in American fantasy. They are the passive and gentle—Holden, Franny and now the flower children—who react to the hard circumstances of modern life by withdrawal and quiescence; or else they are the active and angry—the delinquents and now the radicals—who respond by an assault upon the system.

In these images, and in our tendency to identify ourselves with them, we can discover the alienation within all of us, old and young. We use the young to represent our despair, our violence, our often forlorn hopes for a better world. Thus, these images of adolescence tell us something, something true and something false, about the young; they may tell us even more about ourselves.

What troubles
our troubled youth?

ROY MENNINGER, M.D.

One cannot read the newspapers or the popular weekly magazines, watch television, or even travel about our larger cities without being made aware of our youth. Whether it is in their numbers, their outlandish or provocative behavior, their fads, or their economic influence, they make us conscious of their presence all about us. To be aware of their presence in all its forms is to become aware of something more: much that they do is somehow troubling to members of other generations, even to persons but a few years older than they.

Those who have occasion to see these youths professionally, as do we psychiatrists, become conscious of the fact that the youths who trouble so many of us are themselves troubled people. It is no trick, of course, to decide that their troubles are their own—particular difficulties peculiar to the individual who seeks our help, youth who are troubled because of having come from troubled families. It is not a much bigger step to decide that these special cases of trouble should be referred to a physician, a psychiatrist, a counselor or the like, or perhaps just treated with pills and otherwise disregarded.

To be sure, many of these troubled youths do come from troubled families, and do need psychiatric help. But what are often not considered by adults, or intentionally ignored if perceived, are some of the concerns these troubled young people have about themselves and their place in the world. This they have in common not only with each other, but also with many of their peers who have not gone the route of becoming patients. These concerns are not to be dismissed with a wave of an older and wiser hand and a disdainful comment on "the modern generation." These concerns that trouble our troubled youth require a hearing, particularly a hearing from those of us who say, loudly and publicly, that we are concerned about our youth, that we are working to help our youth, that we

WHAT TROUBLES OUR TROUBLED YOUTH? From *Mental Hygiene*, Vol. 52, No. 3, July 1968. Reprinted by permission of the publisher and the author.

are humanitarian in our interests. I think we have failed our youth by having failed to listen—or, having listened, failed to hear.

The evidences of their trouble are manifold. Statistics have a way of sounding cold and harsh, of often failing to reveal the human tragedy they imply; but let me share a few of them with you. One out of every six teenagers becomes pregnant out of wedlock; one-third to one-half of all teenagers' marriages are prefaced by illegitimate pregnancy; the number of unwed mothers under 18 years of age has doubled since 1940; one teenage marriage in every *two* ends in divorce within five years; 40 percent of all the women who walk down the aisle today are between the ages of 15 and 18.

But it does not stop there. Three youngsters in every hundred between the ages of 10 and 17 will be adjudged delinquent this year. There are nearly half a million children haled into juvenile court every year. There is a tremendous increase in the use of drugs—amphetamines, barbiturates, LSD. It is estimated that in Nassau County, New York—there is no reason to think things are different here than they are there—one youngster in every six has taken marijuana or LSD. Some estimate that up to 50 percent of the youth on college campuses are experimenting with these drugs. The statistics go on, and they do not get better.

To me, these figures are dismaying, they are troubling; they certainly are a sign of troubled youth. One of the first reactions of most adults to these statistics and the tragedies that lie behind them is fear. So much evidence of disrupted living evokes apprehension within most of us.

Will any of these things happen to my children? If they do, am I, the parent, to blame? These are questions we are likely to ask. These chilling statistics, coupled with our own impressions of adolescence as a stormy and turbulent time, contribute to a sense of apprehension about adolescence in general. "Clearly, they are unpredictable, stormy, and potentially violent people," we think. The sudden sound of screeching tires on a nearby street in a quiet neighborhood brings an immediate reaction: "There goes a teenager" —when, of course, we cannot know whether we are right or not. We walk down a city street and see a clustered group on the corner. For all we know, they are a bunch of happy, contented kids on the way home from a movie. But what do we feel? Fear. What do we think? They might attack us. So often is there conveyed by the word "teenager" an image of turbulence, conflict, explosiveness, unpleasantness, uncontrollability.

Not all of us are so consciously aware of this fear; but its workings are nonetheless evident in the reactions of contempt, disdain, disgust, or distaste so frequently expressed in the wake of some teenage act. This reaction or rejection is born perhaps of some conviction that adolescents are volatile combinations of sex and aggression barely under control. For most of us, it is a short and easy step to a reaction of indignant anger. Made anxious by the visible struggles of our teenagers, we are quick to defend ourselves by righteous proclamations, usually emphasizing our adult wisdom, our greater experience. Out of these anxious and angry feelings come unreasonable constraints on our adolescents, vitriolic attacks on their behavior, ready capitulation to their demands, or, perhaps, what is worst of all, turning our backs on them, their concerns, and their needs.

These adult reactions are problems for all sorts of reasons. They enable the adolescent to feel misunderstood (which he is); they allow us to think we have done something constructive, when we have done nothing of the kind; and, even worse, they lead us to miss the whole point of this troubled behavior. In my view, so much of it speaks of the failure of society to deal with the real issues that adolescence poses for the adolescent, and for the society in which he lives. By their very provocativeness, these behaviors draw our attention to the symptoms, obscuring completely the existence of a more serious problem that may underlie them.

For so many adolescents, their challenging behavior is a reaction of frustration to the failure of society to make a reasonable and sensible and appropriate place for them. To put it bluntly, our adult society tends to regard the adolescent as an unfortunate inconvenience, a sort of bad moment that we half wish would go away; a distraction or maybe a disruption that gets in the way of the real business of living for the rest of us; a kind of incidental way-station in life that will surely pass if we wait long enough or hold our breath or look the other way. It is as if adult society regards adolescence as an unattractive extension of childhood that we must somehow put up with, until the magic of time has somehow transmuted that cute little baby of yesteryear into the adult of tomorrow. Most of us feel put upon by the very existence of the adolescent, annoyed with his presence, his unpredictability, his demands, his parasitic nature, and the like, as if we were somehow the victim and he the aggressor. And, as with any victim, the roads of appeasement and bribery are natural resources. So we give him a car when he asks, or a new electric guitar, or an increase in his allowance—anything, just to get him "off our backs" and out of our way.

More than this, we couple our anxious responses with words of moral uplift, sermonizing about how things will have to change when they get out into that cold, cruel world, how they must carry their end of the load, learn to be responsible, put their shoulder to the wheel, and so forth. Often in that vein we tax them with busywork that is meaningless to them and little more than our exploitation of their cheap and available labor.

So it is logical to suggest that our adolescents' provocative behavior may be their way of saying to us, "I object." They may be trying to tell us how they feel about our systematically segregating them from adult society. They may be trying to make us understand how grave is our failure to perceive their legitimate needs for participation, their legitimate needs for genuine challenge and engagement in the real tasks of living.

How is it that adolescents are not greater participants in society? Partly, perhaps, because we look upon the job of the child and the adolescent as a single, narrowly focused task: completing their schooling. No matter how we define it, attending school is their task, and all else is secondary and generally classified under the rubric of play. By virtue of this commitment to schooling imposed by society, the child through late adolescence has no other significant social contribution to make. But beyond this we ask,

"How can he make a contribution?" He is too immature, too irresponsible, or too inexperienced, or a drag on the labor market, or without enough social merit in the aggregate to permit anything more than the most token participation in any of the social processes characteristic of adult living. He is not ready for the privileges and responsibilities of this participation until some magical point has been reached—a particular age or an official change in status.

Without regard to their individual talents, their interests, their perceptiveness, their energy, their idealism, or their enthusiasm, we deny them a significant role in society at large.

Nowhere are the starkness and meagerness of this social isolation more apparent than in the lot of the 15-year-old. Except for going to school, virtually nothing that he can do is legal. He can't quit school, he can't work, he can't drink, he can't smoke, he can't drive in most states, he can't marry, he can't vote, he can't enlist, he can't gamble. He cannot, in fact, participate in *any* of the adult virtues, vices, or activities.

But consider the consequences of this enforced sidelining of the adolescent. There he waits, champing at the bit, full of energy, drive, and curiosity, intrigued and tempted by the publicly advertised advantages of adulthood. Yet, he is asked to forego the pleasures that he sees the adults all around him engaging in freely and often to excess. Is it any wonder that he samples these experiences secretly, or in defiance, or inappropriately? And how does it prepare the adolescent for the world of adult responsibilities when he is given no opportunities to test, to try, to experience, to learn by doing? By what magic do we expect this growing adolescent, denied opportunities for the participation that teaches, suddenly to emerge on the stage of adulthood, full-fledged, capable, mature, and responsible? Small wonder that so few are ready for these responsibilities when the time comes, when their predominant experience has been the frustration of waiting, foregoing, postponing, and standing apart from the society flowing all around them.

How does this come to be? How is it that we view our adolescents as overgrown children, treat them as such, and then are perturbed by their acting that way? How is it that we are face to face with a social phenomenon of discontented adolescence that we can neither understand nor manage?

In a paper "Socio-cultural Dilemmas in the World of Adolescence and Youth," prepared for the pre-congress book for the International Association of Child Psychiatry and Allied Professions, Soskin, Duhl, and Leopold [1] presented several interesting factors about the social phenomenon of discontented adolescence.

One of these factors is the dramatic change in the economic status of the adolescent. The affluence of our society means, in effect, that the adolescent does not have to work, because the money he might earn is not as necessary

---

[1] W. F. Soskin, L. J. Duhl, and R. L. Leopold. "Socio-cultural Dilemmas in the World of Adolescence and Youth." Paper prepared as a chapter for inclusion in Pre-Congress book for the International Association of Child Psychiatry and Allied Professions.

for support of the family as it once was. Affluence provides him with the means for fantastic self-indulgence. It is estimated that last year the aggregate total for allowances and money earned by adolescents came to the staggering sum of $14 billion. This amount of money (plus a large amount of leisure time, plus a lack of significant involvement in the social fabric) inevitably makes for a pattern of living with the character of end-less play. This is a sharp swing of the pendulum to the opposite extreme from the days of child labor of fifty years ago.

Moreover, the affluence in our society provides a devastating contrast between the luxuries available to middle-class youth and the continuing deprivations of the lower class, and particularly to the Negro youth. Undoubtedly this contrast produced part of the inflammatory pressures that led to the riots in the summer of 1967.

This tremendous affluence means, of course, a tremendous consumer market, which develops a self-sustaining and expanding dynamic of its own. And, from the point of view of the adolescent, it could be argued that this self-sustaining market tends to introduce more superficial, materialistic, spurious, shifting, status-centered values that push out the more solid virtues.

A second factor is the upward extension of schooling itself. Compulsory public education for all, initially limited to the elementary grades, was gradually extended to secondary school education, as there was an ex-pansion of knowledge that needed to be mastered and an increasing need for more and better training of people. But out of this virtue of compulsory public education have come a few unexpected disadvantages. Among other things, it has meant an extended period in which the growing adolescent is dependent upon, and controlled by, adults. This spells further delay in permitting him to engage in some of the activities that will teach him how to deal with such ultimate life functions as work and the assumption of citizen and social responsibility. We have watched the age of legal re-sponsibility creep upward from seven, where it used to be, to 16, 18, 21— surely, for very good reasons, but with not so happy consequences. Many years ago, a boy of 16 might well have been head of the household, or a soldier in the king's army. Even in our Civil War there were drummer boys and buglers serving at the age of 15.

What are some of these unhappy consequences? Perhaps the most serious is the extent to which the adolescent is infantilized—"childized" as Soskin and associates [1] have called it. The adolescent becomes more childish, with the room and the permission to stay that way. This state is a deterrent to healthy growth; it provokes and sustains our perceptions of him as imma-ture. It is a magnificent example of a self-fulfilling prophecy. We deny the adolescent some of the responsibilities of maturity; and, when he responds with childish behavior, we say, "See, I told you all along you weren't ready." As we react by giving him still less responsibility and penning him up more, he reacts with still greater evidence of the immaturity, which then justifies another round of adult control and demands for conformity.

I think this infantilizing of the adolescent does something more. I think it probably provokes adventure-seeking, thrill-seeking, serious risk-taking behavior, such as taking drugs, playing "chicken" on the highway, speeding at 90 miles an hour through the city, and so forth. I would suggest that this behavior not only expresses the sense of helplessness and frustration the adolescent feels at being so irrelevant to the adult society all around him, but conveys as well his anger and his resentment for being disregarded and shoved aside by adults.

Adolescents are action-oriented people; they are people seeking a cause and a reason for being. If we fail to supply tasks that are adequate to absorb their energies and relevant to their psychosocial needs, they will do the only thing they can: seek their own outlets, and adults be damned. The fatal combination of their needs plus our indifference necessarily and inevitably leads to behavior that will either embarrass or trouble us and risk being a danger to all.

Our expectations and our presumptions about the adolescent as generally too immature to assume much responsibility embarrass us when he shows unexpected evidence of political or social maturity. Witness our astonishment at the success of the Peace Corps and our amazement at the conviction and effectiveness of the adolescent civil rights worker. We may not always agree with the sentiments adolescents express and work for, but we cannot deny the strength and the effectiveness of their commitment when they are finally given the opportunity to make it.

In our systematic social infantilization of the adolescent, we hang him between the horns of a serious dilemma. By its nature, adolescence forces gradual estrangement of the youth from the support and the nurture that the family gave him as a child, yet does not provide the benefits and supports of adulthood. And there he hangs, able neither to retreat to the warmth and support of the family nor to advance into the companionship of adult society. This limbo in which the adolescent now finds himself was filled in earlier times by the opportunity to serve as an apprentice and by the availability of real work. With these no longer open to him, the adolescent's world is an empty one, populated by church and youth groups and some commercial interests. As others have observed, the former are too selective and exclusive, failing to reach the very youth who may need them most; and the latter only exploit the chaos of adolescence for their own interests, with service neither to youth nor to society.

Even more tragic, enforced schooling combined with enforced infantilization cemented by a systematic absence of real work and real participation in the social process yields an unfortunate fruit. In spite of twelve years of education, the average high school graduate emerges from his educational cocoon with no place to go and nothing to be. He has no occupational identity, no skills worth selling, no systematic practice in the arts of living in a complex society, and not much of a clue about where to go to find what he does not yet have.

The exceptions are the college-bound youths; but they, by that very token, are not average. Even here, though they may continue their schooling through various kinds of higher education, these older adolescents continue to feel isolated from society and are, in fact, excluded from much significant

The most serious complication in designing field studies of these problems is the fact that social and psychological factors may independently have the same adverse effects as malnutrition on learning and behavior and on the anatomical and biochemical development of the brain. Studies with rats, kittens, and monkeys have clearly indicated that animals which are protected from stimulation and prevented from exploring their environments have not only smaller brains with fewer nerve cells but also develop functional impairment of the central nervous system.

Similarly, institutionalized children, well fed and genetically normal, but deprived of affection and stimulation at an early age, may show marked mental impairment. The many kinds of psychological and social deprivation common among malnourished children can exert a direct effect on intellectual performance. Unstimulating home environment, poor educational facilities, isolation resulting from illness, limited recreational opportunities, and lack of incentive due to repeated discouragement are examples of such deprivations.

In industrialized countries, inadequate intellectual or social performance in a child is more likely to be the result of a complex interaction over a period of time between genetic variables and primarily non-nutritional factors in the social or cultural environment than a consequence of malnutrition. In the rural areas of many developing countries, however, and often in city slums and ghettos, variations from family to family in education, economic status, and cultural practices may be relatively slight. In such populations, deficiencies in intellectual performance due to malnutrition and its synergism with infection may be detectable. While genetic factors are important determinants of individual potential, they do not account for most differences between privileged and underprivileged populations.

Very few long-term field studies in human learning and behavior have been completed, and most have failed to separate adequately the effects of malnutrition from those of other environmental factors. In the Capetown study, a series of intelligence tests revealed consistently lower scores in malnourished children when compared with the control group's scores over a period of approximately ten years. The disparity in living conditions between the two groups, however, was equally marked. Wretched housing with no sanitary facilities, alcoholism, unemployment, illegitimacy, and broken homes were the rule for the initially malnourished group. By contrast, the families of the control group lived in clean brick houses with running water and flush toilets; the children were legitimate and their parents employed.

The Capetown observers believe that the smaller body size and brain size in the malnourished group, as well as an increased frequency of abnormal brain waves and impaired visual perception, indicate organic brain damage. Despite this there is no way to separate the nutritional from other environmental influences in evaluating performance on various intelligence tests. Unfortunately, this was also the case in a number of studies of Serbian, American, and Indian children.

Dr. Fernando Mönckeberg of the University of Chile has reported a more critical study of the same type. Fourteen children with severe marasmus diagnosed at ages one month to five months were treated for long periods, discharged, and observed during visits to the out-patient department. As each child was discharged from the hospital, the mother was given 20 liters of free milk per month for each preschool child in her family. Three to six years later the children were clinically normal and some had weight-to-height ratios above normal. Their height, head circumference, and intelligence quotients, however, were significantly lower than in Chilean children of the same age without a history of clinical malnutrition. Significantly, language skill was the most retarded.

The information gathered in the town of Tlaltizapán, Mexico, by Dr. Joaquin Cravioto, Dr. Rafael Ramos-Galván, and their collaborators, is the outstanding pioneering effort in this field. Their studies have played the major role in attracting attention to the association of nutritional retardation of growth and development with performance on tests of learning and behavior. Because the economic, educational, and social status of families in Tlaltizapán was very uniform, these factors were judged to influence the variation within the study population to a lesser degree than the differences in nutritional status.

Retardation in physical growth and development was found to depend upon family dietary practices and on the occurrence of infectious disease. It was not related to differences in housing facilities, personal hygiene, proportion of total income spent on food, or other indicators of social and economic status. Under these circumstances, the investigators found test performance of preschool and school children to be positively correlated with body weight and height.

In order to extend these studies to another population and also to make more prolonged observations, Dr. Cravioto and several members of his team joined forces with INCAP in Guatemala. They selected school-age children living in Magdalena Milpas Altas, Guatemala—a predominantly Mayan Indian village of 1,600. More than 10 percent of the children born in this village died in their first year, and mortality in the one-to-four-year age group was more than forty-five times higher than in North America and Western Europe.

Variations in height and weight among the children of this community were not related to height of the parents or to the minor differences in economic and social status among families. The major reason for short stature was malnutrition at an early age. Two years of intensive work in this village showed once again that retardation in height for age relative to other children in the village was accompanied by poorer performance on psychological tests.

A growing body of evidence indicates that primary learning and the development of adaptive capacity is based on the development of inter-relation among the separate senses. During ages six to twelve years, intersensory relationships follow a well defined growth pattern in normal children. Dr. Cravioto gave principal emphasis, therefore, to tests of intersensory integration. The tests involved manipulating eight differently shaped wooden blocks. The examiner determined visual integration by asking the child to put the blocks into their corresponding holes as rapidly as possible. The integration of visual stimuli with the complex sensory input required by active manual manipulation of a test object was judged by asking the child whether a block placed in his hand behind a screen was the same or different from one in front. Kinesthetic-visual integration was measured by moving the child's hand behind the screen to trace a shape which he had to judge to be the same or different from that of a block in front of him.

Each of these types of intersensory relationship improved with the age of the child. This was true for both children of the study village and those from middle- and upper-income families in Guatemala City. The rural children clearly lagged in the development of intersensory competence when compared with the privileged urban children. Of even more significance, the relationship between poorer test performance and shorter physical stature in the rural village did not apply to the well nourished urban children. Among the urban children there was no correlation between the height of the child for age and test performance.

Dr. Cravioto returned to Mexico and obtained similar information on intersensory integration among school children in Tlaltizapán. He found that here, as in Guatemala, the smallest children in the village show poorer intersensory integration for their age than those who are tallest. Among children of upper-income families in Mexico City, no such correlation exists. Clearly, where the child is more nearly able to realize his genetic potential for growth, differences in height lose their nutritional and social significance.

The most comprehensive and well controlled study to date is now under way in Guatemala under the direction of Dr. Cipriano Canosa of INCAP. Children in three villages are being given adequate supplementary food from an early age. An extensive battery of psychological tests is being used to compare their performance over the next seven years with that of children in three control villages.

There are circumstances in which the effects of early malnutrition on mental development are firmly established. A number of hereditary diseases induce a nutritional deficiency through an inborn error of metabolism. The resulting impairment of brain development is so disastrous that it illustrates dramatically the way in which nutritional factors can influence development and function of the central nervous system if operative at an early postnatal age. These inherited nutritional defects should dispel any doubt that nutritional deficiency, if sufficiently early and severe, can have profound and permanently detrimental consequences for the learning and behavior of children.

It is clear that under circumstances common to developing countries, malnutrition can interact with infection, heredity, and social factors to bring about physical and mental impairment. The social factors responsible are multiple and difficult to correct, but the elimination of malnutrition and infection among underprivileged populations is a feasible goal. For each child in the world, of any race or heritage, of any social or economic background, the events of early childhood determine whether he will suffer some degree of permanent physical and mental impairment. Every child should have the opportunity to attain his full potential. Measures to ensure the maximum mental development and optimum learning and behavior of children deserve a high priority. Among these the prevention of malnutrition is of fundamental importance.

*A*therosclerosis

DAVID M. SPAIN

The incidence of heart attacks among adult white males in relatively affluent occupations in the U.S. has reached epidemic proportions. From such
attacks (coronary artery occlusions) the overall U.S. death rate is now
500,000 a year, and 200,000 more die from strokes. At least 5 percent of
the adult males in the nation show signs of some form of heart disorder.
The basic disease responsible for most of these disorders and deaths is
atherosclerosis. There is every indication that the prevalence of atherosclerosis in the U.S. is steadily increasing.

It used to be thought that atherosclerosis was a disease of old age and
that its rising incidence might be due simply to the lengthening of the
average life-span by the control of infectious diseases. This idea has now
been refuted by a number of studies. My colleagues and I have made a
comparative examination in Westchester County, New York, of two samples
of the population taken 20 years apart. The samples were comparable in
that both groups covered the same age range (from 20 to 60), had records
of good health before a fatal episode, had died of sudden causes not connected with heart disease and had been autopsied after death, so that the
extent of atherosclerosis in their coronary arteries and aortas was known.
The first sample consisted of people who had died of acute infections in
the period between 1931 and 1935; the second was made up of people who
had been killed in automobile or industrial accidents between 1951 and
1955. We found that the second group, representing a period 20 years later
than the first, had a significantly greater amount of atherosclerosis. This
was true for every age level: the young people in the second group had
more atherosclerosis than the young ones in the first. A similar autopsy
study in Sweden yielded the same finding; the degree of coronary atherosclerosis in a population sample in 1958 was greater than in a sample from
1934.

Laboratory studies of experimental animals and postmortem examinations of human infants have established that the development of atherosclerosis often begins shortly after birth. Fatty streaks signaling the beginning of atheromas have been found in many human aortas as early as the age of three. In a group of U.S. soldiers killed in the Korean war whose average age was only 23, examination showed that most had extensive formations of atherosclerotic "plaques" in their arteries. In our study of accident victims in Westchester County we found that many 35-year-old males who had shown no indication of heart disease nevertheless had their coronary arteries so thickened by atherosclerosis that the channels were narrowed by 50 percent. It has become quite clear that atherosclerosis is a widespread disease of the young as well as the old.

Atherosclerosis appears to be at least as old as the civilization of mankind. The aortas of some Egyptian mummies that were entombed more than 3,500 years ago show the typical lesions of atherosclerosis. The modern name of the disease is derived from two Greek words: *athere*, meaning "porridge" or "mush," and *skleros*, meaning "hard." This apparently contradictory combination describes the fact that the lesion begins as a soft deposit and hardens as it ages. Materials that have been deposited from the bloodstream in the inner lining of the major arteries penetrate the arterial wall; they form plaques that gradually grow and thicken the wall, thus narrowing the blood channel. Eventually the thickening may close the channel entirely, or pieces of the plaques may break off and travel with the bloodstream until they are stopped in a smaller artery and thereby plug it. When the blockage occurs in the coronary artery, it produces a heart attack by cutting off the blood supply to the heart muscles; in the brain it produces a cerebral stroke; in the lower extremities it can lead to gangrene.

The circulatory system of the human body is a pipeline through which blood is pumped at a rate amounting to 4,300 gallons a day through 60,000 miles of pipe reaching every cell of the body. We might liken the atherosclerotic deposits in an artery to the rustlike encrustations that may form on the inner wall of a pipe. The living system, however, is vastly more complex than any ordinary pipeline. The fluid coursing through the arterial pipes contains living cells and a mixture of liquids that are continually changing in chemistry and physical characteristics. The flow is pulsatile, varying from moment to moment in velocity, volume and pressure. The living walls of the arteries themselves partake of the same changeability. They undergo a continual metabolism, conduct exchanges with the blood and the fluids bathing them externally and are subjected to various kinds of stress. In this dynamic system, subject to so many internal and external influences, unraveling the process that is responsible for atherosclerosis is akin to trying to solve a many-body problem in astronomy without knowing how many bodies are involved.

The atherosclerotic lesion is a complicated affair. When fully developed, it is composed of a considerable variety of structures and substances: blood and blood products, fibrous scar tissue, calcium deposits, complex carbohydrates, cholesterol (a fatlike, waxy substance normally present in the blood and body tissues), fatty acids and lipoproteins. Apparently the fatty acids and cholesterol are the crucial substances responsible for the development of the lesion, because they provoke inflammation and scarring of the arterial-wall tissue.

How does the process leading to atherosclerosis begin? Examination with electron and light microscopes shows that the first visible event is the invasion of the inner lining of the artery by fatty substances. These substances appear mainly in smooth muscle cells and foam cells found within the lining. In the spaces between the cells small amounts of cholesterol can be detected. Very fine fibers of a material that behaves like fibrin (a natural product of blood coagulation) also show up, both within the lining and on its surface. At this early stage the forerunner of the atherosclerotic lesion can be recognized in the form of fatty streaks, which when stained with a suitable dye are visible to the unaided eye as red streaks or spots on the lining surface.

To solve the mystery of the origin of atherosclerosis one of the first questions we must answer is: How are the fatty materials deposited in the arterial wall? There are several current hypotheses. The one most widely accepted is that the fatty substances are transported into the wall by plasma, the blood fluid, and are trapped within the wall. It is believed that the plasma itself, under the force of the blood pressure, can leak all the way through the wall of the artery in small amounts, which then return to the bloodstream by way of the lymph-circulating system. The large lipoprotein molecules or complexes, on the other hand, cannot filter through the wall so easily; consequently they may tend to pile up within the wall, particularly if the plasma carries an excessive quantity of them.

The known structure of the walls of the major arteries gives support to this view. The wall of an artery consists essentially of three layers: outer, middle and inner. The outer layer and part of the middle one are nourished by a system of fine blood vessels (called vasa vasorum) that come from the outer coat and go inward only as far as the middle layer. The nourishment of the inner portion of the arterial wall is taken care of by nutrients filtering into it from the bloodstream in the channel of the artery. Between the inner and the middle layer of the wall there is a curtain of elastic tissue. This tends to impede the flow of fluids through the wall. Hence it may act to trap substances that follow the gradient of flow, which in an artery is from inside to outside. Significantly, atherosclerosis rarely develops in veins, where the flow gradient is from outside to inside.

That lipids and other large molecules from the bloodstream can penetrate the arterial walls has been demonstrated conclusively by experiments with radioactively labeled cholesterol and other materials. These labeled materials usually turn up in highest concentration in areas in the walls that are already atherosclerotic. It has also been learned that in the early lesions of atherosclerosis the pattern of lipids present in the lesion is strikingly similar to the pattern in the blood.

Are there special conditions that favor the infiltration of lipids into the arterial wall? At least one interesting finding points in that direction.

It was found that the administration of high doses of vitamin C to experimental animals inhibited the accumulation of lipids in the walls of their arteries. Conversely, when animals were fed a diet on which they developed a vitamin C deficiency, the inner lining of their arteries became more permeable: its cells were more widely spaced.

Abel Lazzarini-Robertson, Jr., of the Cleveland Clinic, who has studied the behavior of arterial-lining cells in tissue cultures, suggests that there may be a self-feeding process that generates expansion of an atherosclerotic lesion. Some of these cells, he says, respond to an excess of lipids by requiring more oxygen. When they fail to obtain enough oxygen to satisfy this increased need, the cell membranes become more permeable to lipids. Thus a vicious circle is set up: the more lipid enters the cells, the easier it is for additional lipid to invade them.

As I have mentioned, hypotheses other than the lipid-infiltration theory have been proposed to account for the origin of atherosclerosis. One of these suggests that a disturbance of the blood-clotting mechanism, in combination with an injury to the inner wall of the artery, may result in the formation of a fibrin clot on the surface of the wall. Fatty substances from the bloodstream may then accumulate in the clot, particularly if there is a considerable amount of such substances in the blood, and this focus may generate the atherosclerotic lesion. Another hypothesis proposes that some alteration of the cementing substances (mucopolysaccharides) in the artery wall that occurs after an injury to the wall may open the way to local invasions or synthesis of lipids. It may be, indeed, that there is some truth in all the hypotheses. There is reason to believe that atherosclerosis can originate in a number of different ways.

Once the process has started it develops a kind of life of its own. Enzymes within the artery wall break down the fatty complexes, liberating cholesterol and fatty acids. These act as noxious foreign agents and excite inflammation of the wall tissues. Scar tissue develops. Fragile capillaries growing into this tissue tend to rupture and thus lead to more inflammation. The artery lining may ulcerate, and blood from the bloodstream clots around these breaks. Gradually the atherosclerotic lesion expands in size, and as the scar tissue and calcium deposits accumulate, the lesion stiffens and renders the arterial wall brittle and weak.

Atherosclerosis may occur simultaneously in many of the body's major arteries. There are, however, certain favored sites. Much depends on the shape and position of the vessel. For example, the coronary arteries, which receive the full impact of the pulsatile blood pressure against their walls during systole (the heart's pumping cycle), have a high tendency to develop atherosclerotic lesions; on the other hand, the renal arteries, which branch from the aorta at right angles and have a low resistance to blood flow and therefore do not feel the pulsatile impact nearly as much, are relatively free of the disease. The vessels that are most often, and most critically, attacked are the coronary arteries, the aorta, the arteries in the neck and brain and the iliac and femoral arteries supplying blood to the lower extremities.

When thrombosis (formation of a blood clot) occurs in a narrowed coronary artery, the resulting partial or complete shutoff of blood supply to a portion of the heart muscle may have various effects: angina pectoris (pain in the chest), a myocardial infarct (destruction of part of the heart wall), irregularity or weakening of the heartbeat or sudden death due to complete failure of the heart. If the arteries to the brain become clogged, the result is a massive stroke causing paralysis or death. "Small" strokes, causing only slight or temporary paralysis of particular functions, may arise from fragments that break off from the atherosclerotic lesion and flow on to clog small vessels in the brain, thereby killing small areas of brain tissue. When atherosclerosis and clots clog a major artery to the legs, the result may be severe pain in these extremities and sometimes so much destruction of tissue that the gangrenous limb must be amputated.

In the aorta the lower section, passing through the abdomen, is particularly subject to atherosclerosis. The disease may so weaken the arterial wall that a portion of it balloons out, forming an aneurysm. Aneurysms of the aorta may press on the important organs in this area, interfering with their functions and causing pain. The rupture of one of these aneurysms usually produces massive hemorrhage and death.

One of the peculiarities of atherosclerosis is that even among the susceptible arteries it often selects particular ones for attack. For example, an individual may have severe atherosclerosis in his coronary arteries but very little of the disease in the cerebral arteries, or extensive lesions in the aorta with very little involvement of the coronary arteries. This form of selectivity is reflected in the disease rates of certain peoples. In Japan, for instance, strokes are common but heart attacks are relatively rare.

It is natural to suspect that diet has a great deal to do with atherosclerosis, and for more than a century the primary suspicion has focused on cholesterol. As early as 1847, a German anatomist, J. Vogel, reported that atherosclerotic arteries invariably contained cholesterol. In 1909 a Russian army medical officer, A. Ignatowski, observing that the army officers, who were of the meat-eating class, had many more heart attacks than the vegetarian peasants, undertook an experiment. He fed rabbits animal products and found that their aortas did indeed develop atherosclerotic lesions. A few years later a pair of Russian investigators, N. Anitschkow and S. Chalatow, followed up with a series of careful studies that became classic references in this field. When they fed rabbits fat and cholesterol, they observed that the cholesterol level in the animals' blood rose and atherosclerotic plaques appeared in their arteries. After cholesterol feedings were discontinued, lipids gradually disappeared from these plaques.

Cholesterol is indeed an inevitable suspect, because the formation of the atherosclerotic lesion is essentially an inflammatory response to this substance. The involvement of cholesterol in the disease has been demonstrated in many different ways. Experimenters have produced the disease by cholesterol feeding in many animals, including rabbits, rats, guinea pigs, chickens, dogs and monkeys. In almost every case in which the disease is induced experimentally the animals' serum shows a rise in cholesterol as a prelude to the atherosclerosis. In primates the disease exhibits all the features that occur in human beings. At the human level a cooperative study in Britain and the U.S. found that peptic ulcer patients who were treated with the Sippy diet (rich in milk and cream) had elevated levels of cholesterol in their serum and suffered twice as high a rate of heart attacks from coronary atherosclerosis as ulcer patients who did not use this diet. Conversely, patients with multiple myeloma, a malignant disease that tends to lower the serum-cholesterol level as one of its effects, have an unusually low rate of heart attacks. People who have died of so-called wasting diseases (essentially malnutrition) show a low lipid content in their arteries, which suggests that the loss of fat may have reduced their atherosclerotic lesions. On the other hand, people with diseases or conditions that are usually accompanied by a high cholesterol level (diabetes, nephrosis, hereditary elevation of lipids in the body) tend to develop atherosclerosis at an earlier age and more extensively than usual.

Yet it has become increasingly clear that atherosclerosis cannot be explained simply in terms of cholesterol, or even a fatty diet. Certain species of pigeons spontaneously develop atherosclerotic lesions closely resembling those of human beings although these birds eat no animal fat. (Spontaneous atherosclerosis is also found in dogs, baboons, ostriches, pigs and whales.) Laboratory experiments have shown that exposure to cold, elevation of the blood pressure, antithyroid substances, high doses of vitamin D, lack of oxygen and other factors can contribute to the development of atherosclerosis. On the other hand, the disease process can be inhibited in animals by undernourishment, thyroid hormones, heparin (the anticlotting agent), fat-eliminating agents, unsaturated fats and sitosterol (a precursor of steroid hormones).

Even the evidence of epideminology is not entirely clear. It is true that populations whose diet contains a relatively small amount of saturated animal fats and cholesterol tend in general to have a low blood-cholesterol level and a low incidence of heart attacks. To illustrate with some often cited statistics. The South African Bantu, among whom death from coronary atherosclerosis is exceedingly rare, have a diet very low in fats (average: 17 percent of the total caloric intake) and a mean serum-cholesterol level of only 166. In Europe, where death from this disease is common, the average fat intake amounts to 35 percent of the diet and the serum-cholesterol level is 234. In the U.S., where the coronary death rate is very high, the average fat intake is between 40 and 45 percent and the serum-cholesterol level is about 250. Moreover, there is some evidence that people who migrate from a country with a low heart-disease death rate to one with a high death rate, and adopt the diet and cultural pattern of the latter country, tend to acquire a rise in the cholesterol level and an increase in the rate of heart attacks. This, at least, has been found to be true of Yemenite Jews and Japanese who have migrated to the U.S.

Nonetheless, it is not easy to determine exactly what factors separate the immune populations from the vulnerable ones, or the sheep from the goats. Among the peoples distinguished by exceptionally low rates of heart attack are the farmers of Guatemala, the Yemenite Jews, the South African

Bantu, the Chinese, the Japanese and the Apache Indians living on reservations. Very high heart attack rates, on the other hand, are found among the adult white male inhabitants of New York, New Orleans, England, Sweden and parts of Finland. What do the latter populations have in common that differentiates them from the first group? This is one of the principal problems that today engages the attention of many investigators of the causes of atherosclerosis.

To narrow down the search for the significant environmental, biological or dietary factors, it would be very helpful if we could identify the individuals in each population who have atherosclerosis. Unfortunately this is difficult to do in a live population. Atherosclerosis has aptly been called an "iceberg" disease, because only five to 10 percent of those whose arteries are affected show any clinical sign of illness. Recently a method has been developed for examining the arteries in the body by X-ray. In this method, called angiography, a radiopaque dye is injected into the bloodstream and the artery is then X-rayed to show whether or not the flow is normal. A narrowing or other abnormality of the channel is taken to indicate atherosclerosis. The technique is not, however, sufficiently simple, accurate or safe to be used as a screening procedure for the general population.

The cholesterol level in the blood is not itself a reliable index of the disease. In any population the level varies as a continuous spectrum, and one cannot find a dividing line that separates the atherosclerotic individuals from those with healthy arteries. Indeed, many people with low serum-cholesterol levels have heart attacks whereas many with high levels do not.

The investigation of atherosclerosis must therefore rely mainly on post-mortem examinations and studies of people who clearly show signs of the disorder by their coronary disease or heart attacks. As everyone knows, there is now a very large accumulation of epidemological studies that have sought to shed light on the factors associated with heart disease. These include the worldwide studies of Ancel Keys of the University of Minnesota and his associates, the famous mass studies in Framingham, Mass., Albany, N.Y., and Chicago and our own recently completed study of 10,000 males in Westchester County. All these studies have arrived at remarkably similar conclusions about the high-risk factors associated with coronary atherosclerosis. To sum them up in one profile, the most vulnerable person would be an adult male who has a high lipid content in his blood and high blood pressure, who engages in little physical activity and is markedly obese and who is a heavy smoker of cigarettes.

The difference between men and women in the rate of heart attacks from coronary atherosclerosis is striking. Our observations indicate that, in the age level up to 55, deaths from such attacks are at least 10 times more common among men than among women. It seems that the factor protecting women is the female hormone estrogen. Women who have had their ovaries removed (thus reducing the estrogen output) tend to have more atherosclerosis than those with their ovaries intact. Injections of estrogens have been found to be capable of lowering the cholesterol level in the blood and of altering lipoproteins from the type associated with the development of atherosclerosis. At the Michael Reese Cardiovascular Research Institute in Chicago, Jeremiah Stamler and his colleagues demonstrated that the development of atherosclerosis in the coronary arteries of young male chickens that had been fed cholesterol could be stopped by injecting estradiol benzoate, a variant of the female hormone. On the strength of all the experimental evidence, estrogen injection has been tried as a treatment to inhibit atherosclerosis in men, but it is not promising for widespread use because of its feminizing effects.

High blood pressure is a serious contributor to atherosclerosis only when it is combined with a high cholesterol level in the blood, in which case the pressure forces cholesterol into the artery walls. The Apache Indians commonly have high blood pressure but seldom suffer heart attacks, probably because their blood content of cholesterol is low. Our studies of New York men indicated that the combination of high blood pressure and high cholesterol carries a high risk. In the age group between 36 and 50 men with this combination had a rate of atherosclerotic heart disease more than four times higher than that of men with normal blood pressure and lower serum cholesterol; the respective disease rates were 7.6 percent and 1.8 percent.

In the cases of the other risk factors revealed by the epidemiological studies—lack of physical activity, obesity, cigarette smoking—no direct tie to the atherosclerotic process has been found. Just how these conditions contribute to heart disease remains to be determined.

Many other elements that are suspected of contributing to atherosclerosis have been investigated. Undoubtedly heredity is an important factor. Atherosclerosis is frequently associated with diabetes and hypertension, diseases that are known to stem from genetic causes. Moreover, it seems likely that an individual's relative ability to metabolize and otherwise handle lipids plays a large part in his susceptibility to atherosclerosis. Studies have shown that identical twins tend to have about the same blood-cholesterol level, whereas twins who are not identical are much more likely to differ from each other in this respect. There have also been dramatic cases in which identical twins have had heart attacks at the same time in the prime of life.

Another factor that has had much attention in emotional stress, arising either from the individual's mode of life or his constitutional disposition. Unfortunately most of the studies of this factor have been so poorly conceived or executed that the conclusions are uncertain or questionable. There is no firm information so far to prove or disprove the hypothesis that emotional stress contributes to heart attacks.

We come back finally to the diet, which today holds the center of research attention as the factor most likely to be primarily responsible for the epidemic of atherosclerotic heart disease. There is no gainsaying the fact that this disease is a dominant feature of industrialized, affluent societies. If we look at metropolitan New York, where the disease has increased strikingly in the past 30 years, we can see that in the same period there has been a marked change toward a more luxurious and more passive manner of life, characterized by great increases in the use of the automobile, in automation of occupations and domestic tasks and in the animal-fat content of the average diet. The insurance companies have been compelled at frequent intervals (about 10 times in the past 30 years) to revise upward their statistical tables of average weights.

In a report to the White House Conference on Children and Youth, Stanley Marion Garn of the Fels Research Institute noted a disquieting trend in the eating habits of the younger generation in the U.S. today.

"If 35 percent of his calories comes from fats, is Junior being prepared, starting in nursery school, for a coronary occlusion?" asked Garn. "Reviewing the dietaries of some of our teen-agers, I am struck by the resemblance to the diet that Olaf Mickelsen uses to create obesity in rats. Frappes, fat-meat hamburgers, bacon-and-mayonnaise sandwiches, followed by ice cream, may be good for the farmer, good for the undertaker and bad for the population.... Through the stimulation of advertising, tap water is being replaced by sugared juices, milk and carbonated drinks. Snacks have become a ritualized part of the movies and are inseparably associated with television viewing."

To what extent can the animal-fat diet be specifically incriminated on the basis of the research done so far? The epidemiologist Ernest L. Wynder has suggested four criteria to determine whether or not a given factor can be regarded as a cause of a disease: (1) the incidence of the disease in a population must be proportional to the population's exposure to the factor; (2) the distribution of the disease—in geography, time, by sex and among various population groups—should be consistent with the distribution of the suspected factor; (3) the factor should produce the same disease, or one corresponding to it, in experimental animals in the laboratory, and (4) the removal of the factor or the reduction of exposure to it by the human population should reduce the incidence of the disease in the population.

The animal-fat diet has fulfilled the first three of these criteria for atherosclerosis in many tests. The fourth piece of incriminating evidence—reduction of the disease in man by reduction of the exposure—has not yet been established. It is currently being tested, however, in a massive dietary study, expected to involve ultimately 100,000 men, that is being conducted at five major centers under the auspices of the National Institutes of Health. If this and similar studies demonstrate that the fatty diet is indeed a major cause of atherosclerosis, there may be hope that the epidemic increase of the disease can be halted and reversed.

Of viruses and cancers

LIN ROOT

Do viruses cause cancers? The answer is yes. Viruses cause cancers in plants, fish, frogs, fowl, mice, rabbits, squirrels, deer, monkeys—in almost every species of animal tested, and presumably in most untested species as well.

When bits of cancer from a diseased animal are ground up and forced through an ultra-fine filter, no cell or bacterium can pass. But the virus, smaller than either—too small to be seen with the strongest optical microscope—slips through in the clear, innocent-looking filtrate. Scientists have injected such extracts into healthy animals and watched tumors develop with sufficient regularity to prove that viruses can cause cancer. Until recently, they believed that a specific virus would infect only animals of the same species, or at most, closely related species. Now, by varying the conditions of infection, they are making specific viruses to infect widely separated species. Latest and biggest jump: virus from a chicken cancer produced cancers in monkeys, our next of kin.

What about the highest species of animal life—man?

Many virus diseases—influenza, polio, others—are caused by the same viruses in man as in animals and produce similar symptoms. Likewise, many virus-caused cancers in animals behave exactly like human cancer, cause unknown. Their cellular composition is the same; they arise in the same organs and tissues; spread through the body similarly; are influenced by hormones in the same way; and kill in the same manner.

The opposing theory, long dominant, attributes cancer to somatic mutation (*soma* meaning body, *mutare*, to change), an inherent ability of body cells to change and transmit this change to all their descendants. This theory, dating from pre-virus days, rested solidly on success in transmitting cancers by transplanting cancer cells from one animal to another. It received additional support, after viruses were discovered, when Paul Ehrlich attempted in the early 1900s to transmit a virus from the breast cancers of mice, and failed. He assured his followers that no other scientists need waste time on the quest.

What is cancer? It is the most formidable, the most studied, the most mysterious malady afflicting man.

Cancer itself is an umbrella word. There are as many kinds of cancer as there are organs and tissues where abnormal growths can occur. They are classified into three groups according to the three types of body cell. These form the skin which separates the body and its organs from their surroundings, the supporting structures which keep the body from falling apart, and the circulating cells. Their cancers are: carcinomas of the skin and the mucous membrane lining the lungs, mouth, stomach and other parts; sarcomas of the muscles, bones, cartilage and connective tissues; leukemias of blood cells, red and white, and the bone marrow where they are made.

One thing distinguishes all cancer cells from normal cells: *uncontrolled replication*. A normal cell reproduces itself (scientists say "replicates"— makes replicas of itself) by dividing into two daughter cells. With superb discipline, normal cells replicate to supply exactly what is needed, be it a liver, a leg bone, or a steady replenishment of the cells that die daily in blood, skin or elsewhere. Should later need arise—to heal a wound, for instance—the cells replicate to make just the required amount of tissue. Crucial to the whole process is inhibition, control. Normal cells know when to stop.

Cancer cells have lost that knowledge. They start without need and replicate without limit. Single cells or clumps may break off from the original growth and travel through blood and lymph vessels to other sites (metastasis). Starting in the liver, let's say, the cancer can end in a brain hemorrhage. Some of the invading cells may still be recognized as having originated in the liver, but most, through wild replication, lose their identity, becoming more and more undifferentiated and immature, young cells voraciously consuming adult tissues (except for certain leukemias) in a suicidal process. The secret of uncontrolled replication is the key to the proliferation of cancer. What sets it off?

In early studies, radiation was indicted. Girls who tipped their radium brushes with their tongues as they painted luminous watch dials, doctors who worked with radiation and X-rays died of leukemia and other cancers. Lung cancer was common in uranium and cobalt mines; bladder cancer in the dye industry; skin cancer in the synthetic oil industry. As chemicals were identified, industry and government took corrective measures, and the incidences of cancer in industry dropped markedly.

Advocates of the somatic mutation theory found corroboration in these cancer inducers, which they termed mutagens, that stimulated the cell's inherent property of mutation.

But independent-minded young scientists continued to seek a virus to explain cancer.

Rous's chickens

In 1910, when Dr. Peyton Rous and the Rockefeller Institute were young, he injected the cell-free filtrate from a chicken sarcoma into other chickens. They developed similar tumors. After numerous such experiments, the results proclaimed the fact: the cell-free extract contained a virus that could transmit a highly malignant cancer. The conclusion was inescapable but terrifying, a heresy too grave to utter. All the great pathologists, from Rudolf Virchow, who developed the cell theory in the 1850s, through Rous's own professor, William Henry "Popsy" Welch, of the Johns Hopkins Medical School, preached the gospel that only the cancer cell itself could transmit cancer.

So in his report to the Journal of the American Medical Association, January 21, 1911, Rous did not use the word virus, but referred to it as a "tumor agent" and continued to call it so for many years.

His deference did nothing to mitigate the storm. "Ridiculous!" was the exclamation that echoed through the laboratories when the chicken sarcomas were mentioned, and although Rous kept piling up evidence, no other investigator bothered to corroborate his work for 20 years.

In 1932, Dr. Richard E. Shope, another young Rockefeller researcher ahead of his time, succeeded in transmitting giant warts from wild rabbits (cottontails) to domestic rabbits by cell-free filtrate. But the growths were nonmalignant. "Shope's papilloma" was largely dismissed as just another wart—innocuous. But Shope felt from certain aspects of his experiments that both the wild and domestic rabbit growths might be true cancer. Subsequent experiments proved him right. Most of the innocuous warts developed into cancers after about six months—first demonstration of the viral transmission of cancer in mammals.

Still the mutationists were not impressed. Most researchers argued that each new discovery about viruses made the cancer theory more ridiculous.

Admittedly, their arguments were persuasive. Viruses cause infections—measles, influenza—which can be transmitted from person to person, even producing epidemics. How could isolated cases of cancer come from an infectious disease? And how about the doctors who treat, dissect, handle tumors daily in hospitals without special precautions? Last and most convincing: tumors occur (leukemia excepted) in an aging population whose cell machinery might well be running down, a favorable field for mutations.

Studies of leukemia provided new clues. In the 1930s, leukemia was recognized as cancer. Remembering the early successes with chicken leukemia virus, many investigators set up experiments with mice. The common mouse leukemia is in many ways similar to human leukemia. But all attempts to transmit leukemia by cell-free filtrate failed. Investigators were about ready to concede that leukemia in mice, therefore in mammals, was of a different nature from the virus-caused leukemia of chicken.

Then, in 1951, Dr. Ludwik Gross of the Bronx Veterans Hospital, New York, reported success in transmitting mouse leukemia by filtrates to newborn mice of a low-leukemia strain. These findings were "accepted with reservations," remarks Gross. The virus particles were too few or too weak, and other researchers had difficulty duplicating his results. (To complicate matters, some of the filtrates induced tumors of the salivary gland instead of leukemia; a few animals developed both. The mystery was solved when Dr. Gross identified two viruses present in the leukemic filtrate. He separated them by ultra-centrifugation; one was the leukemic virus, and the other virus caused salivary gland tumors.)

Gross persisted. Finally he found a potent virus strain which he isolated from spontaneous mouse leukemia. After serial passover of this virus through newborn mice, this virus strain became so potent that it induced leukemia in practically 100 percent of newborn mice, and even, to a lesser extent, also in adult mice.

From now on the preferred animal in virus-cancer research would be newborn. For investigators, newborns are useful for two reasons: they have not had time to acquire diseases, and they have not yet developed the immune mechanism which helps their systems fight foreign substances.

A curious transformation

Following Gross's early experiments on leukemia induction, Dr. Sarah Stewart of the National Cancer Institute, Washington, D.C., set herself to duplicate the work. None of her mice got leukemia. Instead they all broke out with tumors of the salivary glands. She, too, had difficulty with virus-poor filtrates. If she could grow the virus particles in tissue culture (a developing and demanding technique at the time, although routine today) she would obtain a richer crop, she surmised. In 1956, Dr. Bernice Eddy, who had been growing polio virus in monkey kidney tissue culture, joined her in a collaborative study. At first, the tissue culture cells grew normally but as the virus growth increased, some of the mouse kidney cells themselves underwent a curious transformation.

Normal cells growing in a glass dish replicate and extend over the glass bottom. When one cell comes in contact with another, it lines up neatly alongside and stops replicating, as though the contact set off a stop signal. Thus the layer grows out into the free spaces until it reaches the boundary walls. Here all replication stops, leaving an orderly wall-to-wall layer of single cells. A cancer cell also multiplies, but when it touches another cell it does not stop, apparently gets no signal. Instead, it grows over the cells and begins to clump on top in tumor formation.

The virus seemed to be transforming some of the normal kidney cells into cancer cells. Yet in most of the cells the virus behaved like any infectious virus producing disease in its host: it penetrated the cell and replicated madly until the exhausted cell died, releasing a myriad of viruses to infect other cells.

The significance of this double-barreled activity was breathtaking. The cancer virus, instead of being a different and mysterious breed, as hitherto believed, was none other than an infectious virus behaving in a different and mysterious way. More surprises lay ahead. Drs. Stewart and Eddy inoculated all the different animals with the salivary gland virus. This virus induced many different kinds of tumors in mice, so many that the virus was christened "polyoma" (many tumors)—and not only different tumors in the same species, but in all the different species of animals that had been inoculated. This contradicted the established belief that a tumor virus was species-specific (one virus induces one kind of tumor in one species of animal) as opposed to the less choosy infectious virus. Here was a cancer virus jumping species barriers as successfully as any infectious virus, and causing infections as if it *were* an infectious virus. No longer need the cancer-inducer be dubbed an agent. The time had come to acknowledge it as a virus, and to reexamine the virus-cancer theory in relation to man.

Dissent in london

These conclusions were too unorthodox to be readily accepted. Some strong voices came to the support of the virus theory, but as late as 1958 other eminent pathologists meeting at the International Cancer Congress in London, continued to discount it.

To some, such persistent theoretical controversy may seem academic, but as a noted virologist explains, "If you speak in terms of somatic mutation, you feel you can never prevent or cure.... The only method you have is radiation or surgery after a tumor develops."

Obviously this fatalism among the experts has contributed to the hopelessness and despair of doctors and patients outside the laboratories, engendering a reluctance to recognize early warning signs as though they bore the features of death.

Commented Dr. Peyton Rous, after the 1958 London conference: "Most serious of all the results of the somatic mutation hypothesis has been its effect on research workers.... For what men think determines not only what they do but what they do not; and numerous workers on cancer are now content to think that it results from somatic mutations. Hence they see no reason to seek in other directions to learn its nature."

While scientific partisans were still defending their positions, new and mighty machines took over the laboratories: the man-size electron microscope which made the invisible visible, magnifying it up to 200,000 times; the ultra-centrifuge, built on the principle of the cream separator, which spun viruses out of cells, and separated them by weight.

For the first time, scientists got an inside closeup of the cell and could photograph its activities. Hitherto puzzling blobs turned out to be complex factories for breaking down the proteins we eat into their basic units. Others reassembled these into body-building blocks for muscles, enzymes, whatever was called for.

Packed into the nucleus in the center of the cell were the chromosomes, seemingly endless threads of genes entwined in pairs, each pair coiled like a bed spring—the double helix structure. One gene (or more) determines a single characteristic of an individual. Thus all the genetic information that makes the individual into a man or a mouse lies stored in the chromosomes.

Virus hunters could see their prey. They still could not see a virus at work, alive, but they could follow its life history by killing it at various stages. They knew from the work, in 1935, of Nobel Laureate Wendell Stanley that viruses consist of nucleic acid and protein in unknown combinations. Baffling information this; normally a cell ejects any foreign protein. Yet the virus somehow manages to overcome this hostility and invade the cell, there to multiply a thousandfold. How?

The virus made visible revealed a core of nucleic acid, neatly and completely wrapped up in a protein coat. On entering the cell, the virus sheds this protein coat on the cell membrane and the naked nucleic acid slips easily into the cell. No wonder. For the genes that control the cell are pure nucleic acid. This was brilliantly demonstrated in 1944 by bacteriologists Oswald T. Avery, Colin M. MacLeod and Maclyn McCarty at the Rockefeller Institute.

Each new solution focused more attention on the underlying riddle: how do chromosomes, containing all the genetic information for the individual and the species, transmit their message from the genes to the cells? How is this message coded to keep it intact down the ages?

Breaking the code

In 1953, James D. Watson, 25-year-old American biochemist, and Francis H. C. Crick, British geneticist, working together at Cambridge University in England, dramatically cracked the genetic code and came up with a model of the nucleic acid molecules that made answers excitingly clear. Suddenly genes became chemical molecules of known structure to be studied like any others with the new technology: no longer need they be verified only in live animals. Cracking the code also solved several unknowns in the virus theory. Let's examine it in this new light.

A virus is a bit of nucleic acid wearing genetic instructions like a gene, but it has no machinery. Biologically, life is a matter of instructions plus the raw materials and machinery to carry them out. Therefore a virus can come to life only inside a living cell where the factories are. Outside, it is as inanimate as an invisible dust mote. Some say the virus is the bridge between life and nonlife. Harmless, inert, with no means of locomotion, it yet travels everywhere—on the wind, on the water, on planes, on people. But let it get into a living cell and it turns dictator. Usurping the cell machinery, it stimulates the cell to frenzied activity toward a single end—replication—making viruses until the exhausted cell dies. For the cell itself has no information but the instructions it receives. It can't tell the difference between the messenger nucleic acid, delivering life-giving orders from the chromosomes, and the virus nucleic acid issuing suicide commands. The cell kills itself obeying orders.

Occasionally, a virus transforms normal into cancer cells. We saw this double play in the polyoma tissue culture experiments. Most commonly, the virus played its infectious role: filling and killing the cell by replication, swarming forth to infect its neighbors. But in some cells no virus particles were formed, the infected cells did not die. They became frank cancer cells.

The change was permanent: daughter cells inherited the cancer factor in every replication throughout hundreds of generations.

This persistence indicates a change within the chromosomes. It is possible, says Watson, "to believe that the essential aspect of viral carcinogenesis is the *introduction of new genetic material* in contrast to somatic mutations which, we suspect, often cause a loss of functional genetic material." The new genetic instructions introduced by the virus change the code and thereby produce a different type of cell: a cancer cell. Exactly how the virus introduces the material is not yet known, perhaps by "crossing over," joining itself to certain genes.

The question is: which genes? To somatic mutationists the increasing incidence of cancer with age proved that the disease resulted from the accumulation of random mutations over the years. We are, of course, exposed to mutagens from the day we come into the world: cosmic rays that bombard us from outer space; traces of radioactive substances in soil, sea, air; ultraviolet radiation from the sun plus man-made radiation; X-rays; fallout. Other mutagens are chemicals, diseases, drugs. We learn more about them every day. Heavy consumption of coffee breaks chromosomes in experimental animals, according to a recent report. Certainly somatic mutations occur and accumulate all along life's way.

Viruses, too, are inside, outside and all around us. We know our body defenses are constantly engaged in the struggle against them—with astonishing success.

Some scientists now think viruses are present in the cell and its nucleus all the time, unattached bits of genetic information with no life of their own, like unattached genes. When enough chromosomal breakage has occurred, the virus can insert itself as part of the heritable mechanism. Then every time the chromosome replicates, its transmits the viral information in its code.

Suddenly the virus-cancer theory has become not only respectable, but also as popular as it was formerly scorned. Every major laboratory is allocating a considerable slice of its research budget to virus studies.

Immune defenses

What of the future?

Vaccines against several cancer-inducing viruses have been successful. Drs. Stewart and Eddy prepared one (called it an immunizing agent) which protected 97 percent of the inoculated hamsters against the polyoma virus. In 1956, Dr. Charlotte Friend, of Sloan-Kettering Division of Cornell Medical College in New York made a killed-virus vaccine that produced antibodies and prevented mouse leukemia about 80 percent of the time.

We have seen that viruses which induce cancer in newborns, "immunologically incompetent" mice and hamsters, usually fail to produce the disease in adults. All this work indicates that immune defenses exist and can be strengthened in animals.

In man, the facts suggest that the human animal, too, may have natural immune defenses. The facts are: some people develop cancers while others do not; cancers may develop at some stages in life and not at others; some cancers develop slowly, others rapidly.

Projects seeking to identify and strengthen such immune reactions are under way in the cancer laboratories across the country. Many projects bearing directly on viral cancer and man are also in progress.

These are but a few of the studies that brilliant virologists across the country are pursuing with new fresh hope.

As Dr. Watson says, "The relevant question is . . . not whether virus can cause cancer, but whether a sizable fraction of cancers are virus-induced. . . . Naturally, we should not underestimate the difficulties ahead . . . nonetheless, most important is the fact that at last the biochemistry of cancer can be approached in a straightforward, rational manner."

The many clocks
of man

JOHN D. PALMER

In most cases the intervals of time we recognize are arbitrary, man-made designations. Periods such as seconds, hours, or weeks, plus the more eso-teric intervals—weekends, the "cocktail hour," vacation time—are obvious cerebral artifacts of our present civilization. Mixed in with all the arbitrary units of time is the period of a day. A day is the interval between successive sunrises and is generated by the rotation of the earth on its axis in relation to the sun. At present, days are 24 hours long, but just a short 370 million years ago (a fleeting instant in the 4.6 billion years that the earth has ex-isted) the earth gyrated more rapidly, and days were only 22 hours long.

At first thought one might decide that the 24-hour day is just another arbitrary interval of time chosen by man because of its ease of recognition and its convenient duration. We sleep at night; work and eat in the daytime. If no other clues were available to know what to do next, we would need only to look for the sun. Still, we know that men isolated from all view of the sun and from man-made timepieces—either deep in a cave or in sound-proof laboratory quarters—still continue to settle down for the "night," to eat, and to regulate their activities around a 24-hour schedule. And while this evidence is often said to reflect our adjustment to a heavenly time in-terval, it may also be interpreted to mean that this 24-hour rhythm is an intrinsic characteristic of man's inner workings.

This period is also found to be a constant feature of plants and animals (*Natural History*, March, 1966; February, 1967). As shown by literally thou-sands of observations, organisms maintained under laboratory conditions in which all time clues are eliminated still continue to measure out 24-hour periods with surprising accuracy, leading some researchers to conclude that a period of approximately 24 hours is a fundamental attribute of protoplasm. It may be that a period of 24 hours is a kind of absolute in the biotic king-dom. Scientists are now aware that within the bodies of all organisms is a "living clock" signaling off these periods.

THE MANY CLOCKS OF MAN From *Natural History*, April 1970. © Natural History, 1970. Reprinted by permission of the publisher.

One concrete example of these rhythms is the sleep–wakefulness cycle in man. About ten years ago, a young speleologist became obsessed with the idea that it was scientifically important for him to live in an ice-filled cave, sans clocks, for a protracted period of time. For sixty-three days he lived 375 feet below ground where the temperature held constant at 32° F., the relative humidity remained unchanged at 100 percent, and the darkness was complete save for a small, battery-powered light. Each time he awoke, ate, or prepared to retire, he called over a field telephone to a surface camp, where the times of the calls were recorded. The inexorable cold and dampness reduced his body temperature to less than 97° F., and he was constantly threatened by avalanches and cave-ins—still he held out for the sake of science and whiled away his time writing a best seller on his subterranean adventures. Throughout his underground stay he tried mentally to keep track of the passage of time on the surface. When the men in the surface camp informed him on September 14 that his experiment was over, he estimated the date at August 20. His judgment of the passage of time had been exceedingly sluggish. Mentally, he had lost 25 days! However, his living clock (as evaluated by the times of his retiring/awakening phone calls) had ignored his mental confusion and guided his body functions all the while, measuring off periods of activity and sleep that totaled just longer than a day: 24 hours and 31 minutes on the average.

A slight deviation from an exact period of 24 hours is the rule rather than the exception when plants and animals are maintained in strictly unvarying conditions. However, a slight inaccuracy should not dethrone the 24-hour period as an absolute, for when one contemplates the possible intervals from less than nanoseconds to the life-span of the universe, a "near-miss" to 24 hours should be leniently accepted. After all, even the atomic clock of the Bureau of Standards, the paragon of accuracy, mysteriously slows down every sunrise.

...Because the period of the cave dweller's rhythm was slightly longer than 24 hours, his sleep–wakefulness cycle fell out of phase with the actual day–night cycle. Only once again during the experiment did it come into phase with the day–night cycle outside, bringing about a rather interesting result. "Daily" during his underground sojourn in this quasi limbo, he entered limited scientific observations and numerous complaints in a log. Save for one entry, the diary is a hodgepodge of chronicled discomforts, misadventures, perpetual intestinal uprisings, cave-ins, and real and imagined terrors. In this particular entry, however, the diary tells us that "for the last few days I have felt very optimistic, I suffer less from the cold; I am better adapted to conditions." During this optimistic period (days 36–39...) his sleep–wakefulness rhythm was again in phase with normal day–night cycles in the French Alps outside the cave.

Since this pioneering venture, more sophisticated, more comfortable, and considerably less dangerous observations of man in isolation have been carried out, especially at the Max Planck Institute in Germany. In these experiments, light and temperature (the major time-signaling cues of our environment) can be held rigorously constant, while subjects remain in isolation for many weeks.

Despite the relative comfort of the modern experimental setup (including kitchens and baths), it is still difficult to obtain a suitable number of volunteers. Few people are willing to subject themselves to the rigors of prolonged isolation and the indignities of continuous medical measurements. Luckily, money can entice some into cooperating, and in the end investigators turn to that always popular experimental subject—the graduate student. His captive willingness is enhanced by his penury, and in exchange for three meals a day, the quiet of constant conditions in which to study, and a temporary escape from the pressures of graduate school, he is more than willing to provide periodic blood and urine samples and to sit impaled on rectal temperature probes for days on end. This traditional exploitation has an additional advantage—the student, as a burgeoning scientist, can relate his experiences to the investigator in a meaningful way after the experiment is over.

In the last few years more than fifty subjects have lived for various lengths of time in these bunkers, and in all cases their internal clocks continued to govern their sleep–wakefulness pattern and other body rhythms in close accordance with the 24-hour time period.

The sleep–wakefulness rhythm does not appear to be present at birth. In a study in which parents of newborns were asked to jot down the times that their babies awakened or fell asleep, it was found that not until the third week of life were signs of a rhythm apparent. During the next few weeks the neonates' nocturnal sleep time increased to an average of ten hours while the day sleep decreased to slightly longer than three and a half hours, beginning to approximate an adult pattern. It is, of course, several years before all day sleep is abandoned. In most of these studies the children were raised in the usual pattern: the parents, for convenience's sake, actively labored to develop sleeping patterns in their newborns that would be similar to their own. However, interesting data came from one set of indulgent parents who allowed their child to determine its own sleeping pattern. In this case, a pattern of sleep geared to a 24-hour day did not develop until the child's eighteenth week of life.

Apparently the major stimulus for the development of a sleep–wakefulness pattern is the parents' concern for getting the child's schedule to conform to their own. However, maturation of the child also plays an important role, as is shown in studies of premature babies. Rhythmicity in these tiny infants develops much more slowly than it does in full-term neonates, despite hospital pressures to get them to conform to a daily pattern.

The living clock may also function in a related aspect of sleep: the ability of some people to awaken at a predetermined time each morning without the aid of an alarm clock. All men are not equally endowed with this capacity, and those who have it show different degrees of accuracy. Various idiosyncratic rituals have been developed by some people to impress the waking time upon their minds: one expert stamps out the desired hour on the floor—much like the old counting horse of vaudeville—before retiring; and another, a politician, slowly raps out the waking hour with his forehead against the bedpost while patriotically whistling "The Star-Spangled Banner."

Temperature rhythms

The body temperature of man is also something of an absolute. Under the control of an elaborate thermostat located in the brain, body temperature is regulated at about 98.6° F. Like the interval of 24 hours, this too is a "relative" absolute in that body temperature is not perpetually 98.6° F., but varies by a few degrees around this average. In 1812 it was discovered that in the small hours of the morning one's temperature is low, rising to a maximum during midday or afternoon. An afternoon temperature slightly over 99° does not necessarily mean that one is slightly feverish, while the same temperature in the morning could indicate febricity.

Since body temperature depends on the balance between heat production and loss, one immediately thinks of the effects of muscular activity, food intake, and sleep as the causal factors of the rhythm. While all these factors exert profound influences on body temperature, they are not the causes per se of the rhythm. Studies in which subjects are confined to bed for several days, eating identical meals at regularly spaced intervals or fasting, show that these treatments do not abolish the rhythm or decrease its amplitude. One man, completely paralyzed with poliomyelitis for sixteen months, still displayed a normal temperature rhythm.

Because body temperature is so easily measured, it is one of the most commonly studied human rhythms. Like other body rhythms it has been shown to persist whether in the constant conditions of deep caves or in the laboratory. For example, before the start of their lonely confinement in the experimental bunkers described earlier, rectal temperature probes were implanted in each volunteer so that deep body temperature could be continuously recorded during the times of wakefulness and sleep without disturbing the subject. Even in these static conditions, all subjects displayed distinct temperature rhythms. A particularly interesting case is [that of a] subject [who] displayed a sleep–wakefulness rhythm with a period of 33 hours, but a temperature rhythm with a period of a more normal 24.8 hours. Therefore, the individual "lost" over 5 days during his stay in constant conditions, while his thermostat lost only half a day. A possible conclusion to such a finding is that the body must have multiple clocks, each controlling a specific function.

Several studies show that man's mental abilities and physical dexterity vary rhythmically over a 24-hour span and that the forms of these rhythms are similar to the form of his personal daily temperature curve. For example, the speed of performing such simple tasks as dealing four hands of cards, sorting a deck of cards by denomination, or multiplying eight digit numbers by each other is studied at various times over the day. These, along with reaction times and steadiness of the hand, are commonly found to be rhythmic. When the subject's temperature curve is simultaneously determined, its form and the forms of the above parameters are usually similar.

Experiments such as these, together with a plethora of similar findings, suggest a causal relationship between body temperature changes and efficiency. The relationship is further strengthened by the finding that "morning" people—those who rise early and work, learn, or perform best in the morning—have temperature curves that reach their daily maximum before noon; while "evening" people have temperature curves that peak in the late afternoon or early evening. The latter case, in which peak performance is delayed until late in the day, discredits the old adage that "sleep recharges the body like a battery" and that body energy gradually runs down during the day.

Rhythmic time perception

A few years ago it was found that one's subjective time perception varies rhythmically. For example, if a subject is asked to estimate the passage of a 60-second interval at different times of the day, he tends to overestimate—indicate periods longer than 60 seconds—when his temperature is lowest and underestimate when it is at its peak, suggesting that the rate at which an endogenous physiological "time-perception" mechanism runs is dependent on body temperature. This is a logical conclusion, for it is well known that all metabolic processes run faster at higher temperatures. Therefore if this clock, which would be expected to be a metabolic entity, was caused to run faster by higher temperatures, then the subjective evaluation of time would be shorter, and vice versa. This deduction was proved experimentally many years ago by an eminent physiologist who capitalized on his wife's bout with influenza. Throughout her illness she indulged him by estimating 60-second intervals while he recorded her attempts with a stopwatch. The higher her fever, the quicker she supposed time to be passing. These findings have now been confirmed many times by artificially augmenting human body temperature with exposure to diathermy or drugs.

The body's chemical rhythms

Many, if not all, of the myriad chemical reactions that take place within the human body are probably rhythmic. Because the end products and excesses of some of these reactions are excreted from the body in the urine, the progress of these inner body reactions can be followed by urinalysis. Just about every component easily analyzable in the urine—potassium, chlorine, sodium, phosphate, and hormones, plus pH and water volume—are found to vary rhythmically, with peaks occurring in the daytime and minima at night. These rhythms make their first appearance in the newborn between the fourth and fifteenth week of life, and are not caused by diet, activity, sleep–wakefulness, or other cycles.

An interesting and unusual series of observations on excretory rhythms has been carried out north of the Arctic Circle. On the Spitsbergen Islands, north of Norway, the sun never sets during the summer months and the days are usually overcast, making it difficult to guess the time of day from the sky. Nineteen subjects—again, mostly graduate students—assisted in an experiment in this desolate region. Before arriving in Spitsbergen many of their rhythms, especially their excretory ones, had been studied at great length. Once in Spitsbergen, complete camping equipment was issued to the students, including sham watches, which ostensibly recorded standard 24-hour days, but which actually (and unknown to the subjects) measured out 21- or 27-hour "days."

Two camps, completely isolated from one another in uninhabited territory, were set up and the subjects, unaware of the timepiece subterfuge, were instructed to carry out their daily activities within the framework of time signaled by their watches. Their routine was interrupted every few hours to take oral temperatures and urine samples (in which potassium, sodium, chlorine, and water content were measured).

It should be pointed out that living within these abnormal time schedules meant that every eight 21-hour days were equal to seven real days; and every eight 27-hour days were equal to nine real days. Halfway through either set of eight experimental days the subjects were exactly 180° out of phase with real time—they were up and active at what would have been nighttime back home. The results of the six weeks' study were surprising.

The temperature rhythm of all but one subject adjusted quickly to the 21- or 27-hour days. Less quickly, the rhythms in sodium, chlorine, and water volume also locked into the artificial days. The potassium rhythm, however, seemed less susceptible to "deceit," and in most cases, maintained its 24-hour periodicity. While some of the body's rhythms can be made to operate according to time intervals of slightly more or less than 24 hours, others (the potassium rhythm for example) cannot. The results suggest that there is probably more than one living clock to control separate body functions, and furthermore, that the dependability of each is variable.

It is biologically necessary for a rhythmic process to be adaptable to change, for man is not sedentary in his habits, but moves restlessly over the face of the earth. Today, jet travel shaves hours off, or piles hours on, the length of a single day as travelers speed eastward or westward, and these geographic relocations place considerable stress upon one's living clock. For example, a person leaving New York at 6:30 P.M. will arrive nonstop in Rome at 8:30 A.M. (local time) just as this ancient city is awakening. However, the traveler's living clock is signaling 2:30 A.M. (New York time) and is informing him that it is time to retire. The clock must readjust to the new local time, and until it does, a person will not feel up to par. It is interesting to note that lack of immediate adjustment to new time zones was first observed in 1860 in an orangutan that was being shipped from Java to Germany. The crewmen noticed that the ape tended to maintain its Java sleep pattern in spite of the ship's westward movement through consecutive time zones. Unfortunately, the observations were cut short at the Cape of Good Hope when the animal died after drinking a bottle of rum.

The diplomatic services, large corporations, and athletic coaching staffs want their representatives to be in peak form when entering into business and competitive events in other countries, and a number of studies have recently been undertaken to this end. The procedure is simple but expensive: enthusiastic volunteers are flown from the United States to all parts of the world, and the rates at which their rhythms adjust to these new localities

271

are measured. In addition to rhythmic processes, other assessments—reaction time, subjective fatigue, and decision time—are made on each subject before and after translocation.

After westerly translocations, for example, from Italy to the United States (crossing six time zones) or from the United States to Japan (ten time zones), subjects had to force their living habits to conform with the new local time. It was found that in general the various rhythms took five to six days to completely rephase to the new local times. Reaction and decision times were impeded, and fatigue was significantly increased the first day in the new location, but settled down to near normal by the second day. Older men showed higher fatigue levels than younger subjects.

On easterly flights—from Japan to the United States and from the United States to Italy—the rhythms rephased to local time much more rapidly: most were completely adjusted to the new local times by the second day. As with westward flight, reaction and decision times were impaired and the level of fatigue increased on the first day. North–south flights in which travelers remained in the same time zone had no effect on the biological rhythms, but again, fatigue was experienced after both outgoing and return flights.

The relative ease with which rhythms adjust after eastward flights as opposed to westward flights can be seen in the following example. A businessman traveling to Rome, and unaware of biological rhythms, would schedule his flight so that he could leave New York at a convenient time and arrive in Rome on the morning of the day of his appointment. He would therefore leave New York at 8:00 P.M. so that after an eight-hour flight he would arrive in Rome at 10:00 A.M. (local time), which corresponds to 4:00 A.M. of his own "body time." Biologically he should still be asleep, but he can force himself to carry out his business (with reduced efficiency, perhaps) and still engage in after dusk social activity there. By bedtime he will be quite tired; his own clock will be registering about 7:00 P.M. (it is already adjusting), and he will easily sleep through the remainder of the Roman night. On the other hand, suppose our businessman is with an Italian firm and must come to America. Leaving Rome at 9:00 A.M. would bring him into New York at 11:00 A.M. (local time) giving him time to conclude his first day of business and join in some social activities, but he will have to force himself to stay awake much of this time. He then tries to retire with New Yorkers just after midnight, but his biological clock is now signaling about 7:00 A.M. Roman time, which is his time to awaken. Even though he has been up for 24 straight hours (assuming he did not sleep in the plane) he now finds it difficult to fall asleep, for while it is easy to avoid sleep by a conscious effort, it is impossible to force oneself to fall asleep through mental persuasion. Thus, adaptation can be expected to require a longer time after a long westward flight than after an eastward flight.

Thus far I have described only a few of the rhythms known to exist in man—there are many more. The list includes pulse rate, blood output by the heart, circulating red and white blood cells, the amount of protein in the blood at any one time, circulating blood volume, blood pressure, the capacity of the lungs, cell division, a variety of psychiatric illnesses, the adaptation of the ear to new sounds, hormone secretions, the retention of memorized material, and about thirty or forty other rhythms. Surprisingly, even one-time or infrequent events in the human life-span also appear to be subject to rhythmicity. For example, the rate of childbirth is greatest between 2:00 and 7:00 A.M. and lowest between 2:00 and 8:00 P.M. (No wonder obstetricians often appear haggard.) Death rate is also highest between 2:00 and 7:00 A.M. Women tend to begin menstruation in the wee hours.

Another natural period on earth is the synodic-lunar month, the time between successive new moons. It is an interval of 29.5 days. There are many organismic rhythms—most of them reproductive cycles in lower marine animals—with periods of 29.5 days. For example, certain insects hatch out of their pupal cases into adults at the times of full moon. Summer egg production in the Mediterranean sea urchin is greatest at the time of full moon as was known by Aristotle, who recommended that gonad *aficionados* collect them at this time to obtain maximum enjoyment of the delicate ovaries.

That the moon was believed to have some influence on man is indicated by the reference to insanity as "lunacy." As it turns out there have been few scientific studies designed to examine the possibility of the effect of the moon on human life. Even the hint of interest in such an investigation would generate condemnation from fellow scientists, for one of the great triumphs of science in the past has been to abandon astrology and the notion that the movements of heavenly bodies in some way influence the lives of man. Some brave souls, however, in the interest of scientific inquiry, are willing to suffer ostracism by their colleagues and look for moon-related influences on human endeavor.

The human menstrual cycle, by its very name, implies a relationship to the month and moon. However, even elementary textbooks promulgate that the menstrual cycle averages 28 days (rather than 29.5—the number of days in a synodic-lunar month), and so ingrained is this belief that the eight and a half million women using the "pill," regulate their menstrual cycles to 28 days. Close re-examination of the data collected by earlier workers (the same data that produced the 28-day interval for the menstrual cycle) has now shown that the true average period of the human menstrual cycle is 29.5 days—the exact length of the synodic-lunar month. It was also found that the average gestation period—the time elapsed between the day of conception and delivery—was exactly nine lunar months (266 days).

Armed with this information it is now possible to count backwards 266 days from a birth date to learn the day of conception. By examining a large number of birth dates, then, it should be possible to learn if there is a synodic-lunar monthly rhythm in the time of conception. After statistically examining the birth dates of over a quarter of a million children born in New York municipal hospitals, it was found that the birthrate, and therefore the conception rate, is highest during the three days around full moon, which gives the "moon-spoon-June" ditty some scientific validity. An increase in conception rate at full moon suggests an increase in mating activity—a phenomenon seen in many lower animals.

Ecologists were quick to postulate that the added light reflected onto earth from the full moon must be the cause for the increased mating activity, although there is no proof of this. Nevertheless the newspapers made head-lines of this "fact" nine months after "Black Tuesday" (November 9, 1965), the day the east coast of the United States was incapacitated by the pan-demic power failure. It was amusingly reported that just nine months after the blackout, birthrates in the New York hospitals had increased. "There-fore," the newspapers proffered, "the ecologists are wrong, it is complete darkness that stimulates mating activity." The papers may have been wrong, for, as can be seen in photos taken that night, Black Tuesday was a night of full moon.

Scientists and others have always wondered if there might not be some sort of a rhythm in the human female's sexual desire. For years it has been tacitly assumed by the medical profession that the female desire for sexual union is greatest around the time of ovulation; however the little literature there is on the subject is a mixture of folklore and fact. Last year a study was done in an attempt to resolve this question. The greatest difficulty in carrying out the study was the selection of suitable subjects. All volunteers who were taking birth control pills had to be eliminated as were those who had undergone hysterectomies, those having intercourse regularly and thus often sated, those who were admittedly frigid, and those who "always felt like sex." The investigator finally assembled thirty women, who all had regu-lar menstrual cycles and no regular sex life. In addition they were in psycho-therapy and could be queried about their sexual feelings during each session with the psychiatrist. In this way a periodic desire for intercourse over 75 menstrual cycles was documented. . . . The women's libido was highest dur-ing the latter half of menses and during the period prior to ovulation. Other studies have shown that women also reach orgasmic climax more often around the middle of their menstrual month.

One of the most intriguing aspects of time-dependent processes is the rhythmic response of recipients to various toxins and medications. For ex-ample, if identical doses of bacterial toxins are injected into mice at various times of day, induced lethality is found to be rhythmic: 80 percent of the mice are killed when injected at 8:00 P.M. while less than 20 percent die from identical injections administered at midnight. Similar studies with ethyl alcohol caused death to 60 percent of a sample mouse population when the alcohol was administered at 8:00 P.M., while 20 percent died after 8:00 A.M. injections. Many drugs used on human beings come only in alcohol solution. Sodium pentobarbital, a commonly used anesthesia, was experi-mentally administered to rats and mice at different times of the day; in-jections given at night produced intervals of unconsciousness 66 percent longer in duration than identical doses given during the daytime. Damage caused by whole body X-irradiation has also been shown to be rhythmic, nighttime exposure being the most dangerous.

It has been shown that the allergic reaction in man varies with the time of day. Injection of common house dust just under the skin causes an in-flammatory reddening and a welt, the severity of which is greatest after 11 P.M. injections, and least after 11:00 A.M. Many patients with asthma have more frequent attacks at night. Another study concerned itself with the length of time that aspirin continues to circulate in the blood. It was found that it remains in circulation a shorter length of time if taken at night, indicating that the analgesic benefits are prolonged when the medication is taken during the daytime.

Some of the most useful and relevant studies on the human living clock should come from the field of medicine. The discovery that the effect of some medications varies with the time of day could alter some of the basic tenets of therapeutic medicine and the test-screening procedures of new drugs. Unfortunately, the medical profession is far behind in the study of human rhythms. There are many questions that need answering in this area. For instance, should the heartbeat rhythm be taken into account before a heart transplant is attempted? Should not surgeons be sure that a donor's kidney is in phase with the excretory rhythms of the potential recipient? Is it wise to subject "evening people," whose temperature cycles and body processes do not reach a maximum until afternoon, to early morning surgery? Are their bodies in a state best able to survive at this hour? Should manned space shots be initiated early in the morning when most men's reaction times and work proficiency have not yet peaked for the day? Would not more world records be broken if athletes were aware of their body rhythms in performance efficiency? There is a great deal left to learn.

Because of the living clock's relentless activity, we are not the same person from one hour to the next; but at the same time each day, we are much like we were the day before and much like we will be tomorrow. Thus far, our studies of time-dependent processes in man are only in the initial, descriptive stages; we are discovering and describing more and more new rhythms. Unfortunately, as yet we have few concrete notions as to how the internal machinery of the living horologe actually functions. This mechanism must be deciphered because of its medical implications, because rhythmic behavior is a fundamental property of all life, and because of the insight it may provide into the personal and social functioning of our species.

Chromosomes and crime: some tentative thoughts

MARY A. TELFER

Chromosomes are threads of DNA (deoxyribonucleic acid), the genetic material which determines all the physical characteristics—sex, build, eye color, etc.—of every individual. They are conveyed through the vehicle of egg and sperm at the moment a child is conceived. But when something goes awry with the chromosomes, the result is genetic tragedy. Mongolism is, by far, the most common of these tragedies. Less well known are two diseases that relate not only to mental retardation but possibly to criminal behavior as well. And these involve mistakes in the number of chromosomes that determine sex in the human male.

Sex in human beings is determined by two chromosomes which have long been designated X and Y; the normal female complement is XX, the normal male XY. Whenever a newborn carries a Y chromosome he appears male, for it is the function of the Y chromosome to produce testes and ultimately male hormones. X and Y chromosomes have served mankind well as sex determinants, but they are by no means infallible.

Once in every 500 male births, for example, the sex chromosome complement is XXY rather than XY, thus erring in the direction of femaleness. The resulting individual, called a Klinefelter male, is usually retarded, unusually tall and sterile.

Erring in the other direction, however, is the XYY complement resulting in the "supermale." He is also unusually tall and somewhat retarded, but appears to be highly, perhaps too highly, sexually motivated. The XYY male is probably a rare creature, found once in 2,000 adult males at large, according to available surveys. From these two figures it can be estimated that one in 400 males or one in 80 tall males in the general population will carry either the XXY or XYY sex chromosome abnormality. The social destiny of such men is the subject of much contemporary study and concern.

While the crime-and-chromosomes theory has been recently handled as a "news" story by the press, it is not entirely new. It was 30 years ago that the eminent criminal anthropologist, Earnest A. Hooton, went so far as to say, "The primary cause of crime is biological inferiority—and that is exactly what I mean," although this is now considered an excessive overstatement.

In 1962, William Court Brown of Edinburgh noted the predisposition of XXY males for "larceny, fire-raising, and indecent exposure." In a perceptive and prescient letter to *The Lancet*, a British medical journal, Dr. Court Brown asked "whether such individuals could be held in law to suffer from a diminished responsibility by virtue of their abnormal constitution."

Dr. Court Brown's colleague, Patricia Jacobs, then pursued the matter one step further. In 1965, she performed chromosomal studies on 197 violently criminal Scots and found seven cases of XYY among them. Given an expected prevalence of only one XYY in 2,000 males, this experience was an eye-opener and laid the groundwork for dozens of genetic investigations of criminals all over the world.

One such study was carried out in our own cytogenetic laboratory at Elwyn Institute, a large private facility in suburban Philadelphia for the evaluation, education and rehabilitation of the mentally retarded. We were intrigued by Dr. Jacobs' contention that an extra Y chromosome results in tall stature, mild mental retardation and severely disordered personality characterized by violent, aggressive behavior. We therefore planned to confirm and extend her studies.

What the studies revealed

For our first experiment, we visited a detention facility for juvenile delinquents in Philadelphia. The results: of 14 tall male delinquents studied, the first one tested, a 6-foot, 2-inch 16-year-old detained for sexual assault and Peeping Tom activities, proved to be XYY.

In the course of our second experiment, we screened 30 tall (71 inches or more in height) males in a state prison for mentally deficient criminals and found two XXY males. A later experiment in a general prison produced one XXY and two XYY males out of 35 tall men studied. Finally, screening of 50 tall patients in a maximum security state mental hospital for the criminally insane, revealed no less than four XXY and two XYY males. As reported in *Science*, we thus found a total of five XYY and seven Klinefelter males, all undiagnosed and all unsuspected, among 129 tall subjects. This resulted in an overall prevalence of one gross chromosomal error among each 11 tall criminal males rather than 1:80 as would be expected from chance alone. Subsequent screening of tall males in relatively "open" state mental hospitals has given negative results, with a single exception—one XXY male who was being housed in a maximum security building. Offenses listed in the records of these males included larceny, burglary, assault, attempted rape, rape, murder, sodomy, corrupting morals, prison breach and robbery.

Syndrome status for the xyy

It is our tentative conclusion, then, that the prevalence of males with gross errors of the sex chromosomes is greater among criminals, particularly the criminally insane, than can be accounted for by chance alone. The XXY male has long been thought to display a constellation of symptoms that makes him diagnosable; that is, he has achieved syndrome status. It would seem that the XYY male is fast achieving similar status. His symptoms, as we and other laboratories tend to think of them, are: extremely tall stature, long limbs with strikingly long arm span, facial acne, mild mental retardation, severe mental illness (including psychosis) and aggressive, antisocial behavior involving a long history of arrests, frequently beginning at an early age.

On reading newspaper accounts of Richard Speck, who murdered eight Chicago student nurses in 1966, we noted all these traits and therefore concluded that Speck was a likely candidate for the XYY disorder. Independently, a cytogenetic laboratory in Chicago confirmed this hunch, reinforcing our inclination to believe that the XYY syndrome is really coming of age. It seems quite possible that in the XYY male, exemplified by Speck, biologists are describing in genetic terms a certain type of defective criminal who has long been explicitly recognized by the forensic psychiatrist.

It should be made clear, however, that studies such as these do not indicate that every criminal has a chromosomal error, or that every victim of a genetic mistake will turn to a life of crime. (A West Coast research team plans to search for well-adusted XYY males—e.g., basketball players, where the height factor is involved.) Nevertheless, these surveys do prove that there are in prisons and hospitals great numbers of males, probably 100,000 all told in the United States, who have detectable chromosomal errors. Furthermore, it is painfully evident that genetic diagnoses are routinely being missed because the staffs of these institutions are physically and intellectually isolated from the sources of knowledge that will enlighten them; they cannot be expected to use tools they cannot even name.

The problem of the future, then, is a familiar one: namely, to apply well what diagnostic tools we already have and to develop new ones. The physician needs more outward and tangible physical clues to detect inward and subtle genetic errors in all abnormal populations—the younger the better.

Having identified a very considerable number of XXY and XYY youngsters, or better yet, newborns, scientists of many persuasions can carefully observe the dynamics of growth and social behavior as a function of age. This will shed light on many vexing problems, including that of the relatively few XXY and XYY males who are known to have stayed out of institutions.

Chromosomes and the law

Should the theory of chromosomes and crime be confirmed, the impact will be felt in fields well beyond the realm of biology and medicine. Psychiatry, particularly psychoanalysis, will be faced with both a challenge and an opportunity—a challenge to accept objective genetic facts and an opportunity to explore the mechanism by which a chromosomal mistake is translated into abnormal behavior.

The legal profession, too, will feel the impact. In Paris, French lawyers cited the chromosome abnormality in the case of Daniel Hugon, a 33-year-old XYY male held on a murder charge, but the jury found him guilty. In Australia, on the other hand, an accused murderer was acquitted after XYY evidence was given on his behalf.

"Irresistible impulse"

Although Anglo-Saxon law made, as early as 1326, provisions for defense by virtue of "madness," and epilepsy has been successfully used as a defense for murder in modern Britain, innocence by virtue of chromosomal constitution puts a new wrinkle in an ancient discipline. Furthermore, should a special biochemical cycle be revealed in XXY or XYY psychopaths—resulting in the periodic buildup of intolerable tension, as suggested by some case histories—the law will have to cope with pleas of "irresistible impulse," even when the defendant is fully aware of right and wrong and of the criminal nature of his act.

The social dilemma has been well-stated by Judge Jerome N. Frank: "Society must be protected against violence and at the same time avoid punishing sick men whose violence drives them beyond their control to brutal deeds. A society that punishes the sick is not wholly civilized. A society that does not restrain the dangerous madman lacks common sense."

One immediate and high-priority goal of this branch of medical genetics should be to promptly identify and treat, by the best means available, every carrier of a gross chromosomal error. To do less is to waste our powers. Ultimately, by use of computerized scanners attached to microscopes, newborns and mass populations of all kinds will be screened rapidly and routinely—the chromosome number will become another facet in that personal profile which already extends from blood type to social security.

Sophisticated techniques will also permit far-reaching studies of epidemics, plotting the occurrences of chromosomal errors as a function of time and place. There is already good evidence that "outbreaks" of mongolism follow viral epidemics by nine months, implicating viruses as damaging agents leading to chromosomal error at the time of ovulation. Greater understanding of the role of viruses and other elements of the environment could help lead to prevention, the long-range goal of all concerned.

Until that remote day arrives, we must identify as many carriers of the XXY and XYY abnormality as possible, covering all degrees of age and intellect, and study them intensively. Such information will provide insight regarding whatever therapy—social, psychiatric or chemical—is helpful in improving the function of these genetic and social misfits. We are a long, long way from a "biochemistry of sin," but it just may be coming.

Recently exploded sexual myths

LEON SALZMAN, M.D.

Over the years, primitive and animistic concepts of nature and of man have lasted far longer than they were needed. Much progress has been made in the last 100 years in sexual attitudes and knowledge, particularly since Freud's revolutionary contributions, but we are still a long way from being truly enlightened. Sexual myths, misinformation, and prejudices are still widespread.

Sexual activity requires not only organs and hormones, but also a complicated set of patterns of interaction which involve the customs, mores, prejudices, and standards of the culture, including the intricate patterns of courting, preliminary sex play, and permissible genital contact. Because sex activity is accompanied by special qualities of pleasure it has occupied a special place in man's activity even though it has not necessarily been the major focus of his interest. Since it is the only biological function that can be postponed for long periods of time or even abandoned permanently, it has played a special role in religious systems which make renunciation a measure of devotion or sacrifice, or a gift to the gods.

Medical history is replete with widely accepted notions which later turned out to be false. Under the influence of brilliant charismatic teachers, man hangs on to fallacious ideas long after they have been shown wrong. This has been particularly true in activities that require not only an understanding of oneself and one's own needs, but also some sympathetic and empathic understanding of the other person in a natural human interaction. Other human physiological functions can be studied in the individual with objective techniques. Sex is the *only* function of man that requires the involvement of another person for its fullest biological expression. Procreation requires only physical intimacy, but some element of relationship is almost invariably present in most humans. Therefore no one's sexuality can be understood by studying one sex or the other, but only by studying both together. In addition, a great deal of data regarding sex behavior is

RECENTLY EXPLODED SEXUAL MYTHS From *Medical Aspects of Human Sexuality*, Vol. I, No. 1, September 1967. Reprinted by permission of the publisher and the author.

subjective and available only through introspection and reporting free from restraint, shame, or guilt. Man's psychology, and particularly his sexual functions, remain the last bastion of ignorance and therefore involve the greatest number of myths and superstitions.

Freud's brilliant contributions, as well as the growth of democracy and personal liberty and the ever-increasing body of knowledge about human physiology, have all helped to explode many sexual myths. In more recent years the contributions of Kinsey, Masters and Johnson, Sherfey, Money, and a host of biochemists and psychoanalysts have produced a major breakthrough in our understanding of human sexuality and our explosion of myths both new and old.

Myths of male primacy

In the monotheistic religions, sex became identified with sin, which severely influenced man's attitudes toward sex and encouraged ignorance and mythmaking about the sex function. Both historically and theologically, the female has been considered inferior to the male as well as more sinful. She has therefore been especially burdened by false, distorted, inconsistent, and damaging views of sex. She is the victim of many myths about her potency, including the feeling that sex is her only interest and simultaneously that she is basically disinterested in sex. She is subjected to myths about man's potency and about her own capacity for orgasm, her sex needs, and her right to be active before and during sexual intercourse. Many myths about femininity (notions of weakness, insecurity, lack of privilege, and absolute dependency on the male) inhibit her from demanding fulfillment in her own right.

The myth of sex-linked character structure: Sexual myths are most abundant in the area of sex differences and the presumed innate psychological qualities in each sex. Freud inadvertently nourished many of the primitive notions of male and female differences which grew out of ignorant and unscientific prejudices of previous ages. He advanced biological hypotheses which supported many of these notions. But recent contributions by psychoanalysts, anatomists, and biochemists have almost completely destroyed these myths and demonstrated that sex and character structure are not biologically ordained, and that many of the differences between male and female are culturally derived and therefore culturally alterable.

In particular, the notion that the female is inherently passive and the male inherently active because of the nature of the sexual organs and sexual intercourse has been shown to be fallacious by detailed physiological studies of sex activity, as well as by the general behavior of man and woman. Far from being passive in the sex act, she is an extremely active participant, to the extent that her vaginal contractions may be more responsible for sperm reaching the ovum than the sperm's own motile powers.[1]

The myth of female coital nonaggressiveness: The assumption that the male must be aggressive in sexual intercourse and the female passive is simply not valid. To achieve maximum gratification, each partner must be passive *and* aggressive, and must participate mutually and cooperatively.

The unfortunate persistence of labels supposedly attributable to one sex but not the other has led to untold misery. Women have been the major victims in the hangover from Victorian morality and scientific infantilism which makes both men and women feel guilty, inferior, inadequate, or even "homosexual" when their inclinations are somewhat different from prevailing prejudices concerning the role of each sex. Since under this notion the mantle of submissiveness falls to the woman, she has been required to wait upon the demands of the male and to be subject to his particular program of sexual activity. To encourage or direct the male's sexual activity was to step outside the female role; to suggest or recommend measures that might enhance her enjoyment would be aggressive, or too "masculine." Consequently, she has been expected to be patient and long-suffering, and to depend upon the man's good will and competence for her enjoyment.

When woman has refused to function in these prescribed ways some theorists have insisted on labeling her behavior as latent homosexuality, masculine protest, penis envy, or a refusal to accept her proper biological role. Such labels are remnants of outmoded conceptions of female psychology.[2]

The myth of penis envy: The notion that envy of the male penis leaves women with indelible scars of inferiority feelings, vanity, and susceptibility to neurotic illness has been shaken by biological studies as well as by psychoanalytic data. Biologically and neurologically the female is not at all inferior to the male. Indeed, in many ways she is better equipped to fulfill her role biologically. She has a more labile nervous system and a more responsive autonomic system, which are probably related to the need for her to handle the recurring crises of menstruation, childbirth, and childbearing.[3]

The myth of male embryological equality: In an excellent anatomical, biochemical, and physiological review of the nature of female sexuality, Sherfey[4] has made use of data assembled by biologists over many years to establish that the female sex is primal, and not the male. The early embryo is female, so that one can no longer speak of a bisexual phase of embryonic development. Genetic sex is established at fertilization, but the effect of the sex genes is not felt until the fifth or sixth week of fetal life. During this period all embryos are morphologically female.

If the genetic sex is male, primordial germ cells stimulate the production of the testicular inductor substance that stimulates the fetal androgens which *suppress* the growth of the ovaries. In this way, androgens induce the male growth pattern.

If the genetic sex is female, germ cells stimulate the production of follicles and estrogen. Even if estrogens are not produced (for example, because of artificial removal of the gonads before the 7th week), a normal female anatomy will develop. Therefore no *ovarian* inductor is required, and the female differentiation is the result of the innate, genetically determined morphology of *all* mammalian embryos.

Thus only the male embryo undergoes differentiation necessary for masculinization, while female development is autonomous. After 12 weeks, male-to-female sex reversal is impossible, since the masculine nature of the reproductive tract is fully established.

Myths of female orgasmic limitation

Despite the extraordinary advances in other areas of medicine during the last 200 years, it is only recently that we have finally learned much about the physiology of the female sexual apparatus, its role in the sex act, and how orgasm is produced.

Orgasms in men and women are biologically identical and consist essentially of the contractions of the responding muscles against the erectile chambers. The contractions expel blood from the woman's erectile chambers, and sperm from the man's.

The female is capable of successive multiple orgasms, while the male requires a refractory period before a further orgasm is possible. This capacity for multiple orgasm and readiness to respond to sexual stimulation requires regular and consistent sexual activity if a woman is to respond most adequately. Probably infrequent or insufficient sexual intercourse is the most common cause of female frigidity and difficulty in achieving orgasm. However, there is also need for continuous stimulation until orgasm, since the sexual tension in the female can fall instantaneously if such stimulation is discontinued. But since the female has a slower arousal time there is often anxiety that the male orgasm will come too soon to permit orgasm in the female. Often the tension produced by the man's anxiety results in too-early ejaculation rather than in the desired delay.[5]

The myth of the vaginal orgasm: The Freudian and post-Freudian sexual enlightenment has had many positive results, but it was also the source of new sexual myths which have only recently begun to be disproved. Physiological misunderstanding produced the notion of separate clitoral and vaginal orgasms, with the vaginal being described as the more mature and therefore more desirable, and the clitoral coming out only second best. The resulting efforts to achieve vaginal orgasms have been the source of enormous mischief. Only recently has the issue been shown to be entirely fictitious.[1,4,6]

There is every reason to believe that female orgasm is normally initiated by clitoral stimulation and that it consists of a series of spasmodic contractions of the vaginal muscles which may extend into the perineal area and beyond, followed by a marked relaxation of the whole genital area. It is a total body response but with marked variations in intensity and timing. Physiologically, it is a physical release from vascongestive and myotonic increments developed in response to sexual stimuli.

The extensive research of Masters and Johnson and the highly informative article by Sherfey have illuminated this problem. From a biological point of view, clitoral and vaginal orgasms are not separate. It is firmly established that the clitoris and the lower one-third of the vagina are the active participants in the female orgasm and are not separate sexual entities. There are indeed quantitative differences in the female response to the sex act, but there is no reason to assume that they are due to a vaginal rather than a clitoral orgasm.

The tendency to reduce clitoral eroticism to a level of psychopathology or immaturity because of its supposed masculine character is a travesty of the facts and a misleading phychological deduction. Embryologically, as Sherfey points out, the clitoris is not a Freudian small penis. In fact, the penis is more properly regarded as a clitoris that has been hormonally enlarged. This makes short shrift of the myths dealing with the immaturity of clitoral foreplay as well as with some assumed normative attitudes in the sex act based on old preconceptions of the role of male and female.

Indeed, the explosion of this myth encourages all kinds of preliminary foreplay through clitoral contact and massage. The presence of the penis in the vagina is a convenient arrangement for the mutual stimulation of the clitoris and the penis. But there is a growing conviction that sex activity should be practiced in whatever manner is conducive to the greatest mutual enjoyment, provided there is no physiological or psychological damage to either partner. The manner of stimulating the penis or clitoris, whether by means of finger, mouth, or vaginal insertion, should not be viewed in terms of either normality or maturity. There is a preferred posture to ensure procreation, but an enlightened attitude toward sex should avoid assigning priorities to particular methods of achieving sexual satisfaction. Laws in many parts of the world still cling to categories of "normal" or "deviant," but those of us with the advantage of modern psychological understanding should try to prevent variations of sex behavior between male and female from being labeled deviant so long as they do not prove physiologically or psychologically injurious to either partner.

The myth of an ideal coital position: Regardless of the anatomical position of the clitoris, the penis rarely comes into direct contact with the clitoral glans. However, the clitoris is continuously stimulated throughout coition even though it retracts during the plateau stage of sexual excitement. The erection and engorgement of the clitoris cause it to retract into the swollen clitoral hood, but the active thrusting of the penis and the traction on the labia minora provide stimulation and energetic friction of the shaft of the clitoris. After some time, the orgasmic contractions begin.

The clitoral reaction is the same irrespective of what is used to stimulate the clitoris and whether the stimulation is direct or indirect. Thus the various positions advocated to increase penile contact with the clitoris are largely superfluous, or else impossible. However, a female-superior or lateral coital position does allow for more direct contact. Such positioning is often discredited and avoided because of the notion that the woman's passive role requires that the man always "be on top." Now, however, we may throw out the myth of masculinity as having anything to do with who is on top.

The myth of simultaneous orgasm: The liberation of the woman was accompanied by her demand for orgasm. She was often encouraged to believe that it should always take place simultaneously with the man's, if indeed the relationship was a mature one.

Simultaneous orgasm soon became a highly valued goal. The enormous complications in the production of the orgasm both in the male and the female were overlooked, as were the extensive education and sophistication which was required to produce simultaneity.

A less idealistic and more realistic understanding of the sex act is now helping to debunk this myth. While simultaneous orgasm is certainly desirable, it is usually possible only under the most ideal circumstances.

The myth of the superiority of the large penis: The lower one-third of the vagina is different morphologically from the remaining two-thirds and is capable of accommodating any size of penis. It is a fallacy to assume that the larger penis will be better able to stimulate the clitoris or more effective in coitus. The notion that the larger penis has greater possibilities for pleasure or for producing orgasm in the female thus also turns out to be a myth.

Myths of the omnipotent libido

The authority of Freud and the readiness to assume that all genital behavior is sexual have permitted other unproved doctrines to persist. Objective observation is made difficult by the libido theory, with its reductionistic hypothesis that all behavior is ultimately libidinal. Doctrines that attribute *everything* to some one cause tend to prejudice the observer by supplying answers and labels for a piece of behavior before a variety of possible explanations has been considered. From the earliest years of Freud's work there have been major disagreements with the notion of the libido as a primal motivating force, and many alternative hypotheses have been presented by Adler, Jung, Rank, Horney, Sullivan, Fromm, Kardiner, Rado, and other psychoanalysts.

The myth of the infant sex drive: The belief that the sex drive is a primary influence on human development prior to gonadal maturation and adolescence is full of half-truths and unproved assumptions. Evidence from the direct observation of children is scanty, and more recent studies tend to emphasize the child's curiosity and other adaptive interests.[7]

Doctrines of infantile sexuality have derived major support from failure to regard the child's penis as a urogenital organ used more often for urination than for sexual purposes. The penis and clitoris have a profusion of nerve endings that make them pleasurable to fondle, but this does not prove that their role in infancy is primarily *sexual*. Penile erections caused by full bladders or rapid-eye-movement dream states need not be called sexual. Sex as such is rarely a human need until adolescence, and it is misleading to apply the adult label "sexual" to genital play, penile or clitoral, prior to gonadal maturation.

Freud's notions about infantile sexuality were an outgrowth of his work with adults. Since it is almost impossible to get direct data from adults about their experiences prior to about age 4, when it is presumed that a great deal of sexual development has already taken place, the information is extrapolated from later years via free association or dream analysis. Some interpretations made in child analyses are heavily influenced by the presupposition that the Oedipal attachment is essentially sexual. All of these observations and adult extrapolations could be understood in a variety of other ways.

Probably the shocked displeasure at Freud's revelations about the infant's sex life was falsely motivated, but it may have had a core of validity. We need not return to the myth of a pure, wholesome, and angelic infancy and childhood. Rather, we might take a naturalistic view of man's early years in which his development is directed at becoming an adaptive and competent organism. There is no privileged biological subsystem with a special motivating force. Instead, the organism develops as a whole under the direction of the needs of the moment.

The myth of sex as the primary cause of emotional disease: The myth that masturbation can cause mental illness is now pretty well on the way out. More persistent is the belief that interference with the full expression of the sex instinct is the primary source of mental disorder.

Most behavioral scientists do not regard sex as an *instinct* in man; rather they tend to view it in the same category as other necessary biological functions, such as cardiac action, ingestion, and excretion. Instinct theorists and sexologists have, in recent years, emphasized the learned elements in human behavior. Generally, sex activity in man takes place in an atmosphere of tenderness and mutual regard and resembles "animal" sex activity only to the extent that it is an act of procreation. Its biological significance in man is only a small part of its total importance. There is no reason to believe that one will develop a mental or physical illness unless one's sex needs are satisfied, or that an individual patient's sex life must be paramount in his emotional adjustment.

Of course disturbances of sex function do occur in mental illnesses, and masturbation, for example, can be used to alleviate anxiety in a distressed person. The greater emphasis on the interpersonal aspects of sex behavior in recent years has drawn attention to the extraordinary capacity of sex to fulfill many of man's needs aside from biological procreation. To this extent sex is important in therapy and may occupy a large or small part of the process.

The myth of "creativity as sublimation": The libido theory has also perpetrated the myth that all creative activities are ultimately the product of sexual sublimation. This notion too is under critical attack by psychologists and social scientists who find evidence that man is motivated—particularly in his esthetic, artistic, and philosophical pursuits—by forces well outside of his sexual interests. Creativity is the outcome of the fullest expression of man's total capacities and ideals, not simply a sublimation of sex.

The myth of universal homosexual latency: Many of the myths of homosexuality are finally being put to rest, but the myth of latent homosexuality and a homosexual stage of development in all individuals still persists. This is tied up with the notion that man is bisexual. These hypotheses can no longer be accepted as fact. The concept of bisexuality is strongly disputed by most biologists, and its application to man is highly doubtful.[8]

The so-called homosexual stage of development may be more adequately understood as a period during which one seeks out one's own sex for a multitude of reasons other than sexual ones. The myth that each of us has both homosexual and heterosexual traits dies slowly. Its demise will be hastened when homosexuality is defined more carefully, and when recent research material is more generally available.

Conclusion

In the past 30 years, and particularly in the last 10, many long-cherished and closely guarded prejudices have been struck down by advances in anatomy and biochemistry. Most credit must be given to those brave and enlightened scientists and public educators who, in the face of public opprobrium and continued self-righteous puritanical criticism, have striven to clarify this most significant aspect of human functioning. It is to them that we owe our enlightenment about the sexual function in man, which has a right to be studied and viewed as any other human activity would be, and to undergo the same rigors of research and investigation as any other human biological function.

When we give these scientists our full and unqualified support, then the myths about sex will disappear just as surely as the myths about man's physical functions and diseases have. This is a worthy goal, for the full and proper functioning of man's sexual activities can greatly expand his pleasure and good will.

References

1. W. H. Masters and V. E. Johnson, *Human Sexual Response* (Boston: Little, Brown and Co., 1966).
2. L. Salzman, "Female Sexuality: A New Look." *Arch. Gen. Psychiat.,* to be published.

3. A. Montagu, *The Natural Superiority of Women* (New York: Macmillan Co., 1953).
4. M. J. Sherfey, "The Evolution and Nature of Female Sexuality in Relation to Psychoanalytic Theory." *J. Amer. Psychoanalyt. Assoc. 14:*28–128, 1966.
5. L. Salzman, "Premature Ejaculation." *Int. J. Sexol. 8:*70–76, 1954.
6. J. Marmor, "Some Considerations Concerning Orgasm in the Female." *Psychosomat. Med. 16:*240–45, 1954.
7. P. Chodoff, "Critique of Freud's Theory of Infantile Sexuality." *Amer J. Psychiat. 123:*5:507–18, 1966.
8. S. Rado, "Critical Examination of the Concept of Bisexuality." *Psychosomat. Med. 2:*459–67, 1940.

Sex and the work of
masters and johnson

HARVEY D. STRASSMAN, M.D.

It is ironic that patients are receiving instruction and guidance about sex from physicians with upper middle class backgrounds and little scientific knowledge of human sexuality. In some instances, their advice is based on myths and fallacies considered to be the cultural and behavioral norms, even though they may not be appropriate for the individual patient. To treat a patient with a sexual problem, the physician must have a sound knowledge of the subject as well as a sophisticated attitude toward this basic human activity. All aspects of human existence, including sexual response, should be within the province of the physician.

The sexual act in lower mammals is triggered by endocrine changes occurring in the female during the estrus. Attracted by the scent of the female, the male prepares for sexual relations and ejaculation for the biologic purpose of procreation. In man, the same function is the basis of sexual union. However, because man has the ability to conceptualize, abstract and symbolize, sexuality means more than just the biologic phenomenon of stimulation through endocrine glands and scent.

Although it has been demonstrated by Benedek that sexual interest in women is related to the preovulatory phase of the menstrual cycle, this is surely not consistent in all women. It is well known that the human female will accept the male at any point during the menstrual cycle if she so wishes. The multifaceted nature of sexual intercourse, tied as it is to the love relationship as well as to pleasure and play, makes sexual behavior a complex matter.

To understand this behavior, three facets of human sexuality must be considered: (1) the societal and cultural aspects, as expressed by the group and subgroup, (2) the psychologic aspects, as developed by the individual within the group, and (3) the biologic and physiologic aspects. In

SEX AND THE WORK OF MASTERS AND JOHNSON From *GP*, Vol. 38, No. 4, October 1968. Reprinted by permission of the publisher and the author.

every individual, sexual intercourse involves all three facets of sexuality. The first two have been studied intensively, the cultural aspects by anthropologists and the psychologic areas by psychologists and psychoanalysts. Two years ago, in *Human Sexual Response*, William Masters and Virginia Johnson reported their 10-year laboratory investigation of the physiology of sexual response.

Cultural and social aspects

American society is governed by the Judeo-Christian tradition as modified by the Protestant ethic. This has created certain attitudes about morality and sexuality that date back to the Puritan origins of our culture. Important elements of the Protestant ethic and Judeo-Christian tradition are the belief in the value of work for its own sake and the assumption that success means worthiness. Clustered with these values are the relation of pleasure to evil and the association of sexual pleasure with the concept of sin. This means that, from the viewpoint of our cultural heritage, sexuality has only one purpose—procreation.

Thus sexual behavior becomes a stereotype for most people, and sexual activities that are solely for the purpose of pleasure and mutual enjoyment become guilt-ridden and interdictive. Some types of sexual behavior are considered deviant by portions of our society but anthropologic studies show that any sexual activity exists with many variations throughout the world. Attitudes of individual groups toward such activities range from complete permissiveness to complete prohibition. It can be demonstrated in various cultural studies that no sexual behavior pattern is universally taboo. It has *not* been shown that what we consider deviations in sexual behavior produce—or are correlated with—any greater incidence of psychiatric disorder in any particular culture. Only a few examples are needed to demonstrate the differences between American values in regard to sexuality and the values governing sexual behavior in other cultures.

Children and sexual experience

Our culture views the involvement of children in sexual intercourse as both physically and psychologically traumatic. In the Society Islands, however, young children are allowed to indulge in sex play and often have some type of sexual contact. Actual intercourse officially starts only at puberty, under the instruction of an older relative of the opposite sex. This is in contrast to the Mojave Indians, who permit intercourse between children before the age of 10 but do not allow them to participate in intercourse with an adult. The Kaingang of Brazil introduce children to intercourse at an early age but always with adults; intercourse is not permitted between children. There is no evidence that these patterns result in any psychologic disorders within these groups.

Mores and response

Individual mores in regard to sexual response are just as variable in many parts of the world. For example, in our culture women are expected to be passive in their approach to sexuality whereas the Muria of India expect women to be as sexually aggressive as men. These variations in attitude have no relationship to cultural sophistication or geography, as demonstrated by three tribes in the New Guinea area of the Pacific. The Munugamur expect women to be aggressive and female orgasm is the expected norm. Among the Manus, women are almost universally frigid and find coitus humiliating. The Arepesh view the sexual act as a comfortable mutual expression of affection but do not admit erotic interest and women do not reach orgasm. In contrast to these attitudes, the Marquesans of the Eastern Pacific, also a culturally unsophisticated society, have erotic patterns similar to those in the United States. For example, sexuality is substituted for tenderness and the breast is the leading erotic symbol.

A recent development in the United States is the need for the man to know that he sexually gratifies the woman; this attitude has long existed in both France and Samoa. In the United States, the man above and the woman below is the common position for sexual intercourse; in many South Sea Island cultures, this is referred to as the "missionary position."

With the knowledge that no sexual activity is forbidden everywhere, that any variation can exist as a normal part of some culture, it is obvious that the individual can adopt whatever he wishes as his own sexual behavior, regardless of cultural setting. What occurs sexually in the privacy of the bedroom between two individuals becomes that which is mutually satisfactory to both, even though it may not meet the stereotype of sexual behavior for their particular culture or subculture.

Sexual intercourse is the most common intimate relationship between man and woman. This biologic act becomes a complex psychologic activity when each individual brings to it the totality of his knowledge, experience and emotional conflicts. Psychologic aspects of sexual relations have their base in the pleasurable bodily sensations discovered in early childhood, in the relationships between child and parents, in the truths, myths and fallacies about sexuality created in the child's mind during his early years and in the actual sexual experiences of adolescence and early adult life.

In early childhood, many tactile sensations are experienced as pleasureable. Sensations arising from irritation of the skin or temperature change are experienced as unpleasant and an inability to relieve the irritation creates tension. When the parent relieves the tension by correcting the situation, the child experiences the relief as pleasure. In the daily care of their children and in play with them, many parents discover the areas of skin that create pleasurable experiences for the child. Some adults quiet a crying child by stroking the genitals. Children also learn through their own experience that pleasant sensations are produced when the genital area is stroked; it is not uncommon to see children playing with their genitals when absorbed in other activities, like watching television. This activity is not perceived by the child as sexual but simply as pleasurable. Some adults view the activity as sexual and punish children for it. The child remembers these areas as the pleasure zones of the skin and in adulthood associates them with sexual pleasure (the erotogenic zones). If tactile pleasure is absent or if the child is punished for these pleasures, negative attitudes are created which will interfere with sexual pleasure in adulthood.

As the child develops, various parts of his body become more significant because the parent pays more attention to them. In the earliest levels of development, the mouth is the most important area because of feeding and weaning; later, during toilet training, the urethral and anal sphincters become the most significant areas. At the age of 4 or 5, children discover for themselves the differences between the genital organs of the male and female and they now become interested in this portion of the body. The differences between the adult's body and the child's body remain an area of curiosity until the child reaches puberty. If his experiences during these various development phases are pleasurable, the child gains healthy attitudes toward his body and its functions. If his relationships with adults have been pleasurable and gratifying, the child looks forward to one day becoming an adult and having adult privileges and pleasures.

Thus sexual interest proceeds from pleasure with one's own body to interest in another child's body, then to interest in the adult's body and, finally, to an adult interest in another adult's body—one of the opposite sex. Affection becomes part of this development very early if the child experiences his mother's love through her constant tender handling and fondling. One can recreate this feeling by looking at any picture of the nursing mother in which the half-satiated child in the mother's arms is looking at her face, while she, with a wonderfully satisfied expression on her face, is looking down on him. This is the primordium of love and requires complete giving on the part of the mother. When an adult is capable of this complete giving of affection and tenderness, he is capable of loving.

Mature sexuality

When sexual intercourse occurs between two mature adults, the act does not begin with carnal sexuality but with a loving interchange in which there is much kissing, tenderness and expression of affection. These expressions generally include touching the partner's skin to provide pleasure. This activity usually proceeds to manual stimulation of the genital area and the beginning of sexual excitement. As sexual excitement rises, each partner becomes more active, using methods known to give the other pleasure. Often this phase may include mild pain but, in normal adults, it is never carried to an unpleasant extent. Each partner, while receiving pleasure, also attempts to anticipate the needs and enhance the pleasures of the other. Each must be willing to give pleasure and postpone gratification for the sake of the other's satisfaction.

In the modern marriage, where sexual intercourse usually occurs at the end of a long work day, in a household where there are a number of children of various sizes and ages, it is apparent that, even under the best psychologic conditions, there are many distractions which can prevent the ultimate in sexual pleasure and love for a married couple.

The psychologic elements indicate that any sexual activity that is acceptable and pleasurable to both partners in the relationship is permissible.

Physiology of sexual response

Most sexual data in the past came from the extensive questionnaires of Kinsey and the reports of psychiatrists based on their examination of the personal lives of patients. A number of theories and fallacies about the sexual act became prevalent among the general public. Masters and Johnson have been able to compile the scientific data necessary to understand and clarify this complex act.

Before the scientific observations of Masters and Johnson are discussed, a few pertinent facts about their research should be emphasized. These investigators were concerned with only the physiologic aspects of human response to sexual stimulation. Their first observations were of men and women during automanipulation and sexual intercourse. They chose subjects who volunteered for the project who were from upper socioeconomic and intellectual strata because they felt these persons could provide the best data. Since their initial studies on individual sexual responses, the authors have investigated husband-and-wife units and individuals with problems of infertility, impotence and frigidity. Although complete medical and emotional histories were taken on all subjects, no attempt was made to correlate emotional problems with sexual response.

Beliefs and fallacies

A common belief is that sexual prowess is related to the size of the genital organ, either the penis or the vagina. It has been shown that the size of the penis is not related to skeletal or muscular development; that erection produces only a relative increase in the size of the penis over its size in the flaccid state, and that the increase is a matter of only 1 or 2 cm. The vagina is infinitely distensible. In fact at one stage of sexual excitement, it actually balloons in the distal portion so that, if intromission occurs at the proper time of sexual excitement, any vagina can accommodate any penis. It is evident, then, that concern about the size and adequacy of the genital organs is based on psychologic factors rather than actual differences in anatomic or biologic function.

Another fallacy is that women experience two different kinds of orgasm. This belief arose from psychoanalytic theory, which held that automanipulation in childhood acquainted women only with clitoral sexual sensations and, therefore, that they could not become aware of vaginal sensations. According to this theory, only the mature woman was able to shift from the awareness of sensation in the clitoris to vaginal sensations and, finally, to experience orgasm arising in the vagina. Scientific investigation demonstrates that sexual stimulation occurs through movement of the clitoris within the clitoral hood, brought about by deep pelvic thrusting of the penis. This stimulation increases sexual excitement and orgasm is finally felt throughout the pelvis. In essence, then, there is only one type of orgasm, no matter how it is produced.

It is also commonly believed that women are able to have only a single orgasm, which leads to satiation. Research shows that women may have many orgasms. The refractory period between them is short and satiation depends on the extent of the woman's fatigue. Women who have had adequate sexual experience and have achieved orgasm many times are often able to achieve orgasm through breast stimulation or even through fantasy. It appears that the lack of orgasm in the female is due to a lack of adequate sexual experience or to a cultural belief that she should expect no pleasure from the act or to psychologic conflicts about sexuality.

Sex and old age

To investigate the belief that sexual activity stops in the geriatric population, Masters and Johnson studied 61 menopausal and postmenopausal women; the oldest was 78 years of age. All those in the study were able to reach orgasm. Kinsey had noted that women who had well-adjusted and stimulating marriages, with adequate sexual gratification, usually continued sexual activity with little or no interruption until old age. Thirty-nine male geriatric subjects were included in the study; the oldest was 89 years of age. These men were able to achieve adequate erection and participate in the sexual act. However, the time necessary to achieve erection increases with aging, from three seconds in the average young male to somewhere between 10 and 15 seconds in the older male. In the older male, there is a longer refractory period between ejaculation and another erection. These biologic facts are the basis for fears of failure and play a definite psychologic role in the sexual prowess of the geriatric male.

The definitive changes in tissues and in the anatomy of reproductive organs at various phases of sexual excitement become important in determining better contraceptive methods and in solving the problems of impotence and frigidity. An interesting finding of Masters and Johnson concerns the production of vaginal fluid during sexual excitement. Although Bartholin's glands were thought to be the major source of vaginal lubrication, it has been shown that lubricating material appears on the walls of the vagina within 10 to 30 seconds after the beginning of sexual stimulation. This fluid is a transudate and comes directly from the venous plexus surrounding the vaginal barrel. When an artificial vagina is created in a woman, by epidermal grafts, a mucoid material appears on the wall of the artificial vagina after adequate sexual stimulation. This transudate increases and becomes an adequate lubricant for coitus. In two of the women evaluated, there was as much vaginal fluid as in the normal female. Masters and Johnson postulated that a venous plexus forms around the artificial vagina and that sexual stimulation assists in the formation of the plexus.

Masters and Johnson identify four phases of sexual response in the human female. The first is the excitement phase, which can last for several minutes to hours; the second is the plateau phase, lasting for 30 seconds to three minutes; the third is the orgasmic phase, lasting for three to 15 seconds, and the fourth is the resolution phase, which lasts 10 to 15 minutes. If no orgasm occurs, this final phase may last as long as one-half to a full day. This research indicates that orgasm is beneficial in female sexual physiology because it assists in draining the venous plexus of blood and helps reduce the tension due to engorgement of the pelvic organs.

Sexual stimulation, sexual response and sexual intercourse are an important part of everyone's life and they deserve the scientific attention they are now receiving. Scientists do not make moral judgments. They determine facts and use them to protect health and prevent disease, whether physical or emotional. Physicians who help persons with medical problems should use the knowledge of sexual response in the identification and treatment of patients' sexual problems.

Drug addiction—facts and folklore

OLIVER GILLIE

"The sufferer is tremulous and loses his self-command; he is subject to fits of agitation and depression. He has a haggard appearance ... as with other agents, a renewed dose of the poison gives temporary relief, but at the cost of future misery." This description is not, as might be thought, an account of the action of heroin or morphine on someone addicted to it, but an account of the effects of coffee given by a distinguished pharmacologist at the turn of the century. Tea was thought to be equally harmful and to cause "hallucinations which may be alarming in their intensity." The now universal habit of drinking tea at breakfast was then considered by many doctors to be hazardous in the extreme. "An hour or two after breakfast at which tea has been taken ... a grievous sinking feeling ... may seize the sufferer, so that speech is an effort. The speech may become weak and vague and by miseries such as these the best years in life may be spoilt." Knowledge of the action of the drugs present in tea and coffee has come a long way since these early years but ignorance, prejudice and fear still haunt our knowledge of many other drugs.

Scientists are not immune to these fears and prejudices and may even have to adopt some of them as working hypotheses before they can progress. There is, for example, a great deal of dispute, still unresolved, as to whether lysergic acid causes mutations (see "LSD and chromosomes," *Science Journal*, September 1968); yet there is very little concern that caffeine—the active drug in tea and coffee—may cause mutations in man. In fact caffeine has been shown to cause mutations very readily in micro-organisms and fruit flies but does not appear to cause mutations in mice. The conclusion that caffeine does not cause mutations in mammals, including man, is in agreement with what most people wish to believe and so the question has been left there. Whereas in the case of LSD very many more experiments have been done and still it seems that no unequivocable statement can be made about its genetic effects in man. If the genetic effects of

DRUG ADDICTION—FACTS AND FOLKLORE From *Science Journal*, December 1969. Reprinted by permission of Transworld Feature Syndicate, Inc.

caffeine on micro-organisms had been known at the turn of the century it is not difficult to imagine how readily the warnings against drinking tea and coffee would have included references to "hereditary degeneration."

This does not mean that there are no hard facts available about drug addiction; on the contrary, facts are available from such a wide range of disciplines—from pharmacology to sociology—that the problem of drug addiction can only begin to be understood by referring to all of them. Efforts have been made in the past by the World Health Organization and other official bodies to define what is meant by the term drug addiction. The term was at first restricted to the "hard" drugs such as heroin and morphine and another term "drug habituation" was said to be the proper way of describing the abuse of "soft" drugs which were believed to induce only psychological dependence. It is now agreed that these general distinctions, while not entirely spurious, are rather misleading. The Expert Committee of the World Health Organization now favors the use of the term drug dependence for all types of "drug abuse." The problem, they now point out, is one for clarification rather than for definition.

The danger to life from drugs can be defined in a rough and ready way by a scale with the hard drugs at one end and the soft drugs at the other. Cannabis has been moving steadily down the scale and amphetamine and barbiturate—drugs only available in the past from the family doctor—seem to be steadily moving up the scale. Alcohol and tobacco are, by tacit agreement, often omitted from this reckoning, yet they possibly constitute the greatest threat to human life in simple numerical terms.

How is it that drugs so grip the body and mind of the addict that they constitute a danger to life? Is there any hope that the seasoned addict can be cured?

Curiosity rather than search for oblivion is the reason given by most heroin addicts for first experimenting with the drug, according to a survey of 106 addicts in the U.K. and U.S. conducted by J. H. Willis of Guy's Hospital, London. These addicts had all been admitted to hospital for treatment and had been administering heroin to themselves daily for at least six months. Other reasons given for first trying heroin were a search for relief of depressed mood or the elevation of mood above normal. About a third of the addicts recalled, however, that their first experience of heroin had been unpleasant.

Nobody knows how many people try heroin once and find this first taste so unpleasant that they do not persist, but the addicts in the sample studied by Willis were found to begin to inject themselves daily within one to six months of the first experience of heroin. A small proportion of the sample injected themselves irregularly for two years before starting to inject themselves daily. Daily injection developed earlier in British subjects than in American subjects, suggesting possibly that the purer heroin available to British addicts produced earlier addiction.

It is almost impossible in the present state of knowledge to separate the picture obtained of drug use from the method of research used to obtain it. Surveys of hospitalized addicts can tell us little about many others who use drugs less frequently and never come to a doctor for help. A different method of investigation which attempts to overcome this difficulty has been used by a group from the Institute of Psychiatry, London; they went to live in hired rooms near the center of a provincial town in England and gained the confidence of addicts who gradually adopted the place as a sort of social center. This enabled them to obtain information by direct observation and interviews.

A picture was built up of the past and present lives of a group of 31 male and six female addicts—the average age of the girls being 18 and the boys 21. They belonged, on the whole, to a higher social class than that of the rest of the town and had had better than average educational opportunities. More than half of them had attended grammar school or the equivalent and about the same number had gone to some form of higher education such as university or technical school. The majority of these, however, failed to complete their courses, although seven were still full time students. Only 14 out of the 37 subjects were in full time employment and they had jobs of a lower level than would be expected with their educational background.

These studies of heroin addicts also showed that heroin is not the only drug which they use. Amphetamines, marijuana, cocaine and LSD were also used by many addicts but this is not evidence that these other drugs lead to heroin. In fact investigations of drug users in general, rather than just heroin addicts, show that there are many people who use other drugs without being entirely dependent on them and without necessarily progressing on to heroin. The evidence suggests that many users of drugs limit themselves to certain kinds of drugs and do not try others which they consider to be too risky.

Turning on and "scoring" are two of the words used by drug takers to describe the different stages of a trip; the world of drugs is characterized by a poetic use of language all its own. The person who knows the words and wears the right clothes belongs to the subculture and is accepted with little question. To consider drug addiction without reference to this aspect of the drug experience would be very misleading. Too often in the past interest in addicts has been limited to the physical aspects of their dependence on drugs and they have been treated as an object to be cured simply by getting them to stop being physically dependent on the drug. Many addicts who have been withdrawn from physical dependence on drugs go back to drugs once more. This is not simply because they "lack will-power," as has sometimes been suggested, but rather because all their friends are "junkies" and they identify strongly with them.

Records show that many addicts have had very disturbing experiences of being rejected or dominated by parents. The drug scene provides a genuine escape into a group which accepts them with little questioning and provides a comradeship which they have failed to find elsewhere. This comradeship is expressed not only by their common clothes and language but also by the sharing of many things, often including the syringe used for injection. The sharing of syringes involves a danger of infection with virus which causes jaundice—so much so that tracing sufferers from jaundice has been found to be a good way of discovering addicts. In a survey in Crawley New Town nine out of 20 people who had had jaundice were found to be heroin users; a further 41 addicts were found during the course of another survey. In all about 20 percent of the addicts found in the area had had jaundice, whereas jaundice is comparatively rare in the general population.

The comradeship of the drug addict sharing his drug and his syringe is similar to the comradeship of the smokers who hand round a packet of cigarettes. Curiously many tobacco smokers are unable to enjoy a cigarette if they are asked to smoke while blind folded. Apparently, for many people, an important part of the smoking ritual is to be able to observe themselves performing. In the same way the rituals of drug taking are important and have some satisfaction in themselves—a conclusion which may seem scientifically dubious to some but one which is in fact supported by experiments on animals described later. This ritual aspect of drug taking may be particularly important amongst addicts in the United States who obtain such small supplies of heroin that they seldom develop the severe physical withdrawal symptoms of the addict on high doses.

As well as providing a ritual, drug use provides a ready identity to the addict. According to Isidor Chein of the Research Center for Human Relations, New York University, the addict's feelings can be summarized like this: "You are a teacher. You are a cop. You are a parent, a man, a woman, a citizen, a voter, a landlord, a housewife. Me, I'm a junkie. A junkie is a person, not a thing." In this way the addict acquires an identity and a set of relationships which have some personal meaning. Available figures show that, the addict is from the earilest part of his life characterized as an outcast, a delinquent or one of a minority group long before he takes to drugs. Out of 100 addicts studied by George E. Valiant of Tufts University, Boston, by 16 years of age 50 percent had lost their fathers and 20 percent their mothers. These figures are three times the national average.

According to folklore the real alcoholic can only be cured by giving up drink altogether; if he touches a drink again he is lost. It was not until a few years ago that this belief was finally disproved, although it still seems to be as strongly entrenched as ever in folklore. Beliefs such as these tend to act as self fulfilling prophecies: an alcoholic who believes that he is bound to return to the bottle when he so much as has a drop is very likely to do so. Alcoholics, like addicts on hard drugs, suffer from withdrawal symptoms which may include hallucinations when they stop drinking. Alcoholism is therefore a physiological as well as a psychological problem.

The experience of four Finnish alcoholics, investigated by D. L. Davies of The Maudsley Hospital, London, first showed that the alcoholic could give up excessive drinking and stabilize on a normal drinking pattern. The four Finns formed themselves into a group which they called the Polar Bears. This group functioned as a self-help group rather like Alcoholics Anonymous but differing from them in their beliefs. The Polar Bears hold informal discussions amongst themselves which are not centered on the question of drink; in fact they believe that Alcoholics Anonymous places too much emphasis on this type of discussion. The Polar Bears have their own views on the cause of alcohol addiction, believing that the addict has suffered "milieu damage" in childhood which leads to maladjustment in adult life. They also believe that normal drinking can be achieved when the addict obtains some insight into his past. The four men were all excessive drinkers and had undoubtedly been alcoholics, but after a number of years of abstinence all resumed normal drinking. Two of them have been drinking normally for two and a half and one and a half years respectively. The other two drink more regularly but less severely, although both enjoy occasional drinking sprees with their friends.

Davies has investigated another 18 cases of a similar kind, 15 of which were drawn from the records of The Maudsley Hospital. Normal drinking habits were achieved in between 15 and 18 cases with only three cases being controlled drinkers still taking in abnormally high quantities of alcohol.

These results show that there is room for a variety of solutions to the problems of addicts. Alcoholics Anonymous has achieved excellent results but their philosophy may be unhelpful to some and quite unsuited to others. The philosophy of the Polar Bears, derived as it is in a more permissive age, may be better suited to other addicts.

The chemical environment of the body is altered by the presence of drugs and this in turn produces changes in the body cells themselves. This is shown by the common observation that heroin addicts, for example, are able to tolerate higher and higher quantities of the drug. The seasoned addict is able to take doses of heroin that would kill the person who takes the drug for the first time. In fact a number of people experimenting with drugs for the first time do die this way and others experience a bodily response which may be very unpleasant and include severe nausea and vomiting.

Experiments have shown that animals can be made tolerant to higher and higher concentrations of drugs in the same way as addicts. Clues about the nature of addiction have come from the discovery that rats and mice do not become tolerant to morphine—an opiate similar to heroin—if at the same time they are given a drug called actinomycin D which inhibits protein synthesis. This suggests that inhibition of the process of protein synthesis by actinomycin D stops the cells from adapting to high levels of morphine. However, the experiments have been criticized because they involve giving animals the very powerful drug actinomycin D over a period of weeks.

These experiments have now been repeated by B. M. Cox and M. Ginsburg of the Chelsea College of Science and Technology, London, who have shown that increase in tolerance to morphine in rats is prevented by administration of actinomycin D for periods of a few hours only. These short periods of administration are such that interference with normal body functions by depletion of proteins is not expected. This suggests that some change in cell proteins normally induced by morphine is prevented by actinomycin D. Actinomycin D does not affect protein synthesis directed by ribonucleic acid (RNA) already produced, but prevents new RNA being formed which carries new instructions from the deoxyribonucleic acid (DNA) blueprint. Further experiments suggest that the site of action of actinomycin D within the body may be in the brain: if the drug is injected direct into the brain then it is effective in much lower concentrations. All this points to the synthesis of a new protein in the brains of people and animals tolerant to morphine, although at the moment it is only possible to guess as to what the functions of this new protein may be.

The action of drugs can also be measured in terms of the effect which they have on nervous activity. Such studies have shown that opiates such as heroin and morphine reduce the amount of "transmitter substance" which serves to carry nerve messages across synapses from one nerve to the next. It is not known definitely that these drugs have the same action within the brain as they do on nerves outside the brain but it seems most likely that they do. If this is so then it is possible to explain withdrawal symptoms as being the result of the sudden release of a lot of dammed up transmitter substance, or as a result of the nerves becoming sensitive to transmitter substances during the period when they receive only reduced quantities of transmitter substance. A variety of theories have been suggested but there is still a lack of facts and still no general agreement as to which is inherently more plausible than the others.

Study of sleep has shown that drugs do not only affect people when they are awake and aware but also that the quality of their sleep is affected by drugs they have taken. The effect of drugs on people is to deprive them of their dreaming sleep—to deprive them of a fantasy world where vital personal problems may be solved. When people accustomed to using drugs are withdrawn from them they begin to sleep abnormally and spend a larger than normal part of the sleep dreaming—often experiencing fearful nightmares.

There are two basic kinds of sleep: "orthodox" sleep and "paradoxical" sleep. During orthodox sleep there are no dreams and measurements of brain waves show a slow "alpha" rhythm. People move their eyes about rapidly during paradoxical sleep and if woken during this period report vivid dreams. The brainwaves of paradoxical sleep are more like those during normal wakefulness.

These two kinds of sleep alternate and there are usually about five periods of paradoxical sleep each night taking up about a quarter of the whole period of sleep. Studies made by Ian Oswald and others at Edinburgh University have shown that people addicted to amphetamines have normal sleep while on the drug, but when the drug is withdrawn they may have periods of paradoxical sleep which last for a whole night or for a long part of it. These abnormalities did not disappear until more than two months after the withdrawal of the drug and were suppressed if the patient returned to drugs. These disturbances of sleep show that even with the "soft" drugs there is a physical basis to drug dependence.

Amongst other things, says Oswald, these experiments have shown that "the distinction between 'physiological' and 'psychological' dependence was a relic of the past in which medical men regarded the body and soul as

301

dichotomous, whereas today we believe that mental events are determined by brain (physiological) events. The most characteristic feature of any abstinence syndrome is the craving. As this was merely psychological it was accorded little importance. It is, however, absurd not to recognize that it has a basis in brain function, as yet unascertainable, just as all drugs which are said to produce 'psychological dependence' do so because they effect brain physiology and change the person's feelings and thoughts."

Barbiturates—the commonly used sleeping drugs—suppress paradoxical sleep and on withdrawal the person may experience a great increase in paradoxical sleep together with nightmares. This rebound increase in paradoxical sleep may continue for months after ceasing administration of the drug, long after all drug has been eliminated from the body. Alcoholics withdrawn from alcohol entering the state of withdrawal syndrome called *delerium tremens* show a great increase in paradoxical sleep, as do addicts withdrawn from morphine. At present it is not known whether these effects on sleep are direct or indirect effects of the drugs themselves; however, they are obviously of the greatest importance in understanding the basis of addiction and withdrawal.

During the course of his experiments on sleep Oswald took heroin for a week and found it to be a miserable experience. This led him to consider seriously for the first time the suggestion that addicts take drugs, at least at first, because they wish to belong to a social group. He described his experience as follows: "The extraordinary thing is that it brings no joy, no pleasure. Weariness above all. At most some hours of disinterest—the world passing by while you just feel untouched. Even after the injection there is no sort of thrill, no mind expansion nonsense, no orgastic heights, no Kubla Khan. A feeling of oppressed breathing, a slight flush, a sense of strange unease, almost fear unknown. You doze, see a daft scene where someone throws something, jump up in sort of panic, and doze again. Hypnagogic hallucinations, they're called. Irritable, lacking something of both patience and libido."

Learning plays an important part in the process of becoming addicted to drugs. The first experience of drugs is often unpleasant yet a person continues to take them because they may be awarded approval or social recognition by a group of people who they aspire to join. Animals, such as monkeys and rats, can also learn to take drugs and become addicted to them when the taking of the drug is associated with some reward.

Animals are made able to inject themselves with drug by the surgical introduction of a tube into a vein which is then connected to a reservoir outside the cage. All the animal has to do is press a lever to obtain an injection. Using this apparatus monkeys will learn to administer drugs to themselves as a means of alleviating withdrawal symptoms induced by the experimenter giving drugs to the animals. Monkeys will also learn to inject themselves with morphine, even if they are not suffering from withdrawal symptoms, although to do this it is often necessary to tape raisins to the lever to begin with to induce the monkey to press it.

Experiments conducted at University College London by Hannah Steinberg and others have shown that it is possible to teach rats to drink solutions of morphine even though they are bitter. Here the rats were given nothing but morphine solution to drink for two days and then on the third day given a choice between morphine and water—this cycle was repeated for 57 days and then the rats were given a choice every day. A clear preference for morphine solution developed so that in the end the rats were taking more than 50 percent of their water as morphine solution.

There was little difference in the amount of morphine solution or water drunk between rats which had been injected with morphine and rats injected with saline before they were presented with morphine to drink; this shows that it was necessary for both groups of rats to learn that drinking the bitter solution was associated with the effects of the drug. A control group of rats offered the similarly bitter solution of quinine developed no preference for it—never taking more than about 15 percent of their liquid in this way. This clearly shows that during the course of satisfying their thirst, the rats learnt to overcome their aversion to a bitter taste and became as a result addicted to morphine. This was confirmed by injecting the addicted rats with morphine which led them to drink less of the morphine solution. When the addicted rats were deprived of morphine altogether they developed withdrawal symptoms which could be measured as an abrupt loss of weight. Rats deprived of the quinine solution showed no such loss of body weight.

If monkeys addicted to morphine are deprived of drugs other types of behavior which they have learned become disrupted, but their behavior returns to normal when they are again given morphine; their learned behavior patterns also show a temporary recovery when the animals are allowed to inject themselves with saline at the same time as the appearance of a colored light which they have learned to associate with the injection of morphine. These studies show many parallels to human behavior with drugs and seem certain to suggest ways of weaning addicts away from the set of conditions associated with drug taking which serve to strengthen their desire to make what they call a "connection."

Cure of addiction to even the hardest drugs is possible but it cannot be guaranteed. It is necessary not only to rid the addict of the physical craving which his body has developed for the drug but to provide rewarding distractions in the hope that the drug itself will become progressively less rewarding. Treatment by subtle forms of punishment, more politely known as aversion therapy, is one possible way of eliminating undesired behavior, but this by itself would probably not be sufficient. Another method is to give the addict large quantities of a different drug which may prevent the first drug from being satisfying. On this principle methadone has been given to swamp the effects of morphine or heroin but the danger of this is that the addict is simply introduced to another drug which may add to his existing repertoire.

There is no simple formula for cure of addiction. In the United States little success has been achieved by subjecting addicts to enforced periods without drugs either in hospital or in prison. Curiously the most effective treatment found in one survey of addicts was imprisonment followed by a year of parole; but the success of this latter treatment may have been because of the parole rather than the imprisonment.

Other experiments in the United States have been made with structured therapeutic communities where each member is committed to do away with antisocial behavior and is encouraged to give to his fellow the emotional support he needs. The Phoenix House community in New York, run by the Addiction Services Agency, has a built-in social status system. Anyone entering the community does so voluntarily and has to work his way up from the bottom; this status system is designed to be always achievable. The addict is given useful work to do, much of which involves maintaining the community. Each day there are meetings of the entire community at which rules, projects and current events may be discussed. Members of the community also have individual psychotherapy with a trained therapist who offers himself to the patient as "a whole person . . . and in doing so establishes commitment." There are also group psychotherapy sessions and, of course, purely social activities. No drugs are used in the community and random checks of urine are made of 20 percent of the members of the community for drug use each week. Phoenix House has had a drop-out rate of only nine percent and there has been no evidence of drug use in the community. This is quite a remarkable achievement as residents had been using drugs for an average of 12 years.

Many different types of therapeutic communities are possible and it seems unlikely that any simpler solution will be successful. The addict is "hung up" on drugs—that is his scene—and nothing short of an alternative scene is likely to satisfy him. He has dropped out of society and rejected all that society has to offer and he feels that society has rejected him. But addiction is a problem not merely of the drop-out on the streets: it is a built-in part of the conventional doctor patient relationship. Estimates show that between 10 and 15 percent of prescriptions given by doctors are placebos: they have no direct medicinal value but are given for psychological reasons. A minimal estimate of the number of patients dependent on the symbolic functions of medication in the United Kingdom is 50,000. Drugs—administered legally or illegally—are a veil which masks the real causes of much psychological illness and distress.

❡Igor stravinsky:
on illness and death

ROBERT CRAFT

May 12, 1966

New York to Paris. Airplane conversations between strangers seem to follow a pattern. The first stage usually begins with a rummage for mutual acquaintances, shared opinions, shared impressions of places. The common knowledge even of a restaurant or hotel will help people to feel weighted together, proving to them that "the world is very small," when in fact it proves only that people of *pro rata* incomes tend to be found in the same places, and hence on the same highways leading to those places. Stage two, distinguished from stage one by the settling-in-of-cocktails, moves on to exchanges of scraps of personal confidences. And sometimes to more than scraps. My remarkably unreticent neighbor, a New Man type—Foundation Representative, I think, or political economist, or Rand mathematician, the sort of person who would chat with you about Quine's set theory or Bohr's complementarity principle if you knew anything about them—manages to deliver himself of a very substantial installment of autobiography, between some twenty or so foot-trampling trips to the lavatory. (When it turns out he is on his way to an important lunch tomorrow in the Congo, I confess that I have had some "contact" with the Congo myself, but not that this was limited to flushing the toilet over it on a flight to Rhodesia.)

Stage two depends on the amount and effectiveness of the libations. Owing to the tensions of flight and the limbo psychology that abrogates not only responsibilities but even the sense of time, the Establishment Narcotic is an especially potent confessing drug in airplanes (to say nothing of its biochemical effects, on blood sugar for example, and the salt content in the hypothalamus). High-altitude alcohol seems to push forward suddenly-remembered connections, stories, comments, all for a moment of supreme importance and all insisting on being voiced, but which turn away as peremptorily as a cat, and a moment later defy recalling. If we are but loosely in control of our thoughts ordinarily, how much less so are we under alcohol and over 40,000 feet?

Stage three, flirtation, depends on individuals, but a great deal of it transpires in airplanes. The reasons reinclude those for stages one and two, with the added factor that flying itself is sexually stimulating, both mentally —all flying dreams are sexual—and physically, if not in tingling sensations aroused by the wheels touching the ground, or in the pressure of braking, then at least in the desire to reembrace life, each landing being a birth. The central sexual ingredient in air travel is none of these, however, but the stewardess, toward whom the male passenger harbors, and often openly attempts to navigate, the most ardent wishes.

The stewardess is not merely a new amalgam of receptionist, party hostess, geisha, waitress, mother, mistress, nurse (bringing napkins every few minutes as if symbolically changing our diapers), but an entirely new aspect, or hitherto unexploited aspect, of Woman. Just as landscape painting did not exist before Giotto, though landscapes evidently did, nor the cult of literary tears before *Manon Lescaut*, though the flow of actual ones must have been fairly constant, so the commercially invaluable combination of beauty and bravery was unknown before the age of air travel. A handsome girl, ever the most desirable traveling companion anyway, is now the most exemplary as well, her valor, or indifference, shaming the passenger and helping him to collar his cowardice.

Our stewardess's lecture on flotation seats and life-raft inflating, on the donning of life jackets and the manipulation of lanyards, sounds like so much fun-filled fashion modeling. But her perpetual cheeriness gives way for a moment nearing the French coast when the plane begins to bump coltishly and to yaw and shake. In fact the sternness of her command to buckle seat belts and gutter cigarettes is then in such contrast to her usual manner that I suddenly become aware of the Holy Bible on the magazine rack, along with *Playboy* and *Time*.

Stravinsky objects to the stewardess tone of voice, nonstop smile, salesmanship ("Your personal airline," she says, repeating the legend of this giant, totally impersonal airline), and interminable translation: "Captain Smith hopes you have enjoyed your flight. Bye now. *"Le capitaine* Smeet . . .*"* I might add that the busy path of the stewardesses to the cockpit with trays of vodka, wine, cognac, champagne, and even Pernod has not greatly increased *my* store of confidence in Hauptmann Schmidt.

December 13, Hollywood

A visit from Yevgeny Yevtushenko, which the I. S.'s much enjoy, the family affection Russians are able to turn on at first acquaintance, even Russians holding such unpromisingly different views as the I. S.'s and Y. Y., amazing me once again. Yevgeny Alexandrovitch—the conversation is immediately on first-name terms—arrives with translator and publicity team in tow, but as soon as he has been pictured peeling his jacket under the tropical glare of his photographers' lamps, the entourage retires to another room. V. (Mrs.

Stravinsky) chats with him about Gorodetsky, Kuzmin, Vladimir Nabokov,[1] and other writers she had known in the Crimea during the Revolution, and of whom, she says later, Yev. Alex. reminded her. He listens carefully to her description of Osip Mandelshtam in the Crimea in 1918. "Mandelshtam was always ardent and always hungry, but as everyone was hungry at the time, I should have said even hungrier than other people. Having very few clothes, he parsimoniously hoarded the most presentable ones, which included an emergency shirt, as he called it, and a pair of almost- fully-soled shoes. Once he called on us wearing a raincoat and nothing else, then paced up and down by our cupboard the whole time like a peripatetic philosopher, not to keep warm but to find out—sniffing like a Platonic philosopher—whether our larder had any food. I also remember a train trip with him to Simferopol. The cars were so crowded with soldiers and refugees that babies sleeping on the floor were helmeted with pails to keep them from being accidentally crushed by people struggling to push through. I sat between Mandelshtam and Sudeikine, who dressed me like a Moslem woman on account of the soldiers." Yevtushenko tops this tale with an account of Mandelshtam's death, "drowned by bread, literally choking on it; his dying request was for *Russian* bread." (Y. Y.'s words, my italics.)

Of all the cultural ambassadors from the U.S.S.R. to have visited the I. S.'s, Yevtushenko is the first to notice the contents of the house. In fact he looks at everything, lifting and inspecting objects as he might do in a flea market, and admiring the paintings, especially one by V., thereby being presented with it on the spot, which is called Russian hospitality. Near the end of the visit he suffers one minor setback, when the talk suddenly turns to music and I. S. gives him a point-blank dismissal of Shostakovitch. But he recovers in time to mention several favorite compositions by I. S. himself.

Why am I recording this not very momentous encounter? I had not intended to, in any case, nor was I very attentive during it until I saw how animated the I. S.'s became speaking their *lingua materna* not, for a change, with other *émigrés*, but with a representative of the Russian political state. It seems to me that they were more natural with Yev. Alex. than they are with their closest American friends.

January 9, 1967, New York

A breath-fogging night. Dinner with Marcel Duchamp, who is tight-lipped and *sec*, but in aspect only. And what an aspect! The profile might have been used for a Renaissance numismatic or medallion portrait, and the posture, the backward tilt of the head, is characteristic of equestrian heroes such as Pisanello's Leonello d'Este, which farfetched comparison I attribute partly to something equine about Duchamp himself, partly to his table talk about the armor of scorpions. He is neat, well-barbered, tightly tailored. He sports a daunting pink shirt and blue necktie, too, though when complimented on the natty combination dismisses it as a Christmas present. A conversational opening is provided by mention of Giacometti, but when someone remarks

[1] Her English tutor in Paris was the novelist's brother, Serge Nabokov.

that this mutually lamented friend must have been "a *triste* person," Duchamp objects to the word: "Not *triste*, tormented." Certainly neither description could ever have applied to the raptorial intelligence of Duchamp himself.

But what *are* the feelings of a man who when the talk gravitates to airplane crashes—I am flying tomorrow—contributes the thought that "Death in the air is a good way to go because you explode"? (Or death in bed from a heart attack because you implode?) They are not morbid feelings, certainly, the thought being purely logical to him, with no more emotional coloring than one of his chess moves. What may seem untrue to type in a crystallizing intellect such as his is the easy susceptibility to outside amusements. He tells a story of the Queen of England visiting an exhibition of his work at the Tate Gallery and questioning an embarrassed curator about an object that, as Her Majesty did not seem to see, was ithyphallic. But this drollery is quickly followed with the observation that, "A freedom we are all much in need of at present is freedom from bad wit."

May 17, Toronto

A CBC concert in Massey Hall, I. S. conducting the *Pulcinella* Suite, after which I conduct *Oedipus Rex*. Leaving the hotel, I. S. happens to pass before a crowd come to stare at Princess Alexandra; what compounds the irony is that no one in it can be aware that the unscheduled parade of the little old man is a far rarer sight than the one they are waiting for, artistic geniuses being much harder to come by than merely well-born ladies.

For the first time in his life I. S. conducts sitting down, but this probably gives him more trouble than he avoids by not standing. He *is* very unsteady on his feet, though, and in spite of the chair, he grips the podium railing with his left hand during much of the performance. V. is alarmed watching him and remembering how vigorously he conducted in Chicago a mere five months ago. Worse still, as she can plainly see, the orchestra is not really following him but the *tempi* of my morning run-through of the piece.

The performance over, I. S. moves to a chair at the front of the stage, averts his eyes from triple-pronged TV exposure, listens to the accolades in French and English of two dignitaries, is bemedaled. This ceremony very evidently affects him, as it would not have done a year ago; in fact he would have been contemptuous of it then. It is not merely the ceremony, either, but the special warmth of the audience whose applause and reluctance to let him go have distinctly said, "This is the last time we will ever see Igor Stravinsky." No one is more aware of this than I. S.

I am unable to sleep after the concert, seeing, as if on one side of a divided movie screen, the I. S. of the past skipping across the stage to the podium, his movements twice as fast as anyone else's, and in this as in everything he did, his energy, physical and mental, leaving everyone around him far behind; and on the other side, I. S. tonight, old, frail, halting, and, I fear, conducting in public for the last time in his life. What makes his case the more disturbing is his terrifying self-awareness. A long decline and withering away would be a great cruelty to him.

May 24, New York

The findings of an electroencephalogram and of other tests performed on I. S. yesterday are amazing, says his physician, Dr. Lewithin. There is no sign of senility, of the brain-softening normal in a man of his age, nor any onset of brain sclerosis. But then, I. S. lives entirely in his brain. The receptivity tests have in fact shown his responses to be as rapid as they are in a man of thirty. I. S. is greatly interested in the encephalogram, which he compares to "an electronic score, with six-line staves and unreadable avantgarde notation," adding that the eighteen electrodes attached to his head made him look like "a bald woman trying to scare up a mane of hair."

At the same time, says the doctor, the composer's body is a ruin. Two blood-lettings and three Roentgen-ray treatments are scheduled for the week, and they are a matter of life and death, as I. S. knows—he is in fact already processing and overcoming the knowledge in his formidable psychological machinery. Armed with an understanding of the apprehensible biochemical facts, he will thus begin to "think positively," harnessing his powerful "esemplastic will" to all the favorable factors and ignoring the unfavorable. But the most difficult enemy to subdue is another part of the same mind, that powerful intelligence which has not aged with the body and remains so ruthlessly aware of it.

June 18, Hotel del Coronado, Coronado Beach, California.

"Are you Mr. Stokowski, the conductor?" the receptionist asks, and I. S. nods affirmatively. He is less amused later seeing his own name in a letter from Public Relations asking whether he would mind being photographed....

I. S.'s birthday party [2] is launched with slugs of Stolychnaya vodka and docked with a cake, baked by Milène, Stravinsky's daughter, and brought into the room by her in a parade with V., who carries a tray with eighty-five lighted candles. We sing "Happy Birthday" and I. S. says that that makes it *"Son et lumière."* But he says little else, and it is hard to know his feelings.

After I. S. has cut the cake, we open some of the four hundred cables and telegrams that have been piling up all week from all over the world. But whereas, for example, the President of Germany has sent a two-page homage, no word has come from any public official in America, where "The poor procession without music goes." Nor, of course, has any message come from that despoliation of the desert in which I. S. has lived for twenty-seven years. In fact the only acknowledgment of the anniversary in his home community was a concert by the "Beverly Hills Symphony," conducted by himself four months ago at a greatly reduced fee not yet received. So let the record stand. While the greatest living composer's eighty-fifth birthday is being celebrated all over the world by entire festivals, and countless individual concerts and performances, no organization in the vale of smog-induced tears that *he* has so long honored by his residence so much as thought

---

[2] He was born June 18, 1882, near St. Petersburg.

of dedicating a program to the event. In fact, the *art* critic of the Los Angeles *Times* alone recognized the necessity, for Los Angeles's sake, of a concert, but when permission was sought for the musicians to contribute their services for it, the Musicians' Union refused on grounds that it would "set a precedent." A precedent for whom? Is a deluge of Stravinskys imminent? In Los Angeles?

July 15, Hollywood

Nureyev and Fonteyn come for aperitifs—directly from rehearsal, which partly excuses his getup: white tennis shorts, white sweater, white sandals. From the front he may be "faun-like," as is said, but seeing the back first, with the long, shaggy Beardsley-period hair, one could take him for a tousled woman. He is quite unlike the thrasonical exhibitionist of newspaper copywriters, nevertheless, and in fact I have rarely seen anyone more gracious and gentle with I. S., to whom his first words are: "This is a very great honor for me; I only hope I am not taking your time."

He talks about Bronislava Nijinska's revival of *Les Noces*, saying he had learned a great deal from it himself. The I. S.'s then talk about their red-carpet reception in the U.S.S.R., and this makes him uneasy. When V. quotes Nancy Mitford on the "clean feeling in the Soviet Union that money doesn't matter," he cannot help breaking in: "Of course it doesn't. There is nothing to buy: no automobiles, no houses, not even food." But he speaks gratefully of Madame Furtseva, the Culture Minister, who discovered him during the Bolshoi Ballet's season in Paris. "One afternoon at a reception for the dancers she pointed to me and told one of her minions, 'Next time this one will dance the solo.' That did it." Explaining his defection shortly after, he says that "The Soviet dancers were quartered in a very poor hotel near the Place de la Bastille, where we never saw anything of Paris. Then one day I learned how to use the Métro and took it to the Champs-Elysées. Walking from there to the Seine, I resolved never to leave; Paris seemed to me the most wonderful place on earth. But tell me, why are Russian *émigrés*, in Paris and California and everywhere else, so nostalgic for a Russia most of them have never seen?" V. suggests that part of the reason is in Russian literature, and it is true that many of the refugees she knows exist in a world of Russian books and have never learned other languages. Nureyev's rejoinder is that "A refugee should live according to the way of life in the country of his adoption." Just as *he* lives?

Next to I. S., who is as thin and shrunken as Mahatma Gandhi, Nureyev is impertinently healthy-looking. Entering the room, he identifies a post-card-size Klimt, and he continues to study the art objects on tables and walls, glancing back and forth from them to I. S., as if trying to crack the "object language" of the house—people being implied by their possessions, after all—which is simply I. S.'s obsession with the minuscule.

July 27, Hollywood

Seeing the I. S.'s again after even a short separation moves me nowadays almost more than I can bear. They are the two most marvelous people in

the world, the last survivors of a richer and better humanity, a whole continent in themselves. But they are so old and creaky and fragile now, and so
terribly alone. They knew the hour of my flight, and when to expect me; if
I am late they will go to the window again and again and play their rounds
of solitaire more anxiously. When I do arrive, the sight of them in the door-
way, to which they come at the sound of my taxi, is upsetting. They seem,
especially after that ride through the junkyard and the dreck of Los Angeles,
so desperately out of place as well as out of time, for I tend to think about
them, when I am away, as they were in the past. To see them after an interval, therefore, is a sudden acute reminder of age, a reminder full of the
pain of impending loss.

August 21, New York

An alarming call from V. during my recording session tonight saying it has
been discovered that I. S. has a bleeding ulcer, that he has been taken to the
Cedars of Lebanon, and that he has lost more than half of his blood. I
arrange to fly back immediately.

September 13, Hollywood

The fourteen days in the hospital and nine subsequent days in bed at home
have been extremely weakening. I. S. has lost eighteen pounds—one wonders from where, since he was so tiny anyway—not much of which can be
regained on his present frugal diet. His rib cage reminds us of photographs
of Buchenwald, and he complains that every nerve ending in his skin-and-
bones body is raw and painful. The hematocrit still stands at only 35, too,
whereas the platelet count has risen to 1,200,000. The one component of the
blood is anemic, in other words, and the other too rich, and to complicate
matters further, the indicated medication for each is "counter-indicated"
for the other. His uremic acid level is high, as well, and each finger of the
left hand throbs like toothache from what has now been diagnosed as gout.
Worst of all, and unspeakably depressing to observe, is the defeat, I pray
only temporary, of that powerful will. He does not even read today, and
when I switch on the television for him to watch his favorite African animal
program, he refuses to turn toward the screen, saying, "I only like to look
at it in Vera's room." He tells V. that he saw his birth certificate in a dream
last night, and it was "very yellow."

September 25

A marked upturn today symptomized by an old-time tantrum over some of
the contents of the mail: a fulsome fan letter; a self-paying *Who's Who*
form; a request to fill in a sexual questionnaire (I. S. is regularly circularized
for this); a tape of a "ballad composed on a harmonica by an airline pilot
during flight," herewith submitted for I. S.'s opinion, which is: "I will be
afraid to fly again." Reaching for a Kleenex and finding it to be the last in
the container, he flings the empty box to the floor. V. gently admonishes
him, as one would a small child, telling him that the box will probably have

311

to remain where it is until a pile accumulates: "Then perhaps the thrower will realize that we have no one to pick up such things."

George Balanchine comes for dinner, snorting and sniffing as if from hay fever, twitching as if he might be getting the *tic douloureux*. In check pants, silver-buckle shoes, double-breasted blue jacket with gold buttons, sideburns to the ear lobes, he looks a spiv, but on arrival puts in a half-hour of very conservative piano practice. He describes the *Salome* ballet now planned for Suzanne Farrell, using mudra-like movements, and asks me to suggest music for it by Berg; but *Reigen*, the only possibility I can think of, is too large orchestrally, and like the Variations and Adagio from *Lulu*, which he has also been considering, is too brooding in character and too explicit dramatically. I suspect Balanchine's conception hinges on the circumstances that the seven-veil striptease, like that of Astarte-Ishtar, would nowadays conclude in a complete disrobing, and that the dance would be able to show Salome, like the Queen in *Alice* ("Off with his head"), really wanting a different part of the victim than the one she gets.

When Mr. B. first enters I. S.'s bedroom, I. S., very self-conscious about his loss of weight, says: "As you see, like all Americans I am reducing."

October 8

At about 4:00 P.M., I. S. complains of a chill, and his teeth, as he says, begin to *"klapper."* By 5:00 P.M. he has a 101° temperature, which, in his weakened state, is very alarming; he can hardly navigate across the room now, and his shoulders and torso are as fleshless as a coat hanger: pneumonia or even influenza could kill him. His lungs seem to be clear, however, and the fulminant pains he complains of are obviously abdominal. But when I ask him to describe them, he sits bolt upright and says, "FEAR." Soon after this he begins to micturate every few minutes, which could indicate an infection from bladder crystals formed by the high uric acid.

Reentering the room at 7:00 P.M., I find him praying, *Gospodi, Gospodi,"* over and over, with his head turned to the wall. At length a doctor arrives and prescribes Gantrisin. At the beginning of the doctor's examination I. S.'s pulse is fast, but as soon as he is convinced that a bladder infection is the true complaint, the pulse rate drops to normal and the temperature to a bit below; he has had a death scare, and was as frightened of flu and pneumonia as we were. All night long, says V., who spends it on a couch at the foot of his bed, he twists, turns, fumbles with the sheets trying to make a nest, but is unable to forget the specter.

I realize now that in recent years I have so often hidden my true feelings for him precisely because of the dread of this moment. Yesterday evening those feelings came irrepressibly flooding out as the result of an extraordinarily clear hour with him, during which he talked to me and discussed his ideas with me in the way it used to be between us years ago. I understood then that he has no thoughts of *not* going on. And he can go on of course, in that undamaged and undaunted mind of his, but only there, which is the tragedy.

Ever since I have known them, I. S. and V. have kissed each other at first sight of every new moon, a promise of renewal. The moon is new tonight, but they do not see it, and there does not seem to be *any* future.

November 2

I. S.'s "gouty" left hand has suddenly turned black. A new team of doctors, after consultation early this morning, attributes the discoloration to circulatory blockage from a sludge of platelets, a rate of some 2,000,000 at last count, versus a normal 200,000. The finger pains of the past eight weeks were caused not by gout, in other words, but by circulatory failure, and the anti-gout medicines were not merely powerless to relieve the hand but were dangerous for the ulcer. The discovery is infuriating as well as frustrating. Why was a gout specialist not called two months ago, and a competent vascular cardiologist?

It is decided to try to dilate the coagulated capillaries by blocking the nerve with Novocain injections, and as this entails a risk in a man of I. S.'s age, the operation can only be performed in the hospital. Choking with tears and fears, I pack his bag and take him there in early afternoon, practically carrying him from his room to the car, for he is heavily drugged and scarcely able to walk.

The injection is not administered until seven o'clock, after a second *consilium* with a second vascular cardiologist, but when we return to the hospital at eleven, the fingers are even more horribly black. The surgeons now speak of it as gangrene and mention the gruesome possibility of amputation, further warning us of a high danger of pneumonia, I. S. having been in bed for so long. I take V. home, then go home myself, but I cannot pass I. S.'s studio and bedroom, or look at his dark window from my room, or, of course, sleep, and when going to bed I remember and use all of my childhood prayers.

November 3

The finger color has improved slightly after the third Novocaine injection, but the hand is still gangrenous. Sick as he is, however, and despite the haze of pain-killing sedation, I. S. shines like a beacon, replying precisely, ironically, originally, I. S.-ishly, to the forensic inquisition of his doctors, and replying to them in English and German, moreover, and to myself and V. in French and Russian, without once mixing or confusing the languages or fumbling for a word.

His extreme fastidiousness is giving him no end of trouble. He insists on staying in the *gabinetto* unaided, and even on brushing his teeth unseen, and he charges me to explain to the nurse that he does not mean to be rude, but is unable to converse with her. To me he says, "I can offer you nothing here but *ennuis*." As we leave him, the nurse, noticing my anxiety and probably seeing me trying to stifle my feelings, follows me into the corridor with the advice that "It is a mistake to get so involved," as if "involving"

313

oneself were a matter of choice, and as if a noninvolved life, if it were possible, would be worth living.

November 5

The index finger is slightly less black this morning, and the palm of the hand is a little rosier; the nerve will not be blocked today. As the amelioration is ascribed in some degree to a trickle of alcohol in the intravenous fluid, it is further decided that I. S. should be allowed to taste the stuff, if it *can* be tasted through the milk he would have to swallow before and after. Accordingly he is to receive three half-jiggers of Scotch, at wide intervals, and each one blended to obliteration with milk. The prescription provokes a great flap among the floor nurses, who say that it is the first time in the history of the hospital that "drink" has been administered in the social fashion.

Returning to the hospital in the afternoon, I spoon-feed I. S., and hold his bad hand: he says the warmth diminishes the pain. Always a naturally affectionate, as well as a deeply lonely man, feeling now pours out of him. And not a little of it pours into me, for we are very close now, as we were in our first years together; he asks me to sit by him all the time, and will allow me to leave only if I promise to return immediately.

To what extent death is in his thoughts I have no idea; that will appear later, if he lives. But it is clear that much of his mental suffering in late years is caused by the absence of a proper sense of himself as aged. In his own mind he is not eighty-five....

A resurrection has occurred between our second and third visits tonight, and of all providential ironies the whiskey may have turned the tide. His face has more color, his hand-grasp is firmer, his voice is stronger, his conversation is quicker, and his criticisms of the nurses are as caustic as they would have been a year ago. He wants to know the date, and, on hearing it, seems as surprised as Rip Van Winkle was on being told how long *he* had slept; only yesterday I. S. was uncertain he was even in the hospital, at one point asking the name of the hotel and the city. The finger is clearer tonight, and as the doctors concur in ascribing at least some of the improvement to whiskey, we tipple once more.

November 11

I. S. has a new nurse today, a tough old trout with scabrous tongue and the personality of a warden. She treats him as if he were a very ancient, puling baby, and deeply offends his decorum with remarks such as, "Do you use Poly-Grip on your dentures?" and "I've wiped more bottoms in my time...." The patient is a lever of compensation in her own life, as I have come to think most patients are for most nurses; she clearly resents V.'s place next to the bed and the rapt gaze of I. S. toward V., as if she were a peri from another world. "Can you see this?" V. asks, holding up a book of photographs for him to peruse, and he says, "I think so, but I would rather look at you." I am now beginning to fear that V. will collapse, unless I can find a way of spreading her burden.

November 13

A *Dies Irae*, the worst since August. A new abscission must have occurred in the index finger, which is blacker than ever. Equally upsetting is I. S.'s semi-delirium. His sense of time and sense of distance are virtually inoperant, and his memory has become a total jumble. He repeatedly asks where he is, and confounds names and places, partly because of verbal resemblances; thus "Dr. Marcus" starts him off on Markevitch. He talks to the nurses in Russian, too, mistaking them for V. Worst of all, he says he cannot see, and he is clearly unable at times to identify objects in the room, and even ourselves. Once he tells me that "I have left my passport behind and cannot return."

Fearing he has had a major stroke I ask for a consultation, convene the two neurosurgeons, and return to the hospital in the evening to witness their examination. The result is an amazing display of an always amazing and still very much intact mind. It is true that I. S. has always been fond of medical interrogations, but tonight he rises to the occasion with some impish *mots d'esprit* as well. Dr. Rothenberg: "Will you answer a few silly questions, Mr. Stravinsky?" I. S.: "No." But the questions come. "Do you see double, Mr. Stravinsky?" "Yes." "How long has this been going on?" "All my life, when I am *soûl*." "What month and year is it?" Here the best I. S. can say is "autumn." "Did you see people or animals in the room at any time today, and realize later that they weren't there?" "Yes. Two boys were sitting in that chair all afternoon." "Did you see a black cat?" "No." But he claims to see vivid mixtures of color in the curtain even now, at the same time telling us that he knows the curtain was a drab brown yesterday. Dr. Rothenberg proceeds to examine his eyes with lights and to test his ability to read a paragraph from a book, but the reading proves to be very laborious, because he sees the letters a half-inch to the left of the print at the same time as the print itself. What distresses him still more, he confesses, is his inability to relate events. "Something is wrong both in my sense of time and in the reasoning faculty," he says, and goes on to describe the symptoms of this mental state with an awareness and a power of reason that a philosopher a fourth of his age and in perfect health might envy. In fact one of the doctors, in the interests of an analogy I fail to follow, puts a question to him about time in music, but bungles his concepts, whereupon I. S. sets him straight by distinguishing "time as a matter of speed, and rhythm as a matter of design."

The doctors seek to assure him that his new complaints are due entirely to the effects of his new drugs. "I am *consolé*," he finally concedes, adding that "I looked hard in myself for the cause of the failure, and was anguished because I was unable to reason about it exactly enough. I want to be more exact in my thoughts." But *is* he *"consolé"?* He pleads for "a more powerful pill, so that I do not have to think about it any more tonight." But stronger

315

sedatives are forbidden because of the danger of pneumonia if he fails to move enough.

November 14

Finally, eight weeks late, I. S. is injected arterially with radioactive phosphorus, by a doctor wearing a rubber suit and what looks like a welder's helmet. Three nurses wheel the patient to a lead-lined room in the basement, making me think of the three queens accompanying Arthur to Avalon. Afterward, a thrice-daily series of abdominal and subcutaneous heparin injections is begun.

The mental wanderings are worse than yesterday. Before the trip to the X-ray room, he asks us to look after his wallet, which of course he has not had on his person in months; the mistake probably betrays a habit of concern about his pocket valuables when disrobed for X-rays in the past. On the return to the room, however, he asks if we have "enough *Frantsuzki Geld* to tip the porters." Then, when dinner comes, he insists on eating from his own tray, thinking he is in his room at home, and when V. says it isn't there, he points to where she can find it. As we leave for dinner ourselves, he asks to come to the restaurant with us. I tell him he will be able to very soon, and after considering this for a moment, he replies, heartbreakingly, "I realize I am not able to eat with you, but I could watch." He also begs to be taken for a "promenade" in the car, and no doubt troubled by his mistake in thinking he was home, asks how it is there now. Very bad, I say, for we miss him all the time.

He has a bad period of hallucinations, a side effect of the heparin, the doctors say. He apprehends people who are not present but fails to see us and his nurses when we are only inches away, and once he asks why there are two watches on his right wrist from which even the one has now been removed. V. says that his Russian comments are "nonsensical" and "delirious," which greatly upsets her, of course, nor is she impressed by my argument that this unreality is better for him now than truth. Then suddenly, in the midst of the rambling, he drops a remark showing such a perfect sense of reality that we know his mind is holding on tight. Overhearing us mention a certain music critic, whose name has not come up in years, he wants to know whether the said critic is dead or alive. "Dead," says V., but I. S. is doubtful. "No, he is probably alive and in Argentina."

The mind seems to be divided into two parts, of which only that part dealing with the outer world and the present is confused. And surely this is natural, considering the disruption of the time sense by drugs and medicine schedules, and the dislocation in consequence of staring at hospital walls, which are not so unlike the walls of his bedroom at home.

The other, the creative part of the mind is undisturbed. In the evening, during one of his lucid spells, I tell him that the BBC wants him to compose six to ten seconds of music to be used with a multicolored eye by Picasso as the signature of a new color-television channel. The creative mind instantly seizes the idea and moves ahead with it like a prow. "The time problem interests me, the six seconds ruling out chords and rhythms in any conventional sense, but of course many notes can be used at a time. An eye means transparency, too, and that the sound should be produced by very high instruments, possibly by flutes, compared to which oboes are greasy and clarinets oily."

November 18

The depredations are showing; I. S. is so thin now that his nose seems to have grown, and his long-untrimmed moustache overhangs his lip, suggesting a walrus or fox terrier. But the finger remains blue-black, and it is painful, less so in the mornings when he is still comatose from the sedatives of the night before. As for the intensity of the pain, the doctors assure us that he performs for our sympathy, which is normal patient behavior, and that he has often dispatched a nurse for codeine or Darvon, only to fall asleep before she has had time to give it to him. Some pain he has, nevertheless, and he moans from it throughout the afternoon. Once the nurse gives him a pill, warns him it is a big one, goes to fetch water to help it down, but when she returns I. S. says, "Already done."

The result of yesterday's midnight consultation, which introduced a new vascular surgeon into the medical-opinion pool, is a compounding of new ingredients in the intravenous, the commencement of arm and hand exercises, and the application of mild heating therapy to the entire integument of the forearm and hand.

November 19

The new intravenous formula, with the new anti-coagulant, Priscoline, has not changed the finger color, but it makes I. S. so drowsy that we get only a few words out of him the whole day. The blindness is far more frightening than the finger. He identifies us by our voices, hardly turning his head to left or right, while what he *does* see—the anti-corona of someone walking past the bed—is not there.

November 20

"Where are you?" he asks, hearing me enter the room this morning, and as I reach the bed he puts his good hand to my face as if he were totally blind. He is so heavily drugged, too, that speech occurs only at great intervals. Once he wakes up saying, "How long will it last?" and again, "How much longer?" Then for the first time in all these months, "I don't want to live this way." I try to make him believe that he will soon be home and composing, but he nods his head weakly toward his hand saying, "I need my hand; I am maimed in my hand." I am more worried about his eyes, nevertheless, and most worried of all about the amount of fight left in him; already, as Lear says, "The oldest hath borne most."

November 23

It is Thanksgiving Day in the most wonderful possible way: the long-prayed for miracle has happened. Not once in seventy-two hours has I. S. complained

317

of pain or taken a pain-killer, and the finger color has returned almost to normal. His sight is not normal, and he is still unable to distinguish faces in what seems to be, as he describes it, a dioramic blur; but his eyes turn much more rapidly toward, and focus more quickly on, us than a few days ago. He sits in a chair for awhile, which makes him look much thinner than in the bed. Milène reads to him, too, and he is quick to pounce on her mistakes in Russian pronunciation. Incredible man! Only three days ago he was in a semicoma, his left hand a half-silted estuary of gangrene, his body worn out by months of pain. And he has come out of it, actually recrossed the Styx. "How much is it costing?" he asks me suddenly, and in all these weeks no words have sounded so good. I. S. is back in decimal-system reality. Thank God.

He is pepped up from glucose and jumpy, brittle, anxious, ready to fly off the handle at any and everything. "I have had enough medical philosophy," he tells one of his physicians, and to a nurse who advises him to "relax," his retort is: "What? And leave the driving to *you?*" He is suffering drug withdrawal, of course, and a mountain of aftereffects, but I like the friction.

V. is ill and in bed today, with flu, she says, though it is more likely battle fatigue. The crisis of last weekend was too much for her, and she has kept her fear inside too long.

November 28

I go at noon to bring I. S. home, but his departure is delayed by requests for autographs from every nurse on the floor, which he gives, even embellishing some with musical notations. Outdoors, out from that stultifying hospital at last, he is as pale as junket; dressed in a suit, he looks terribly thin, shrunken, and frail.

As I lead him from the car into the house, he says that it must seem to me as if I am "towing a wreck," but weak as he is, he props himself on the couch and will not go to bed. He is contemptuous of his medicines and balks at his doses of milk, saying, "Milk is the Jesus Christ of the affair," to which profanity V. responds with: "Now at least we see how much better you are." But he will not have any of that. "Not better, bitter," he corrects. But when V. plays some games of patience to divert him and asks him to keep the tally for her in his head, his scores, she says, and meaning no pun, are perfect.

He asks about the newspapers (which say that Zadkine, another coeval, has died) and the post. The latter contains a package from André Malraux, a copy of *Anti-Mémoires* with the author's dedication: *"Pour Igor Stravinsky, avec mon admiration fidèle."* But I. S. jumps on this. "When was he ever *fidèle?* He once said that music is a minor art." And so I. S. is still I. S.

Later in the day the doctors call to congratulate themselves, but he flummoxes them, too, as he has done at every stage, telling them that "The finger and the eyes are from the same cause." In fact the chief neurosurgeon corroborates this to me privately, saying that there have been not one but three thromboses, and that some peripheral vision in the left eye is permanently lost. I. S. himself is less distressed by his poor sight, at the moment, however, than by a gas pain, and when the doctors attempt to remind him that he has not suffered alone, he snaps at them with, "Maybe, but you don't have this gas pain." (Apostrophizing them later, he adds that "It was very well-paid suffering for them.") But he is beginning to talk like a doctor himself. "Is the pain merely spasmodic," he asks at one point, "or could it be organic?" One of the medics tells him, in parting, that "Healing takes longer at eighty-five, Mr. Stravinsky," but I. S. turns on this with "Damn eighty-five."

He watches Daktari in V.'s room tonight, but tosses and turns in his bed afterward, tormented, he says, about the state of his mind. At eleven o'clock I go to V. to see if she is all right, and find her room dark and herself quietly crying, the tears streaming down her face. Not once during the whole horrible ordeal did she ever lose control, and only now is it clear that she was losing belief and only continued to pray that he would ever be home again. After an hour of trying to talk her into some "peace of mind," I am summoned by the night nurse to help with I. S., who is not sleeping in spite of his pills. I try to fake some more good cheer with him, but he says he is "in a bad way psychologically." When finally I leave him, he answers my last inane "Please stop worrying" with "I am not worrying any more, only waiting," which wrenching remark kills the possibility of any sleep of my own. "Old people are attached to life," says Sophocles, condemning it as a fault.

Man's
future

Babies and mothers love peek-a-boo games. The games are good training for handling surprise and change, but things are never allowed to get out of hand. Anxieties are built up only to be quickly relieved. Everybody who plays peek-a-boo needs to know what is going to happen. A certain amount of that need to know never leaves a person.

But today nobody knows enough of what is going to happen. Things can't be counted on any more. For grown-ups, the atom bomb ruined forever all the peek-a-boo games and they have been replaced by what John Platt calls "nuclear roulette." To make matters worse, man's problems have changed greatly but his institutions to handle them have not. They are mired in "a wide sea of glue." And about them the winds of change keep blowing.

More praying is probably going on these days than is generally suspected. A list of today's predicaments has the quality of a litany: population, pills, pollution, plutonium, poverty, proliferation, priorities, politics, procrastination, planning . . . or babies, bulldozers, bombs . . . and so on. But the string of repeated words, like a string of worry beads, always adds up to the same crisis.

In "The Scientific Urgencies of the Next Ten Years," John Platt discusses what the future holds and suggests what the present generation will have to do to survive their crises. As Donald Fleming tells about some of the more recent and most startling biological discoveries in "On Living in a Biological Revolution," he adds to a deeper understanding of the meaning of these discoveries. "He that increaseth knowledge increaseth sorrow" is written in Ecclesiastes. Fleming is concerned that human significance may be drowned in the flood of biological knowledge; his thoughts about depersonalization are especially worth pondering. Charles Winick, in "The Desexualized Society," suggests that sexual permissiveness is a bore. Who can doubt that the sex symbols of this era are boring? It is not the first time. A generation ago, a movie queen sued her husband for divorce because he wouldn't come home at night. That same week, a national magazine featured her as the "sex symbol of the era." It would appear that her sexual attributes, by themselves at least, were not of enough interest to her husband to bring him home. Today who really cares about what the current movie queens are doing? Yet many people still look at sex symbols more than they participate in sex. They fear involvement. What this suggests for the future is incisively explored by Winick, who considers these times "The Age of Voyeurism."

This book closes with a letter. Some will reject its contents in whole or in part; others will accept it completely. No one can ignore it. It is included here to provoke needed discussion. The letter can and does stand alone. An explanation of the circumstances of its writing is, however, necessary and is presented with it.

The scientific urgencies of the next ten years

DR. JOHN PLATT

In the present generation, mankind is passing through the greatest turning point in history. Within the last century, we have increased our speeds of communication by a factor of 10^6; our speeds of travel by 10^2; our energy resources by 10^3; our power of weapons by 10^6; our speeds of computers by 10^6; our power over diseases by 10^2; and our rate of population growth by 10^3 over what it was a few thousand years ago. Can anyone suppose that human relations around the world have not been affected to their very roots by these changes? Within just the last 30 years, the Western world has moved into an age of jet planes, missiles and satellites, nuclear power and nuclear terror, computers and automation, a service and leisure economy, superhighways, superagriculture, supermedicine, mass higher education, universal TV, oral contraceptives, environmental pollution, and urban crises. We have explored to the ends of the earth and are reaching for the moon and the planets. We have come to the end of 3 billion years of evolution by natural selection, and we are now beginning the era of evolution by human selection, as our breeding, protection, predation, or pollution begins to affect the numbers of every plant and animal species on earth.

It is striking to realize how enormous these changes are. But it is almost equally striking to see that many of them are now approaching certain natural limits, determined by such things as the speed of light or the finiteness of the earth or the limits of overkill or the tolerable densities of human population. Because of these limits, it is very hard to see technically how the human race can ever again have such another vast and sudden explosion of new potentialities.

The result is that the present generation is the hinge of history. The young people under 30, who have grown up from childhood in the presence of these new ways of doing things and who are now reaching voting age in great numbers, are the first generation of what might almost be called

THE SCIENTIFIC URGENCIES OF THE NEXT TEN YEARS From *Rehovot*, Vol. 5, No. 3, Winter 1969/70. Reprinted by permission of the publisher.

a new breed of man. No wonder they do not trust the older generation! As Margaret Mead has said, the people over 30 today are like the immigrants to a new country who were too old when they arrived and who will never learn to speak the new language or understand the new customs very well. It is the children who are the natives and who laugh at our fumbling and bewilderment.

These vast changes of pace and attitude are not peculiar to America or to capitalist countries. The new developments affect every country—as we can see by looking at student revolutions around the globe!—and it seems likely that every corner of the world will share in these powers and problems within 30 years or less, when we consider how rapidly Japan, Russia, China, and Israel have already made the technological jump.

These new developments have brought many good things for human beings, such as decreasing work loads and death rates, and increasing consumer goods and communication and education and the possibility of abundance and diversity. But now they are also bringing crisis after crisis everywhere. The reason is that the institutions that we have for dealing with these new powers are frequently 19th-century institutions, if not older, and they are usually grossly inadequate for handling these order-of-magnitude changes—when they are not simply irrelevant or positively dangerous. It is surprising that they have done as well as they have, so far! But the old structures and attitudes and privileges, the old ideas of hierarchy and authority and hatred and revenge and war, are incompatible with our new densities and intensities of human interaction. Unless these outmoded ways and structures can be adapted more rapidly to the new powers and dangers, the rapidly increasing strains and crises of the next 10 years may kill us all. They will make the last 20 years look like a peaceful interlude.

Three types of crisis may reach explosion-point in the next 10 years—nuclear escalation, famine, and the crisis of administrative "legitimacy." In the continued absence of adequate stabilizing peace-keeping structures for the world, we continue to live under the daily threat not only of local wars but of nuclear escalation with overkill and megatonnage enough to destroy all life on earth. In addition, many agricultural experts think that within this next decade the great famines will begin, with deaths that may reach 100 million people in densely populated countries like India and China. There will be food riots, troops called out, governments falling, and international intervention that will change the whole political map of the world. And what will make all our situations worse is that there will be continued crises of "legitimacy" of all our overloaded and dehumanized administrations, from universities and unions to cities and national governments. Every crisis will be unstabilized further by the frequent repudiation of administrations and negotiators by their own distrustful constituents.

The human race today is like a rocket on a launching pad. We have been building up to this moment of take-off for a long time, and if we can get safely through the take-off period, we may fly on a new and exciting course for a long time to come. But at this moment, as the powerful new engines are fired, their thrust and roar shakes and stresses the whole structure, and their vibrations may cause the whole thing to blow up before we can steer it on its way. Our problem today is to harness and direct these tremendous new forces through this dangerous transition period to the new world of abundance instead of to destruction. Our problem is to use all our science and common sense and everything we know, in an urgent program to help make the old structures work or to design new ones that will help get us through this next decade without killing all of us.

Science, in the next 10 years or so, may bring to fruition several important contributions to human welfare. In biochemistry, the solution of the "central problem" of the relation between sequence, structure, and function in protein molecules may make possible the mass production of improved enzymes or catalysts for many purposes. In the case of the endemic tropical disease, bilharzia, some anti-snail drugs and chemicals now show great promise. In the problem of cancer, the identification of environmental agents causing cancer, and the exploration of the virus hypothesis with the possible development of vaccines or repressors, may lead to a 10-fold reduction in the disease. In the case of schizophrenia and some other mental diseases, the identification of the strong genetic component that is now indicated by many studies may make possible early diagnosis and possible prevention or cure by suitable drugs or diets.

The trouble is, however, that the best of these hopes for the conventional kind of scientific achievements have little relation to the major dangers today. Most of our expensive physics and chemistry and engineering research, including fusion power and the Man in Space program, together drawing in hundreds of thousands of our best young scientific and engineering brains, could be postponed for 50 years without making any great difference to the welfare or survival of the human race. Even in the biological field, the things that will destroy human society, or exacerbate most dangerously our social and structural problems, are not our ignorance about enzymes, or cancer or schizophrenia, on which thousands of scientists are working—but overpopulation, pollution, and famine, on which there are hardly a handful of our best scientific minds.

In the case of the population explosion, for example, it is clear that our present most effective methods of birth control—the oral pill and the intrauterine coil—are almost ineffective in the countries that need them most, because they require individual prescription or treatment as well as considerable education for reliable use. Several years ago, Homi J. Bhabha, the Indian Atomic Energy Commissioner, suggested that a much better method would be to develop safe and effective contraceptive chemicals that could be put into widely used factory-processed human foods, such as salt. Obviously such a measure would have to be adopted by democratic vote, and antidotes or untreated foods would have to be available for couples who wanted to have children. But it is easy to show that such a method would be thousands of times cheaper, and might level off population growth 20 years sooner—a billion mouths sooner!—than any of our present methods. But the fear of political or religious opposition seems to be preventing anyone from working on such methods at present. Twenty years ago there was the same kind of fear of opposition to any kind of oral contraceptives, until two dedicated men, Gregory Pincus and John Rock, developed a chemical that worked—and suddenly the opposition melted away, and the production of these chemicals became a hugely profitable industry, with 13 million daily users already. The same thing might happen today if this much more effective method could be developed. Considering how much we know already about different contraceptive chemicals and their sites of action and side-effects, it might take only a few years for a few men in one or two small laboratories to develop acceptable compounds that would change the whole dimensions of the world population problem. Who will dedicate himself, or what government will assign teams, to such a task, more important for the human race than almost any other research today?

If population could be leveled off, it becomes essential to feed, clothe, and educate every human being that is already here. Feeding the world may be helped by the new high-yield grains, if farmers can be taught to plant them and consumers eat them. Intensive development of marine resources may help, as well as the synthetic production of protein and carbohydrates from coal. This would take only a fraction of our coal production, and it is estimated that if it were done on a large enough scale, it would cost no more per pound than chicken or fish today.

Great increases in meat production might also come from "genetic copying" of champion cattle, hogs, sheep, or chickens. Some studies indicate that this might be done by controlled parthenogenesis, or "virgin birth," with the daughter animals being identical to the mother. But most biologists believe that it can also be done by "nuclear transplantation," taking nuclei from cells of a champion animal and putting them in fertilized egg cells in a foster mother. The eggs would develop into identical twins of the champion, and could give thousands of "instant champions" in a single breeding season, with 50 to 100 percent increases in meat, milk, or egg production in any country. So far this process has only been done with frogs, by J. B. Gurdon and others, but several of the steps in transplantation have now been carried out successfully with mice, and it seems likely that two or three years of concentrated development work might easily permit extending it to all our food animals. This is the most revolutionary change in animal propagation in the last half-billion years. It is like the propagation of plants by cuttings, and would revolutionize animal husbandry in the same way that revolutionized fruit growing. The consequences for the world may be imagined—but less than a dozen scientists are working on this problem at the present time.

The environmental pollution problem is one where physicists, chemists, biologists, engineers, industrialists, legislators, administrators, and community representatives all need to contribute to successful solutions. But the scientists can and should make central contributions, from the invention of better low-level measurement methods, new and more economical disposal methods and less toxic insecticides and herbicides, all the way up to the education of everybody about the interdependencies of the whole ecological system of the planet on which we live.

Our immediate and urgent need for scientific contributions that will head off or help to solve our crisis problems is of course not limited to natural scientists and engineers. We need mathematical systems scientists to do operations research, and to study information handling and improve communications and administrative design. We need social scientists and behavioral scientists to show us how to use the new and powerful methods of behavior theory and of game theory, how to get more responsive and effective social groups and organizations, and how to understand and reduce the "lock-ins" of conflict situations between groups, races, and nations. We need scientists to work out new feedback and stabilization designs for peace-keeping structures and cooperation-increasing mechanisms. Stabilization-design might be a complex modern counterpart of the systematic use of stabilization "checks and balances" in designing the constitution of the United States 200 years ago.

But when we see the scope and urgency of our world-wide human problems today, the idea of "science as usual" is so irrelevant and wasteful of our best brains that it almost approaches criminal frivolity. It is no longer enough to go on working in the labs just to "build another brick in the temple of science," hoping it will fit into some great intellectual synthesis in 30 years. Nor is it enough to be politically concerned, working by circulating petitions or trying to influence the government in some current 3-month crisis.

Neither of these time scales is appropriate to the dimensions or the scientific needs of the crises that might destroy us in the next 10 years. Our urgent social problems now are more like wartime problems, such as anti-submarine warfare or the development of atomic energy. These are cases where we must get different experts and inventive minds together to make interdisciplinary operations-analysis and action-oriented designs and pilot studies, but where the time scale is that of a crash program, permitting, say, a few months or a year or two of study before we must come up with some much more effective solutions. Wartime task forces of this kind, as in the anti-submarine and radar and atomic energy projects, have often produced order-of-magnitude changes in effectiveness within a short time.

It would not be as impossible as it may seem for some social task forces of this kind to make social or socio-technical inventions that could also have large effects in a 1–5–10-year time span. Oral contraceptives were in widespread use in the U.S. within 8 years after they were developed. The Pay-As-You-Go Income tax transformed the U.S. taxing power within two years. On the international scene, the Test-Ban Treaty, the "hot-line" between Washington and Moscow, the Peace Corps, and the Antarctic Non-Nuclear Treaty, were all implemented within less than a decade.

Long-range science is useless unless we survive to use it. Today the most urgent need is for scientists, with their interdisciplinary knowledge, and their library and laboratory resources, to pull themselves together into action-oriented task forces, working on a 1–5–10-year scale of urgency, to reduce and avert the imminent crises facing humanity before they destroy us all. This year, next year, this decade, is the time of decision. If we can work out the problem of making stable and responsive structures to manage our vast new powers for the benefit of all mankind in the next 10 years or so, we can look forward to a long fruitful future for our children in the 21st century and for their descendants. If not, the human experiment will shortly come screaming and whimpering to an end.

*O*n living in a
biological revolution

DONALD FLEMING

Here are a dozen things that we have discovered in the last fifteen years.

1. We have discovered   the structure of the genetic substance DNA—the double helix of Watson and Crick—the general nature of the process by which the chromosomal strands are replicated.

2. We have discovered   in viruses how to achieve the perfect replication of DNA molecules that are biologically effective.

3. We have discovered   the code by which DNA specifies the insertion of amino acids in proteins.

4. We have discovered   how to produce hybrid cells between the most diverse vertebrate species, including hybrids between man and mouse; and some of these hybrids have gone on multiplying for several (cellular) generations.

5. We have discovered   the power of viruses to invade bacterial and other cells and to insert the genes of the virus into the genome of the host; and we have good reason to conjecture, though not yet to affirm, that this phenomenon is involved in cancer.

6. We have discovered   hormonal contraceptives and grasped in principle the strategy for devising a contraceptive pill for *both* sexes, by knocking out certain hormones of

ON LIVING IN A BIOLOGICAL REVOLUTION From *The Atlantic Monthly*, February 1969. Reprinted by permission of the author.

the hypothalamus, the master sexual gland of the body.

7. We have discovered on a large scale in the livestock industry that deep-frozen mammalian sperm, suitably mixed with glycerol, can be banked indefinitely and drawn upon as desired to produce viable offspring.

8. We have discovered in human females how to produce superovulation, the release of several eggs into the oviduct at the same time instead of the customary one, with the possibility on the horizon of withdrawing substantial numbers of human eggs for storage, culture in test tubes, or surgical manipulation, without destroying their viability.

9. We have discovered in rabbits how to regulate the sex of offspring by removing fertilized ova from the female before they become implanted in the wall of the uterus, "sexing" the embryos by a technique entailing the deletion of some 200 to 300 cells, flushing embryos of the "wrong" sex down the drain, and then in a substantial minority of cases, successfully reinserting in the uterus embryos of the desired sex that proceed to develop normally.

10. We have discovered drugs, above all the hallucinogens, that stimulate psychotic states of mind; and have thereby rendered it plausible that the latter are the product of "inborn errors of metabolism" and as such remediable by the administration of drugs.

11. We have discovered in principle, and to a certain extent in practice, how to repress the immunological "defenses" of the body.

12. We have discovered a combination of immunological and surgical techniques by which the kidney, liver, or heart can be transplanted with fair prospects of the recipient's survival for months or even years—the first constructive proposal for turning our death wish on the highways to some advantage.

Each of these is a major discovery or complex of discoveries in itself, but they add up to far more than the sum of their parts. They constitute a veritable Biological Revolution likely to be as decisive for the history of the next 150 years as the Industrial Revolution has been for the period since 1750.

Definitions of what constitutes a revolution are legion. An undoctrinaire formulation would be that every full-scale revolution has three main components: a distinctive attitude toward the world; a program for utterly transforming it; and an unshakable, not to say fanatical, confidence that this program can be enacted—a world view, a program, and a faith.

In this sense, Darwinism did not usher in a full-scale biological revolution. Darwinism was a profoundly innovating world view, but one that prescribed no steps to be taken, no victories over nature to be celebrated, no program of triumphs to be successively gained. Indeed, one of the most plausible constructions to be put upon it was that nothing much *could* be done except to submit patiently to the winnowing processes of nature.

This defect was not lost upon Darwin's own cousin Sir Francis Galton, who tried to construct an applied science of eugenics for deliberately selecting out the best human stocks. But Galtonian eugenics was sadly lacking in any authentic biological foundation. Once the science of Mendelian genetics came to general notice about 1900, a more promising form of eugenics began to commend itself, the effort to induce artificial mutation of genes in desirable directions.

This was long the animating faith of one of the most extraordinary Americans of the twentieth century, the geneticist Herman J. Muller. He was the actual discoverer in 1927, of artificial mutation through X-rays. But this great achievement, for which he got the Nobel Prize, was a tremendous disappointment to Muller the revolutionary. There was no telling which genes would mutate in which direction, and he came to suspect that the vast majority of mutations were actually harmful in the present situation of the human race.

Muller at the end of his life—he died in 1967—was thrown back upon essentially Galtonian eugenics. He did bring this up to date by his proposal for sperm banks in which the sperm of exceptionally intelligent and socially useful men could be stored for decades and used for artificial insemination. He also envisioned, in the not too distant future, ova banks for storing superior human eggs. But none of these modern touches, these innovations in technique, could conceal the fact that this was still the old eugenics newly garbed, but equally subjective and imprecise.

Biological engineering

The Biological Revolution that Muller failed to bring off was already in progress when he died, but on very different terms from his own. There is a new eugenics in prospect, not the marriage agency kind, but a form of "biological engineering." When this actually comes to pass, chromosomes, segments of chromosomes, and even individual genes will be inserted at will into the genome. Alternatively, germ cells cultured in laboratories will be enucleated and entire tailor-made DNA molecules substituted. Alternatively still, superior genes will be brought into play by hybridization of cells.

The detailed variants upon these general strategies are almost innumerable. They all have in common the fact that they cannot be accomplished at present except in viruses and bacteria or in cell cultures. But it would be a bold man who would dogmatically affirm that none of these possibilities could be brought to bear upon human genetics by the year 2000.

That is a long way off for the firebrands of the Biological Revolution. The Nobel Prize winner Joshua Lederberg in particular has been pushing the claims of a speedier remedy, christened by him "euphenics," and defined as "the engineering of human development." The part of human development that fascinates Lederberg the most is embryology, seen by him as the process of initially translating the instructions coded in the DNA into "the living, breathing organism." Embryology, he says, is "very much in the situation of atomic physics in 1900; having had an honorable and successful tradition it is about to begin!" He thinks it will not take long to mature— "from 5 to no more than 20 years." He adds that most predictions of research progress in recent times have proved to be "far too conservative."

The progress that Lederberg has in mind is the application of new embryological techniques to human affairs. He is at once maddened and obsessed by the nine-months phase in which the human organism has been exempted from experimental and therapeutic intervention—such a waste of time before the scientists can get at us. But the embryo's turn is coming. It would be incredible, he says, "if we did not soon have the basis of developmental engineering technique to regulate, for example, the size of the human brain by prenatal or early postnatal intervention."

Sex control

Nothing as sensational as this has yet been attempted, but the new phase in embryology that Lederberg heralded is undoubtedly getting under way. The most conspicuous figure at present is Robert Edwards of the physiology laboratory at Cambridge University. In 1966 Edwards reported the culture of immature egg cells from the human ovary up to the point of ripeness for fertilization. He made tentative claims to have actually achieved fertilization in test tubes. The incipient hullabaloo in the newspapers about the specter of "test tube babies" led Edwards to clamp a tight lid of security over his researches in progress.

In the spring of this year, however, he and Richard Gardner announced their success in "sexing" fertilized rabbit eggs before implantation in the wall of the uterus and then inducing 20 percent of the reinstated eggs to produce normal full-term infants. The aspect of these findings that attracted general attention, the prospect of regulating the sex of mammalian offspring, is not likely to be of permanent interest. For this purpose, Edwards and Gardner's technique is obviously a clumsy expedient by comparison with predetermining the "sex" of spermatozoa—presently impossible but certainly not inconceivable within the next generation.

The real importance of Edwards and Gardner's work lies elsewhere. They have opened up the possibility of subjecting the early embryo to microsurgery, with the deletion and "inoculation" of cells at the will of the investigator, *and* the production of viable offspring from the results. The manufacture of "chimeras" in the modern biological sense—that is, with genetically distinct cells in the same organism—is clearly in prospect.

Work in this vein has just begun. The only branch of euphenics that has already become something more than a promising growth stock in science is the suppression of immunological reactions against foreign tissues and the accompanying, highly limited, successes in the transplantation of organs.

Biological revolutionaries

The technical details and immediate prospects in eugenics and euphenics, however fascinating, are less important than the underlying revolutionary temper in biology. The most conspicuous representatives of this temper are Lederberg himself, the biochemical geneticist Edward L. Tatum, and Francis Crick of the model—all of them Nobel Prize winners, with the corresponding leverage upon public opinion. Robert Edwards, though slightly singed by the blast of publicity about test tube babies, is clearly in training for the revolutionary cadre.

One of the stigmata of revolutionaries in any field is their resolute determination to break with traditional culture. For a scientist, the most relevant definition of culture is his own field of research. All of these men would angrily resent being bracketed with biologists in general. Biology has always been a rather loose confederation of naturalists and experimentalists, overlapping in both categories with medical researchers. Today even the pretense that these men somehow constitute a community has been frayed to the breaking point.

At Harvard, for example, the revolutionaries have virtually seceded from the old Biology Department and formed a new department of their own, Biochemistry and Molecular Biology. The younger molecular biologists hardly bother to conceal their contempt for the naturalists, whom they see as old fogies obsequiously attentive to the world as it is rather than bent upon turning it upside down.

In one respect, the molecular biologists do overlap with the contemporary naturalists and indeed with most creative scientists in general—in their total detachment from religion. In a way, this is a point that could have been made at any time in the last seventy-five years, but with one significant difference. Herman Muller, for example, born in 1890, had no truck with religion. But he was self-consciously antireligious.

The biological revolutionaries of today are not antireligious but simply unreligious. They give the impression not of defending themselves against religion but of subsisting in a world where that has never been a felt pressure upon them. They would agree with many devout theologians that we are living in a post-Christian world, to such an extent that some of the most doctrinaire biological revolutionaries are able to recognize without embarrassment, and even with a certain gracious condescension, that Christianity did play a useful role in defining the values of the Western world.

The operative word here is in the past tense. Francis Crick says that the facts of science are producing and must produce values that owe nothing to

Christianity. "Take," he says, "the suggestion of making a child whose head is twice as big as normal. There is going to be no agreement between Christians and any humanists who lack their particular prejudice about the sanctity of the individual, and who simply want to try it scientifically."

This sense of consciously taking up where religion left off is illuminating in another sense for the revolutionary character of contemporary biology. The parallel is very marked between the original Christian Revolution against the values of the classical world and the Biological Revolution against religious values.

All the great revolutionaries, whether early Christians or molecular biologists, are men of good hope. The future may or may not belong to those who believe in it, but cannot belong to those who don't. Yet at certain points in history, most conspicuously perhaps at intervals between the close of the Thirty Years' War in 1648 and the coming of the Great Depression in 1929, the horizons seem to be wide open, and the varieties of good hope contending for allegiance are numerous. But the tidings of good hope don't become revolutionary except when the horizons begin to close in and the plausible versions of good hope have dwindled almost to the vanishing point.

For the kind of good hope that has the maximum historical impact is the one that capitalizes upon a prevalent despair at the corruption of the existing world, and then carries conviction in pointing to itself as the only possible exit from despair. Above everything else, revolutionaries are the men who keep their spirits up when everybody else's are sagging. In this sense, the greatest revolutionaries of the Western world to date have been precisely the early Christians who dared to affirm in the darkest days of the classical world that something far better was in process and could be salvaged from the ruins.

Both of these points are exemplified in the Biological Revolution that has now begun—despair at our present condition, but infinite hope for the future if the biologists' prescription is taken. Anybody looking for jeremiads on our present state could not do better than to consult the new biologists. "The facts of human reproduction," says Joshua Lederberg, "are all gloomy—the stratification of fecundity by economic status, the new environmental insults to our genes, the sheltering by humanitarian medicine of once-lethal genes."

More generally, the biologists deplore the aggressive instincts of the human animal, now armed with nuclear weapons, his lamentably low average intelligence for coping with increasingly complicated problems, and his terrible prolificity, no longer mitigated by a high enough death rate. It is precisely an aspect of the closing down of horizons and depletion of comfortable hopes in the second half of the twentieth century that conventional medicine is now seen by the biological revolutionaries as one of the greatest threats to the human race.

Yet mere prophets of gloom can never make a revolution. In fact, the new biologists are almost the only group among our contemporaries with a reasoned hopefulness about the long future—if the right path is taken. There are of course many individuals of a naturally cheerful or feckless temperament, today as always, but groups of men with an articulated hope for the future of the entire race are much rarer. The theologians no longer qualify, many Communists have lost their hold upon the future even by their own lights, and the only other serious contenders are the space scientists and astronauts. But just to get off the earth is a rather vague prescription for our ills. Few people even in the space program would make ambitious claims on this score. In a long historical retrospect, they may turn out to have been too modest.

This is not a charge that is likely ever to be leveled against the new biologists. It is well known by now that J. D. Watson begins his account of his double-helix double by saying that he had never seen Francis Crick in a modest mood. But after all, modesty is not the salient quality to be looked for in the new breed of biologists. If the world will only listen, they *know* how to put us on the high road to salvation.

Custom-made people

What exactly does their brand of salvation entail? Perhaps the most illuminating way to put the matter is that their ideal is the manufacture of man. In a manufacturing process, the number of units to be produced is a matter of rational calculation beforehand and of tight control thereafter. Within certain tolerances, specifications are laid down for a satisfactory product. Quality-control is maintained by checking the output and replacing defective parts. After the product has been put to use, spare parts can normally be supplied to replace those that have worn out.

This is the program of the new biologists—control of numbers by foolproof contraception; gene manipulation and substitution; surgical and biochemical intervention in the embryonic and neonatal phases; organ transplants or replacements at will.

Of these, only contraception is technically feasible at present. Routine organ transplants will probably be achieved for a wide range of suitable organs in less than five years. The grafting of mechanical organs, prosthetic devices inserted in the body, will probably take longer. Joshua Lederberg thinks that embryonic and neonatal intervention may be in flood tide by, say, 1984. As for gene manipulation and substitution in human beings, that is the remotest prospect of all—maybe by the year 2000. But we must not forget Lederberg's well-founded conviction that most predictions in these matters are likely to be too conservative. We are already five to ten years ahead of what most informed people expected to be the schedule for organ transplants in human beings.

The great question becomes, what is it going to be like to be living in a world where such things are coming true? How will the Biological Revolution affect our scheme of values? Nobody could possibly take in all the implications in advance, but some reasonable conjectures are in order.

It is virtually certain that the moral sanctions of birth control are going to be transformed. Down to the present time, the battle for birth control has been fought largely in terms of the individual couple's right to have the number of babies that they want at the desired intervals. But it is built into the quantity-controls envisioned by the Biological Revolution, the control of the biological inventory, that this is or ought to be a question of social policy raher than individual indulgence.

Many factors are converging upon many people to foster this general attitude, but the issue is particularly urgent from the point of view of the biological revolutionaries. In the measure that they succeed in making the human race healthier, first by transplants and later on by genetic tailoring, they will be inexorably swamped by their own successes unless world population is promptly brought under control. The irrepressible Malthus is springing from his lightly covered grave to threaten them with cata-strophic victories.

Licensed babies

The only hope is birth control. The biologists can contribute the techniques, but the will to employ them on the requisite scale is another matter. The most startling proposal to date for actually enforcing birth control does not come from a biologist but from the Nobel-Prize-winning physicist W. B. Shockley, one of the inventors of the transistor. Shockley's plan is to render all women of childbearing age reversibly sterile by implanting a contraceptive capsule beneath the skin, to be removed by a physician only on the presentation of a government license to have a child. The mind bog-gles at the prospect of bootleg babies. This particular proposal is not likely to be enacted in the near future, even in India.

What we may reasonably expect is a continually rising chorus by the biologists, moralists, and social philosophers of the next generation to the effect that nobody has a right to have children, and still less the right to determine on personal grounds how many. There are many reasons why a couple may not want to be prolific anyhow, so that there might be a happy coincidence between contraception seen by them as a right and by states-men and biologists as a duty. But the suspicion is that even when people moderate their appetite in the matter of babies, they may still want to have larger families than the earth can comfortably support. The possi-bility of predetermining sex would undoubtedly be helpful in this respect, but might not be enough to make people forgo a third child. That is where the conflict would arise between traditional values, however moderately in-dulged, and the values appropriate to the Biological Revolution.

This issue is bound to be fiercely debated. But some of the most profound implications of the Biological Revolution may never present themselves for direct ratification. In all probability, the issues will go by default as we gratefully accept specific boons from the new biology.

Take, for example, the role of the patient in medicine. One of the principal strands in Western medicine from the time of the Greeks has been the endeavor to enlist the cooperation of the patient in his own cure. In certain respects, this venerable tradition has grown much stronger in the last century. Thus the rising incidence of degenerative diseases, like ulcers, heart trouble, and high blood pressure, has underscored the absolute necessity of inducing the patient to observe a healthful regimen, literally a way of life.

This has been the whole point of Freudian psychiatry as a mode of therapy, that cures can be wrought only by a painful exertion of the patient himself. We often forget, for good reasons, how traditional Freudianism is after the one big shock has been assimilated. In the present context, it actually epitomizes the Western tradition of bringing the patient's own personality to bear upon his medical problems.

Where do we go from here? The degenerative diseases are going to be dealt with increasingly by surgical repair of organs, by organ transplants, and later on by the installation of mechanical organs and eventually by the genetic deletion of weak organs before they occur. The incentive to curb your temper or watch your diet to keep your heart going will steadily decline.

As for mental illness, the near future almost certainly lies with psychopharmacology and the far future with genetic tailoring. Though the final pieces stubbornly decline to fall into place, the wise money is on the proposition that schizophrenia and other forms of psychosis are biochemical disorders susceptible of a pharmacological cure. If we are not presently curing any psychoses by drugs, we are tranquilizing and antidepressing many psychotics and emptying mental hospitals.

Neuroses, the theme of Freudian psychoanalysis, are another matter. It is not easy to envision a biochemical remedy for them. But even for neuroses, we already have forms of behavioral therapy that dispense with the Freudian tenet of implicating the patient in his own cure. For the *very* long future, it is certainly not inconceivable that genetic tailoring could delete neurotic properties.

Everywhere we turn, the story is essentially the same. Cures are increasingly going to be wrought upon, done to, the patient as a passive object. The strength of his own personality, the force of his character, his capacity for reintegrating himself, are going to be increasingly irrelevant in medicine.

Genetic tailoring, boon or bane?

This leads to what many people would regard as the biggest question of all. In what sense would we have a self to integrate under the new dispensation? The Princeton theologian Paul Ramsey has now been appointed professor of "genetic ethics" at the Georgetown University Medical School, presumably the first appointment of its kind. He thinks that genetic tailoring would be a "violation of man." To this it must be said that under the present scheme of things, many babies get born with catastrophic genes that are not exactly an enhancement of man. Our present genetic self is a brute datum, sometimes very brutal, and anyhow it is hard to see how we can lose our identity before we have any.

As for installing new organs in the body, there is no evident reason why the personality should be infringed upon by heart or kidney transplants per se. Brain transplants would be different, but surely they would be among the last to come. States of mind regulated by drugs we already possess, and obviously they do alter our identity in greater or lesser degree. But even here we must not forget that some identities are intolerable to their distracted possessors.

We must not conclude, however, that the importance of these developments has been exaggerated. The point is that the immediate practical consequences will probably not present themselves as threatening to the individuals involved—quite the contrary. Abstract theological speculations about genetic tailoring would be totally lost upon a woman who could be sure in advance that her baby would not be born mentally retarded or physically handicapped. The private anxieties of individuals are likely to diminish rather than increase any effective resistance to the broader consequences of the Biological Revolution.

One of these is already implicit in predicting a sense of growing passivity on the part of patients, of not participating as a subject in their own recovery. This might well be matched by a more general sense of the inevitability of letting oneself be manipulated by technicians—of becoming an article of manufacture.

The difficulty becomes to estimate what psychological difference this would make. In any Hegelian overview of history, we can only become articles of manufacture because "we" have set up as the manufacturers. But the first person plural is a slippery customer. We the manufactured would be everybody and we the manufacturers a minority of scientists and technicians. Most people's capacity to identify with the satisfactions of the creative minority is certainly no greater in science than in other fields, and may well be less.

The beneficiaries of the Biological Revolution are not likely to feel that they are in control of the historical process from which they are benefiting. But they will not be able to indulge any feelings of alienation from science without endangering the specific benefits that they are unwilling to give up.

The best forecast would be for general acquiescence, though occasionally sullen, in whatever the Biological Revolution has to offer and gradually adjusting our values to signify that we approve of what we will actually be getting. The will to cooperate in being made biologically perfect is likely to take the place in the hierarchy of values that used to be occupied by being humbly submissive to spiritual counselors chastising the sinner for his own salvation. The new form of spiritual sloth will be not to want to be bodily perfect and genetically improved. The new avarice will be to cherish our miserable hoard of genes and favor the children that resemble us.

The
desexualized society

CHARLES WINICK

The next few generations are likely to be involved in sexual choices and situations that are unprecedented, certainly in American history. These new developments reflect such contradictory factors as the culture's libidinization, depolarization of sex, the flourishing of voyeurism on an unprecedented scale, and the perfection of the technology of genetic engineering. They will pose and are already raising a number of ethical issues of great consequence.

Decline in libido

Our social and cultural climate is currently so libidinized that sexual energies, which are probably finite, are being drained to an extraordinary extent by the stimuli in our surroundings. As a result, there could be less and less libido available for traditional kinds of sexual activity involving relationships with people.

Paradoxically, our age of so much libidinization of mass media could be the beginning of an epoch of declining sexual behavior. Why? The few studies that have explored the relationships between sexual attitudes and behavior suggest that a society with liberal attitudes toward sexual expression is likely to have less sexual behavior than a culture that places sanctions on such expression. We may identify as the Godiva Principle the proposition that people will be attracted to sex in proportion to the extent to which it is prohibited. As our society accepts sex more casually, its members may engage in less sexual behavior.

Christiansen and Carpenter in their study, "Value Discrepancies Regarding Premarital Coitus," compared the relationship between sexual behavior and attitudes in a group of college students among three matched groups in: (a) the intermountain region of the United States; (b) the

THE DESEXUALIZED SOCIETY This article first appeared in *The Humanist*, Nov.–Dec., 1969, and is reprinted by permission.

341

Midwest; and (c) Denmark. One conclusion of the study was that the Danes had the most liberal attitudes but the least premarital activity. The intermountain students disapproved most explicitly of premarital relations but engaged in such relations more frequently than either of the other groups. We can speculate that the Danes were under the least pressure and therefore engaged in the least sexual behavior.

Additional evidence on the inverse relationship between sexual attitudes and behavior comes from still another survey by Wheeler, who claims that persons of lower socioeconomic status are much more likely than those of the middle or upper classes to express disapproval of nonmarital intercourse. However, male Kinsey interviewees with a grade-school level of education engaged in 10.6 times as much nonmarital intercourse as college men.

It would seem that more liberal sexual attitudes are likely to be correlated with less expression of libido. As we develop such permissive attitudes, we shall probably be less interested in sexual pursuits.

Further clues to the decline in the amount of libido that is available for sexual relationships can be found in studies of the effect of the various forms of the contraceptive pill on the incidence of sexual intercourse. It would be logical to expect the nine million women who currently use the pill would engage in substantially more sexual intercourse than they did before this new contraceptive technique became available. In fact, we find that there is no substantial increase in intercourse on the part of women users of the pill. This nonincrease is occurring even though many women are able to remind themselves each day of their potential as sexual partners and freedom from pregnancy, at the time they ingest the pill.

We can speculate that the pill will ultimately lead to a decline in sex relations because like so many other aspects of our culture it routinizes such relations.

Depolarization of sex

Certainly, one of the most extraordinary aspects of American sex roles for the last 25 years has been the extent to which masculinity and femininity are becoming blurred and a strange neutering is moving to the center of the stage of at least middle-class life. As sex becomes increasingly depolarized, its ability to excite and incite is likely to decline.

Documentation is hardly needed to confirm that men and women increasingly are wearing each other's clothing. Their leisure activities tend not to be sex-linked. In the home, a husband is often a part-time wife, and vice versa. Furniture related to either sex is disappearing, e.g., the leather club chair or the boudoir chair. American men use three times as much fragrance-containing preparations as their wives. Men have been wearing more jewelry at the same time that women are sporting heavy chain belts.

The shoe is the one item of costume that reflects gender most sensitively, perhaps because the foot's position in the shoe is so analogous to the position of the sexual organs during intercourse. As men's shoes have been looking more tapered, higher, and delicate, women's shoes have become stubbier, heavier, and lower.[1]

The blandness of social-sex roles is reinforced by the neuter quality of much of the environment in our beige epoch. Scotches, beers, and blended whiskeys succeed to the extent that they are light or bland. The convenience foods, which have revolutionized our eating habits, are bland. Even the cigar, once an outpost of strong aroma, has become homogenized.[2] In a society in which, as Mies van der Rohe said, "less is more," our new buildings tend to be neuter.

This blurring lessens the range of satisfactions available to people and leads to a decline in the quality and quantity of experience available to them. But an even more pressing source of concern for the humanist is the ability of our society to survive at all, if the current trend toward depolarization of sex continues. We can state this proposition paradigmatically: (1) A society's ability to sustain itself and to grow creatively is based on the ability of its members to adapt to new situations. (2) Such adaptability is intimately related to the strength of the feelings of personal identity of the people in the society. (3) At the core of any person's sense of identity is his or her awareness of gender. (4) To the extent that a man's sense of masculinity or a woman's feelings of femininity are blurred, such persons will possess a less effective self-concept and be less able to adapt to new situations.

If this paradigm is correct, the depolarization of sex, which is now endemic in this country, could be a prelude to considerable difficulty for us. It could bring about a situation in which the United States may have to choose between our laissez-faire sexual ethic, with its seeming potential for social disaster, and the kind of rigid sex-roles that are associated with authoritarianism. It is interesting to note that China and the Soviet Union have adopted a Puritan ethic which, if our hypothesis is correct, may actually encourage sexual expression *because* it is so anti-sexual.

The humanist philosophy is clearly opposed to authoritarianism and its attendant rigidity of roles and quashing of individual differences and personal style. Yet, studies of the mental-health implications of various kinds of family structure have tended to conclude that almost any male-female role structure is viable, provided that there is clear division of labor and responsibilities. It is disconcerting to consider the possibility that our open society's ambiguous sex roles may be almost as pathogenic as the rigidities of authoritarianism.

What can the humanist do about this situation? If he agrees that masculinity and femininity should be preserved, he can realize that a number of decisions available to him may contribute to this end. Certainly, we can control the costume and appearance which we present to the world. We can choose the shapes and colors with which we surround ourselves. The toys and dolls which we get for children can reflect gender differences.

---

[1] Charles Winick, "Status, Shoes, and the Life Cycle," *Boot and Shoe Recorder*, 156, October 15, 1959, pp. 100–01.

[2] "The Mellow Cigar," *Barron's*, September 5, 1960, pp. 1–3.

The names that we give children can communicate maleness or femaleness quite explicitly. We can select leisure activities that make possible an expression of masculinity and femininity. In many other ways, we may exercise options that permit us to avoid being locked in to the traditions of the past while still expressing modern forms of masculinity and femininity.

Voyeurism

Of the many pop-sociological descriptions of the period since the end of World War II, certainly one of the most apt is the Age of Voyeurism. We see and look and ingest with the eye to a degree that is perhaps unparalleled in human history.

If we hypothesize that an increase in one form of sexual expression is related complementarily to other outlets, we can speculate that the great increase in voyeurism is taking place at the expense of coitus and other interpersonal kinds of sex expression.

We know from several studies of readers of peep magazines like *Playboy* and *Confidential* that masturbation is a very popular, and perhaps the most frequent behavioral response to the magazines. It is probable that movies that explicitly present some form of sexual intercourse (e.g., *I Am Curious, Blowup, I A Woman*) will become ever more popular. Such movies and the plethora of print materials presenting sexual or erotic content, may be expected to move people in the direction of masturbating activities rather than interpersonal relations involving sex.

Voyeurism not only is satisfying in itself, as can be inferred from the extraordinary success of *Confidential* and *Playboy*, but it can also inhibit socially constructive action. Thirty-seven New Yorkers heard Kitty Genovese being attacked and murdered and yet did not respond in any way. It is likely that the satisfactions provided by fantasying about Miss Genovese were sufficiently strong to block any impulses toward going or looking outside or phoning the police. Voyeurism is seemingly rewarding enough to inhibit more socially constructive action. There is every reason to expect that our culture will be doing more peeping and less of other kinds of sexual behavior.

Genetic engineering

Yet another sexual deterrent is the perfection of procedures for freezing sperm and storing it for extended periods. Many routinely successful impregnations with sperm that had been frozen for several years have occurred, and the children show no defects traceable to the manner in which they were conceived.

Procedures are being perfected for removing an unfertilized egg cell from a woman's ovary, fertilizing it in a laboratory flask, and keeping the resulting embryo for an extended period. Such procedures will make it possible for a woman to have a baby by proxy. The egg cell from A could be fertilized in a test tube by sperm from B and nurtured in the body of C, as is taken for granted in breeding sheep and rabbits.

Genetic engineering is an almost inevitable result of the availability of such procedures. What would the humanist position on such matters be? Let us assume that the application of principles of genetic engineering leads to a decision to minimize breeding by a specific ethnic group. How could a humanist deal with such a situation? There would be a clear conflict between the presumed needs of society and unwillingness to label any group as intrinsically and permanently inferior.

Yet if we are to abide by principles of genetic engineering, we presumably shall have to make such evaluations. One of the reasons that the United States is the only civilized country without a system of financial allowances for children is the fear of some legislators that the major beneficiaries of such help would be members of some ethnic groups that are believed to be inferior.

Once the genetic counselor begins to advise potential mates and combines his skills with computer capabilities, romantic love as we know it is doomed. Life will not only be different, but it will be considerably delibidinized.

Why sex?

The several trends noted above would seem to be working toward an overall decline in sex expression. A key ethical issue, then, in the next several decades would seem to be why people should engage in the various kinds of sexual behavior that involves others. The strength of the sexual drive is not self-sustaining, and as the culture drains more and more lidibo, people will have less occasion for engaging in sexual relations. It certainly will not be necessary for purposes of procreation. Presumably other levels of personal satisfaction will become important.

The affirmation and expression represented by sexual relations with others are human values that are too fulfilling to abandon. A humanist view of the sexual scene could encourage its adherents to make every effort to counter the trends that threaten to make sexual expression, in terms of relations with others, an historical subject. The very ability of our society to survive is at stake.

The
beckwith letter

Nature, *an English "International Journal of Science" has long been one of the world's more literate and respected scientific magazines. In over a century of existence it has published many distinguished articles. One of the most impressive of these articles appeared in the issue of November 22, 1969. In it, a Harvard research group of young people, headed by Dr. Jonathan Beckwith, reported the isolation of a pure sample of a gene. As* Nature *editorialized, it was a "technical tour de force," a scientific first of major proportions. The feat made world headlines. Receiving more newspaper space than the achievement itself were the statements of the young scientists. How did they feel about their work? They doubted man's wisdom to use scientific discovery to human advantage. Too often was pure science put to destructive purpose. Man, they said in effect, is not yet ready.* THE FRIGHTENING FACT OF LIFE, *screamed the* Daily Mail *in England. And that newspaper ran this front-page subhead: "Scientists find secret of human heredity—and it scares them." When Einstein heard that an atom bomb had been dropped on the Japanese, he raised both hands in horror. "Man is not yet ready," he agonized quietly. Beckwith and his group said essentially the same thing. But they were young and not so used to loneliness and suffering. Less withdrawn than the aging physicist, they talked more. Yet in one respect, at least, they were older than the Einstein of those early atomic days. They knew that they had grown to manhood with strontium in their bones. And this knowledge makes some men old before their time.*

The following week Nature *published a reproving editorial called "More Alarums and Excursions."*

"In the past few months," the editors wrote, "the legitimate concern with problems such as pollution has spilled over into a phrenetic anxiety about the survival of the human race. . . ." Referring to the Boston press conference at which Beckwith and the other Harvard researchers had been interviewed, they continued:

> *A part of the trouble seems to have been a confrontation between the authors of the research and newspaper correspondents in Boston at the*

weekend; what seems to have caught the popular fancy is the awesome prospect of what might be done with genetic engineering if ever such a practice were possible. . . . There is, however, no assurance that manipulations like these presage the manipulation of the inheritance of E. Coli [the involved bacterium] in any deliberate way, and it is of course a far cry from even that to the deliberate manipulation of genetic inheritance in more complicated organisms than bacteria. . . .

So why are people anxious to read sinister messages in this new development? The question is perplexing because it reflects an implicit change in the public mood. A century ago, for sure, few people would have been tempted to look for such sinister outcomes. For all the opposition of the Victorians to what they called Darwinism, few people feared (as they might have done) that the discovery of the importance of natural selection would make it possible for eugenicists to transform the character of living things. Indeed, the tendency to seek sombre consequences for scientific discoveries is a comparatively recent event, a thing of the sixties and not simply of the nuclear world. Two dangers lie concealed in this. First, the progress of science itself may be interrupted or even halted by excessive fears of the consequences. Second, as in the tale of the shepherd boy who cried wolf too often, exaggeration may blunt the sensibilities of society to real dangers. It is for scientists to help to distinguish between a responsible concern for the social consequences of what they do and an exaggerated fear of them.

About a month later Nature *published the scientists' answer. It follows.*

SIR,

We wish to reply to your comments (*Nature*, **224**, 834; 1969) on the publicity surrounding the appearance of our article on the isolation of pure *lac* operon DNA (*Nature*, **224**, 768; 1969). To a certain extent your comments were perfectly correct. The press greatly inflated the importance of our particular piece of work. This was due in part to some of our own statements, which were misleading. It is true, however, that progress in the field of molecular genetics in the last few years has been extraordinary. We felt that the isolation of pure *lac* operon DNA was a graphic, useful and easily understood example of that progress.

We did not publicize our work in order to add to our own or Harvard's prestige or to make a plea for more money for basic research. In a country which makes a prodigious use of science and technology to murder Vietnamese and poison the environment, such an enterprise would be at best terribly irrelevant, at worst criminal. On the contrary, we tried to make the following political statement. In and of itself, our work is morally neutral—it can lead either to benefits or to dangers for mankind. But we are working in the United States in the year 1969. The basic control over sci-

THE BECKWITH LETTER: MORE ALARUMS AND EXCURSIONS From *Nature*, Vol. 224, December 27, 1969. Reprinted by permission of the publisher and the authors.

entific work and its further development is in the hands of a few people at the head of large private institutions and at the top of government bureaucracies. These people have consistently exploited science for harmful purposes in order to increase their own power.

The reality of the dangers we and others point out should not be minimized. Social agitation does not arise in a vacuum, as you seem to think. In Los Angeles, air pollution is often so bad that school children are prevented from taking physical exercise. Breast feeding in the United States, Sweden and Britain has become a serious health hazard because of the high concentration of DDT and other pesticides in human milk. The American Indians, the Jews, the Biafrans, the Vietnamese and the Palestinians are no strangers to the use of technology as an instrument of genocide. The survivors of Hiroshima and Nagasaki and the parents of thalidomide babies can testify to the horrors of the uncontrolled use of science by governments and private corporations. The list is virtually endless. We do not need to expand on it here. Let us simply point out to those who feel we have ample time to deal with these problems that less than 50 years elapsed between Becquerel's discovery of radioactivity in 1896 and the use of an atomic weapon against human beings in 1945. As to the specific issue of genetic engineering, we cannot predict the future. But who in 1896 could have foreseen the weapons of mass destruction which now threaten us all?

What we are advocating is that scientists, together with other people, should actively work for radical political change in this country. If we do not, we will one day be a group of very regretful Oppenheimers. Scientists have no right to claim a special position of intellectual leadership in this political effort. We differ from other members of society only in that our working conditions are generally more free than theirs. This is so because governments and industry realize that science and technology develop more efficiently without stringent controls. As we see it, scientists are obligated to inform the public about what is happening in their secluded fields of research so that people can demand control over decisions which profoundly affect their lives. If our arguments mean that "the progress of science itself may be interrupted," that is an unfortunate consequence we will have to accept. It certainly should not inhibit us from speaking out on crucial issues.

Permit us to contradict one of your statements ("Miscellaneous Intelligence," *Nature*, **224,** 842; 1969). You said that you published our article as it was received. This is not so. On our manuscript there were nine authors listed at the head of the article. You saw fit to relegate three of them to the acknowledgments without informing us: Bill Reznikoff, Rita Arditti and Ronnie MacGillivray. (On the manuscript the authors were listed as "Jim Shapiro, Lorne MacHattie, Larry Eron, Garret Ihler, Karin Ippen and Jon Beckwith after discussions with Bill Reznikoff and Rita Arditti and with the technical assistance of Ronnie MacGillivray.") We see now that it was a mistake to make any distinction at all between various authors in our manuscript. It is an almost universal fiction in modern science that the only people responsible for a given piece of work are the professionals and students who sign the article.

The signatories of this letter were responsible for the various statements which appeared in the press. This letter represents their views. Some of the other authors of the original article agree with these views, some disagree, and some have not been contacted.

Yours faithfully,

JIM SHAPIRO
LARRY ERON
JON BECKWITH

Department of Bacteriology and Immunology,
Harvard Medical School,
25 Shattuck Street,
Boston, Massachusetts 02115, U.S.A.

Author-title index

Adelson, Joseph, 197
Aichinger, Ilse, 231
Alexander, Tom, 36
Alienated Youth, 216
Allen, James R., 183
Angel, Klaus, 189
Atherosclerosis, 249

Beckwith, Jonathan, 346
Beckwith Letter, The, 346
Bound Man, The, 231
Brauner, Charles C., 105
Breaking Isn't Everything, 224
Brown, William Neal, 216

Chromosomes and Crime: Some Tentative Thoughts, 276
Craft, Robert, 305
Culture of Poverty, The, 160

Dernburg, Ernest A., 77
Desexualized Society, The, 341
Drug Addiction—Facts and Folklore, 296
Dubos, René, 28

Eron, Larry, 346

First Probe, The, 105
Fleming, Donald, 331
Fog, The, 5

Gillie, Oliver, 296

Health of Haight-Ashbury, The, 77
Herron, William G., 146
Human Ecology, 28

If Hitler Asked You to Electrocute a Stranger, Would You?, 133
Igor Stravinsky: On Illness and Death, 305
Infant Malnutrition and Adult Learning, 241
Informal History of Love U.S.A., An, 169
It's Time to Turn Down All That Noise, 46

Kantor, Robert E., 146
Kaufman, Joshua, 183

Lewis, Oscar, 160
Luce, John, 77

351

Many Clocks of Man, The, 267
Mecklin, John M., 46
Medicine in the Ghetto, 68
Menninger, Roy, 207
Meyer, Philip, 133
Mortgaging the Old Homestead, 17
Mukhopadhyay, Subhas, 224

No Marijuana for Adolescents, 189
Norman, John C., 68

Of Viruses and Cancers, 259
On Living in a Biological Revolution,
  331

Palmer, John D., 267
Paranoia and High Office, 146
Platt, John, 325
*Psychohistorical Perspective of the
  Negro, A,* 152

Rapoport, Roger, 58
Recently Exploded Sexual Myths, 280
Ritchie-Calder, Lord, 17
Root, Lin, 259
Roueché, Berton, 5
Roy, Kshitis (translator), 224
Runaways, Hippies, and Marihuana,
  183

Salzman, Leon, 280
Schlesinger, Arthur, Jr., 169
*Scientific Urgencies of the Next Ten
  Years, The,* 325
Scrimshaw, Nevin S., 241
Secrecy and Safety at Rocky Flats,
  58
*Sex and the Work of Masters and
  Johnson,* 289
Shapiro, Jim, 346
Sharpley, Robert H., 152
Smith, David E., 77
Smith, Roger C., 93
Spain, David M., 249
Steinbeck, John, 127
Strassman, Harvey D., 289

Telfer, Mary A., 276

West, Louis Jolyon, 183
What Generation Gap?, 197
What Troubles Our Troubled Youth?,
  207
*Where Will We Put All That Gar-
  bage?,* 36
Winick, Charles, 341
World of Migratory Workers, The,
  127
*World of the Haight-Ashbury Speed
  Freak, The,* 93

A	1
B	2
C	3
D	4
E	5
F	6
G	7
H	8
I	9
J	0